Advances in the Diagnosis and Management of Pediatric Diseases

Advances in the Diagnosis and Management of Pediatric Diseases

Guest Editor

Elena Tarca

MDPI

Basel • Beijing • Wuhan • Barcelona • Belgrade • Novi Sad • Cluj • Manchester

Guest Editor
Elena Tarca
Department of Surgery
II—Pediatric Surgery
University of Medicine and
Pharmacy "Gr. T. Popa"
Iasi
Romania

Editorial Office
MDPI AG
Grosspeteranlage 5
4052 Basel, Switzerland

This is a reprint of the Special Issue, published open access by the journal *Diagnostics* (ISSN 2075-4418), freely accessible at: https://www.mdpi.com/journal/diagnostics/special_issues/P8042Q80I2.

For citation purposes, cite each article independently as indicated on the article page online and as indicated below:

Lastname, A.A.; Lastname, B.B. Article Title. *Journal Name* **Year**, *Volume Number*, Page Range.

ISBN 978-3-7258-7651-8 (Hbk)
ISBN 978-3-7258-7652-5 (PDF)
https://doi.org/10.3390/books978-3-7258-7652-5

Contents

About the Editor

Elena Tarca

Elena Tarca is an Associate Professor at the Department of Pediatric Surgery and Orthopedics, Grigore T. Popa University of Medicine and Pharmacy, Iași, Romania. She completed her PhD studies at the Grigore T. Popa University of Medicine and Pharmacy. Dr. Țarcă is also a consultant in pediatric surgery and orthopedics, with clinical activity in the "Sfanta Maria" Children's Emergency Clinical Hospital in Iași, a tertiary hospital for pediatric patients in the southeastern region of Romania. Her research interests focus on pediatric surgery, pediatric orthopedics and trauma, neonatal surgery, congenital malformations, pediatric oncology, and pediatric urology, with more than 150 publications in international peer-reviewed journals. Dr. Tarca serves as a Guest Editor for international scientific journals and books, participates in national and international research projects, and is a member of professional pediatric surgical and orthopedic societies.

diagnostics

Editorial

New Improvements in Pediatric Disease Diagnosis and Treatment

Elena Țarcă

Faculty of Medicine, Grigore T. Popa University of Medicine and Pharmacy, 700115 Iași, Romania;
tarca.elena@umfiasi.ro

Pediatric patients can present significant diagnostic and therapeutic challenges, as their pathophysiology differs substantially from that of adults. The pediatric population encompasses a vast spectrum, ranging from premature newborns to adolescents up to eighteen years of age and from extremely low-birth-weight infants to patients weighing up to one hundred kilograms. This wide variability underscores the complexity of pediatric care. Although substantial progress has been made in understanding the biological mechanisms and management of several congenital and acquired pediatric diseases, such as mucoviscidosis, Niemann–Pick disease, and celiac disease [1–3], outcomes for other conditions remain suboptimal. These include genetic and metabolic disorders, severe congenital malformations, and neonatal sepsis, highlighting the ongoing need for research and innovation in pediatric medicine [4].

This Special Issue includes original research articles, reviews, and case reports that collectively highlight the breadth and depth of contemporary pediatric diagnostic research, addressing several important key topics. Chromosomal anomalies, extremely low birth weight, and prematurity are frequently associated with congenital deformities, representing a broad and clinically significant area of study. Accurate syndromic classification, supported by imaging, genetic testing, and clinical correlation, remains essential for guiding management and counseling families [5]. This is particularly relevant in cases of anorectal malformations and congenital anterior abdominal wall defects, which are often associated with cardiac or pulmonary anomalies, further complicating surgical management and worsening prognosis [6–9]. Surgical techniques also must be tailored not only to the patient's age and weight but to specific requirements related to anesthesia, medication dosing, and blood transfusions [10,11].

Another important pillar of this Special Issue is the development of genetic analysis and molecular diagnostics. The increasing availability of next-generation sequencing, improved cytogenetic techniques, and refined genotype–phenotype correlations has transformed the diagnostic landscape for inherited and metabolic diseases [1]. Despite these advances, many disorders continue to have limited therapeutic options, underscoring the importance of early diagnosis, supportive care optimization, and ongoing translational research. Neonatal intensive care, pediatric oncology and gastroenterology similarly present challenges distinct from those encountered in adult populations, requiring specialized approaches to care [12]. Advances in medical sciences and technology have enabled increasingly individualized treatment strategies, allowing clinicians to tailor interventions to achieve optimal outcomes.

The breadth of research topics addressed in this Special Issue on pediatric pathology, as outlined in the Contributions list, reflects the comprehensive nature of pediatric medicine. The studies included employ a range of methodological approaches, including systematic

https://doi.org/10.3390/diagnostics16040542

and literature reviews, as well as prospective and observational designs. The findings yield significant insights that can be extrapolated beyond the original study contexts, and their dissemination contributes to the advancement of the scientific and medical community. Notably, some articles and case reports address practical challenges commonly encountered in clinical practice, providing readers with valuable insights into current research on genetic, congenital, neonatal, and pediatric pathology, as well as their application to routine clinical care [13–15].

Conclusions

Congenital abnormalities, maternal–fetal medicine, and genetics are among the most rapidly advancing fields in modern medicine. Technological innovations, novel imaging techniques, and the development of new therapeutic strategies have significantly improved our understanding and management of neonatal and pediatric conditions. Considering patient age, weight, anatomy, disease biology, and developmental stage, predictive and preventive medicine, as well as personalized medical approaches, are becoming increasingly integral to pediatric diagnosis and treatment.

Aiming to improve clinical outcomes in pediatric populations, this Special Issue highlights the complexity of pediatric and congenital disorders and underscores the importance of multimodal diagnostic approaches that integrate clinical evaluation with advanced imaging techniques, laboratory biomarkers, and histopathological assessment. It further emphasizes the value of individualized therapeutic strategies and multidisciplinary, translational research.

Future innovations in wearable technology, regenerative medicine, genomics, and artificial intelligence have the potential to improve long-term outcomes, early diagnosis, and treatment in children, particularly in rare, genetic, and severe congenital conditions.

Funding: This research received no external funding.

Conflicts of Interest: The author declares no conflicts of interest.

List of Contributions:

1. Donos, M.A.; Ghiga, G.; Trandafir, L.M.; Cojocaru, E.; Țarcă, V.; Butnariu, L.I.; Bernic, V.; Moroșan, E.; Roca, I.C.; Mîndru, D.E.; et al. Diagnosis and Management of Simple and Complicated Meconium Ileus in Cystic Fibrosis, a Systematic Review. *Diagnostics* **2024**, *14*, 1179. https://doi.org/10.3390/diagnostics14111179.
2. Ionescu, A.; Mihăilescu, A.; Chiriță-Emandi, A.; Munagala, N.; David, V.L.; Dumache, R.; Săndesc, D.; Bedreag, O.; Folescu, R.; Bratosin, F.; et al. Assessing Differential Transfusion Requirements for Children with Congenital Malformations vs. Pediatric Acute Abdomen Emergencies. *Diagnostics* **2024**, *14*, 2216. https://doi.org/10.3390/diagnostics14192216.
3. Marković, B.; Gazdić Janković, M.; Igrutinović, Z.; Medović, R.; Stojadinović, N.; Ljujić, B. Monosomy 18p with Unbalanced Translocation Between 13 and 18 Chromosomes: First Reported Case in Serbia. *Diagnostics* **2025**, *15*, 358. https://doi.org/10.3390/diagnostics15030358.
4. Al Namat, D.; Roșca, R.A.; Al Namat, R.; Hanganu, E.; Ivan, A.; Hînganu, D.; Lupu, A.; Hînganu, M.V. Correction: Al Namat et al. Omphalocele and Associated Anomalies: Exploring Pulmonary Development and Genetic Correlations—A Literature Review. *Diagnostics* 2025, *15*, 675. *Diagnostics* **2025**, *15*, 3210. https://doi.org/10.3390/diagnostics15243210.
5. Vlad, R.M.; Dobritoiu, R.; Pacurar, D. From Genes to Treatment: Literature Review and Perspectives on Acid Sphingomyelinase Deficiency in Children. *Diagnostics* **2025**, *15*, 804. https://doi.org/10.3390/diagnostics15070804.
6. Hencke, J.; Staubach, R.; Loff, S. Manometric Evaluation of the Sphincter Complex in Anterior Anus and Mild Anorectal Malformations—An Important Diagnostic Tool. *Diagnostics* **2025**, *15*, 1078. https://doi.org/10.3390/diagnostics15091078.

7. Fang, H.-H.; Lee, C.-L.; Chuang, C.-K.; Chiu, H.-C.; Chang, Y.-H.; Tu, Y.-R.; Lo, Y.-T.; Wu, J.-Y.; Chou, Y.-Y.; Wang, C.-H.; et al. Functional Independence of Taiwanese Children with Silver–Russell Syndrome. *Diagnostics* **2025**, *15*, 1109. https://doi.org/10.3390/diagnostics15091109.
8. Cetin, T.; Cinar, G.; Ucan, B.; Memis, F.; Irgul, B.; Aydin, S. Incidental Calcifications of Carotid and Vertebral Arteries: Frequency and Associations in Pediatric Population. *Diagnostics* **2025**, *15*, 1263. https://doi.org/10.3390/diagnostics15101263.
9. Hincu, M.-A.; Gheorghe, L.; Dimitriu, C.; Paduraru, L.; Zonda, G.; Andronic, D.-C.; Vasilache, I.-A.; Baean, L.-M.; Nemescu, D. Procalcitonin, Presepsin, Endocan, and Interleukin-6 in the Early Diagnosis of Neonatal Sepsis—A Prospective Study. *Diagnostics* **2025**, *15*, 1341. https://doi.org/10.3390/diagnostics15111341.
10. Zelenova, E.; Belysheva, T.; Sharapova, E.; Barinova, I.; Fedorova, A.; Semenova, V.; Vishnevskaya, Y.; Kletskaya, I.; Mitrofanova, A.; Sofronov, D.; et al. Atypical Manifestations of Cowden Syndrome in Pediatric Patients. *Diagnostics* **2025**, *15*, 1456. https://doi.org/10.3390/diagnostics15121456.
11. Pfeifer, J.; Poryo, M.; Fries, P.; Abdul-Khaliq, H. Plastic Bronchitis: Extensive Cast Expectoration in a 6-Year-Old Boy with Fontan Circulation. *Diagnostics* **2025**, *15*, 2864. https://doi.org/10.3390/diagnostics15222864.
12. Çirkin, G.; Taskin, R.B. Evaluation of Nailfold Capillaroscopic Findings in Pediatric Patients with Celiac Disease: A Cross-Sectional and Comparative Study. *Diagnostics* **2025**, *15*, 2102. https://doi.org/10.3390/diagnostics15162102.
13. Nguyen, T.T.H.; Le, K.M.; Tran, T.A.T.; Nguyen, K.N.; Can, T.B.N.; Bui, P.T.; Tran, D.T.; Vu, C.D. Growth Assessment and Nutritional Status in Children with Congenital Adrenal Hyperplasia—A Cross-Sectional Study from a Vietnamese Tertiary Pediatric Center. *Diagnostics* **2025**, *15*, 1534. https://doi.org/10.3390/diagnostics15121534.

References

1. Guyot, E.; Deygas, F.; Belhassen, M.; Berard, M.; Van Ganse, E.; Sermet-Gaudelus, I.; Tiaiba, S.; Dubus, J.; Durieu, I.; Reix, P. Newborn Screening for Cystic Fibrosis Is Associated with the Lowest Healthcare Costs: A 10-Year Observational Follow-Up Study in France. *Pediatr. Pulmonol.* **2025**, *60*, e71134. [CrossRef] [PubMed]
2. Scarpa, M.; Diaz, G.A.; Giugliani, R.; Jones, S.A.; Mengel, E.; Guffon, N.; Witters, P.; Ganesh, J.; Armstrong, N.M.; Srivastava, S.; et al. Long-Term Safety and Clinical Outcomes with Olipudase Alfa Enzyme Replacement Therapy in Children and Adolescents with Acid Sphingomyelinase Deficiency. *J. Inherit. Metab. Dis.* **2025**, *48*, e70086. [CrossRef] [PubMed]
3. Valitutti, F.; Cavalli, E.; Leter, B.; Leonard, M.; Alessio, F.; Cucchiara, S. Coeliac disease and microbiota: Is it time for personalised biotics intervention? A scoping review. *BMJ Nutr. Prev. Health* **2025**, *8*, e001100. [CrossRef] [PubMed]
4. Sokou, R.; Lianou, A.; Lampridou, M.; Panagiotounakou, P.; Kafalidis, G.; Paliatsiou, S.; Volaki, P.; Tsantes, A.G.; Boutsikou, T.; Iliodromiti, Z.; et al. Neonates at Risk: Understanding the Impact of High-Risk Pregnancies on Neonatal Health. *Medicina* **2025**, *61*, 1077. [CrossRef] [PubMed]
5. Adam, H.; Ghenimi, N.; Minsart, A.F.; Narchi, H.; Al Awar, S.; Al Hajeri, O.M.; Elbarazi, I.; Al-Rifai, R.H.; Ahmed, L.A. Impact of major congenital anomalies on preterm birth and low birth weight. *Sci. Rep.* **2025**, *15*, 24872. [CrossRef] [PubMed]
6. Smith, C.A.; Rialon, K.L.; Kawaguchi, A.; Dellinger, M.B.; Goldin, A.B.; Acker, S.; Kulaylat, A.N.; Chang, H.; Russell, K.; Wakeman, D.; et al. Classification and Surgical Management of Anorectal Malformations: A Systematic Review and Evidence-based Guideline from the APSA Outcomes and Evidence-based Practice Committee. *J. Pediatr. Surg.* **2024**, *59*, 161598. [CrossRef] [PubMed]
7. Dadoun, S.E.; Shanahan, M.A.; Parobek, C.M.; Burnett, B.A.; King, A.; Ketwaroo, P.; Donepudi, R.V.; Adams, A.D. Prenatal Prognosis of Omphalocele Using Magnetic Resonance Imaging Measurement of Fetal Lung Volumes. *Am. J. Obstet. Gynecol. MFM* **2024**, *6*, 101457. [CrossRef] [PubMed]
8. Tarcă, E.; Aprodu, S. Past and present in omphalocele treatment in Romania. *Chirurgia* **2014**, *109*, 507–513. [PubMed]
9. Pitaka, R.T.; Fauzi, A.R.; Makhmudi, A. Gunadi Comparison and impact of associated anomalies on the anal position index in neonates with anorectal malformation. *BMC Res. Notes* **2022**, *15*, 294. [CrossRef] [PubMed]
10. Wells, M.; Goldstein, L. The utility of pediatric age-based weight estimation formulas for emergency drug dose calculations in obese children. *J. Am. Coll. Emerg. Physicians Open* **2020**, *1*, 947–954. [CrossRef] [PubMed]

https://doi.org/10.3390/diagnostics16040542

11. Mokhtar, G.; Adly, A.; Baky, A.A.; Ezzat, D.; Hakeem, G.A.; Hassab, H.; Youssry, I.; Ragab, I.; Florez, I.; Sherief, L.M.; et al. Transfusion of blood components in pediatric age groups: An evidence-based clinical practice guideline adapted for the use in Egypt using 'Adapted ADAPTE'. *Ann. Hematol.* **2024**, *103*, 1373–1388. [CrossRef] [PubMed]
12. Okello, D.A.; Masiga, M.; Muasya, M. Dental Caries and Oral Mucositis Among Children Undergoing Cancer Therapy at Kenyatta National Hospital, Kenya: A Cross-Sectional Study. *Cureus* **2025**, *17*, e94417. [CrossRef] [PubMed]
13. Pfeifer, J.; Poryo, M.; Fries, P.; Abdul-Khaliq, H. Plastic Bronchitis: Extensive Cast Expectoration in a 6-Year-Old Boy with Fontan Circulation. *Diagnostics* **2025**, *15*, 2864. [CrossRef] [PubMed]
14. Marković, B.; Gazdić Janković, M.; Igrutinović, Z.; Medović, R.; Stojadinović, N.; Ljujić, B. Monosomy 18p with Unbalanced Translocation Between 13 and 18 Chromosomes: First Reported Case in Serbia. *Diagnostics* **2025**, *15*, 358. [CrossRef] [PubMed]
15. Donos, M.A.; Ghiga, G.; Trandafir, L.M.; Cojocaru, E.; Țarcă, V.; Butnariu, L.I.; Bernic, V.; Moroșan, E.; Roca, I.C.; Mîndru, D.E.; et al. Diagnosis and Management of Simple and Complicated Meconium Ileus in Cystic Fibrosis, a Systematic Review. *Diagnostics* **2024**, *14*, 1179. [CrossRef] [PubMed]

https://doi.org/10.3390/diagnostics16040542

diagnostics

MDPI

Systematic Review

Diagnosis and Management of Simple and Complicated Meconium Ileus in Cystic Fibrosis, a Systematic Review

Mădălina Andreea Donos [1,2], Gabriela Ghiga [2,*], Laura Mihaela Trandafir [2,*], Elena Cojocaru [3], Viorel Țarcă [4], Lăcrămioara Ionela Butnariu [5], Valentin Bernic [6], Eugenia Moroșan [3], Iulia Cristina Roca [7], Dana Elena Mîndru [2] and Elena Țarcă [8]

1 Saint Mary Emergency Hospital for Children, 700309 Iasi, Romania; madalina.donos@umfiasi.ro
2 Pediatrics Department, "Grigore T. Popa" University of Medicine and Pharmacy, 700115 Iasi, Romania; mindru.dana@umfiasi.ro
3 Department of Morphofunctional Sciences I—Pathology, "Grigore T. Popa" University of Medicine and Pharmacy, 700115 Iasi, Romania; elena2.cojocaru@umfiasi.ro (E.C.); eugenia_morosan@yahoo.com (E.M.)
4 Department of Preventive Medicine and Interdisciplinarity, "Grigore T. Popa" University of Medicine and Pharmacy, 700115 Iasi, Romania; viorel.tarca@umfiasi.ro
5 Department of Medical Genetics, Faculty of Medicine, "Grigore T. Popa" University of Medicine and Pharmacy, 700115 Iasi, Romania; ionela.butnariu@umfiasi.ro
6 Department of Surgery II, "Saint Spiridon" Hospital, 700115 Iasi, Romania; bernicvalik@yahoo.com
7 Department of Surgery II, "Grigore T. Popa" University of Medicine and Pharmacy, 700115 Iasi, Romania; iulia.roca@umfiasi.ro
8 Department of Surgery II—Pediatric Surgery, "Grigore T. Popa" University of Medicine and Pharmacy, 700115 Iasi, Romania; tarca.elena@umfiasi.ro
* Correspondence: ghiga.gabriela@yahoo.com (G.G.); laura.trandafir@umfiasi.ro (L.M.T.)

Abstract: The early management of neonates with meconium ileus (MI) and cystic fibrosis (CF) is highly variable across countries and is not standardized. We conducted a systematic review according to the Preferred Reporting Items for Systematic Reviews and Meta-analyses statement. The protocol was registered in PROSPERO (CRD42024522838). Studies from three providers of academic search engines were checked for inclusion criteria, using the following search terms: meconium ileus AND cystic fibrosis OR mucoviscidosis. Regarding the patient population studied, the inclusion criteria were defined using our predefined PICOT framework: studies on neonates with simple or complicated meconium which were confirmed to have cystic fibrosis and were conservatively managed or surgically treated. Results: A total of 566 publications from the last 10 years were verified by the authors of this review to find the most recent and relevant data, and only 8 met the inclusion criteria. Prenatally diagnosed meconium pseudocysts, bowel dilation, and ascites on ultrasound are predictors of neonatal surgery and risk factor for negative 12-month clinical outcomes in MI-CF newborns. For simple MI, conservative treatment with hypertonic solutions enemas can be effective in more than 25% of cases. If repeated enemas fail to disimpact the bowels, the Bishop–Koop stoma is a safe option. No comprehensive research has been conducted so far to determine the ideal surgical protocol for complicated MI. We only found three studies that reported the types of stomas performed and another study comparing the outcomes of patients depending on the surgical management; the conclusions are contradictory especially since the number of cases analyzed in each study was small. Between 18% and 38% of patients with complicated MI will require reoperation for various complications and the mortality rate varies between 0% and 8%. Conclusion: This study reveals a lack of strong data to support management decisions, unequivocally shows that the care of infants with MI is not standardized, and suggests a great need for international collaborative studies.

Keywords: meconium ileus; cystic fibrosis; diagnostic; management; neonates

1. Introduction

Cystic fibrosis (CF) is an autosomal recessive disease caused by a defect in a gene on the long arm of Chromosome 7 which codes for the cystic fibrosis transmembrane conductance regulator (CFTR), a chloride channel on epithelial surfaces [1]. Among the thousands of mutations that can be involved, the best known is *delta F508*, being responsible for unregulated epithelial sodium channels (ENaCs), decreased chloride secretion, and increased sodium resorption on epithelial surfaces. Other known mutations responsible for the appearance of CF manifestations are *G542X*, *W1282X*, *R553X*, *G551D*, and other modifier genes, all explaining approximately 17% of the phenotypic variability [2]. The risk for a patient to present with meconium ileus (MI) is 24.9% if he has two copies of *F508del* mutation, 16.9% if he has one *F508del* paired with another mutation and 12.5% for two other CFTR mutations [3]. While individual studies have found various modifier genes that either increase or decrease the risk of MI, there has been limited capacity to reproduce these findings [4–6].

CFTR is in charge of the excretion of both Cl^- and HCO_3^- in the small intestine. The tight matrix of exocytosed mucins in the gut lumen is mediated by HCO_3^-, which is essential for chelating Ca^{2+} to generate normal, loose, well-hydrated mucus [2]. Abnormal HCO_3^- secretion decreases luminal pH and creates an acidic, dehydrated environment and thick mucus. Increased mineral content, protein-bound carbohydrates, and greater amounts of stool albumin are further encouraged by the excessively acidic luminal environment. Together with the viscous mucus, these result in viscid meconium, which physically obstructs the terminal ileum [3].

Meconium ileus occurs in between 12% and 20% of neonates diagnosed with CF and is usually the first manifestation of the disease; it is defined as a mechanical small bowel obstruction in the perinatal period, caused by inspissated meconium within the terminal ileum [7]. When there is only the occlusion created by the thickened meconium, meconium ileus is classified as "simple". In cases with antenatal manifestation, MI can coexist with meconial peritonitis, intestinal atresia, perforations, and necrosis or ileal volvulus; in this case, MI is "complicated". In neonates with CF, simple and complex MI happen at comparable rates [3]. The early management of neonates with MI is highly variable across countries and is not standardized [8]. Also, the optimal surgical technique remains controversial, and because primary anastomosis may result in complication rates between 21% and 31%, ileostomy and delayed anastomosis is recommended by some authors [2,9], while others recommend primary anastomosis to avoid electrolyte losses and the need for surgical reintervention to close the stoma [10].

This article sets out to explore a difficult topic that completely lacks standardization, diagnosis, and management of simple and complicated meconium ileus in cystic fibrosis. The aim of our review is to summarize the latest data from the specialized literature regarding the treatment of simple and complicated meconium ileus, in the hope of discovering and applying uniform treatment norms.

2. Materials and Methods

This systematic review was conducted according to the Preferred Reporting Items for Systematic Reviews and Meta-analyses (PRISMA) statement [11]. The protocol was registered in PROSPERO under the Registration Number: CRD42024522838.

2.1. Search Strategy of Electronic Databases

Between 15 March 2024 and 30 April 2024 we performed a systematic review of the data available with regard to the management of MI in cystic fibrosis. We evaluated articles from three providers of academic search engines (PubMed, EMBASE, and Web of Science) using the following search terms: meconium ileus AND cystic fibrosis OR mucoviscidosis. We then used a combination of MESH terms like neonatal intestinal obstruction OR meconial peritonitis OR constipation OR distal intestinal obstruction syndrome AND cystic fibrosis

OR mucoviscidosis to find the most relevant articles about the diagnosis and management of this neonatal occlusion syndrome.

2.1.1. Including and Excluding Criteria

Studies included in this review met the following criteria: full-text available online, published in the last 10 years, clearly stated methodology, human subjects, and articles available in English. We searched the reference lists of the included articles in order to identify other potentially relevant articles. We excluded the duplicated, non-relevant studies and the ones treating non-human subjects; after the title and abstract assessment a total of 112 studies were excluded.

Regarding the patient population studied, the inclusion criteria were defined using our predefined PICOT framework: studies on neonates with simple or complicated meconium who were confirmed to have cystic fibrosis and were conservatively managed or surgically treated. These two groups were compared for the need of surgery and placement of an ileostomy (main outcomes). The secondary studied outcomes were the imagistic findings, the number of days until weaning from total parenteral nutrition (TPN), days of hospitalization, the number of days until stoma closure, and mortality rate.

2.1.2. Selection of Studies and Information Extraction

Three authors [M.A.D., E.T., and L.M.T.] independently selected the articles included in the review by searching databases. They independently screened all titles and abstracts of identified studies for eligibility. If disagreement between the reviewers existed, consensus was formed or a fourth reviewer [G.G.] acted as referee. Duplicate references and non-human studies were eliminated. Title and abstract assessment were performed by V.T., E.C. and L.I.B. References review of the relevant articles were reviewed by V.B. and D.E.M. for pertinent articles that would meet inclusion and exclusion criteria; 112 articles were initially selected, then excluded by E.M. and I.C.R. as being non-relevant.

3. Results

From Web of Science, 890 articles were found discussing meconium ileus AND cystic fibrosis OR mucoviscidosis; 63,111 were selected from PubMed and 89,676 from EMBASE. After applying the filters (full-text available online, published in the last 10 years, English language, humans, age: birth-1-month, publication types: articles, reviews, meta-analyses), 454 studies remained to be screened for eligibility. During the second step, we reviewed the titles, abstracts, and the full texts of the papers and selected the studies reporting neonatal intestinal obstruction OR meconial peritonitis OR constipation OR surgery to extract pertinent data for our review (Figure 1). A total of 566 publications were verified by the authors of this review to find the most recent and relevant data, and only 8 met the inclusion criteria (Table 1). Forty-seven relevant studies with their citations were included in our reference list.

Table 1. Procedural treatments for neonates with MI.

Author and Publication Year and Study Design	Purpose of the Study	Simple MI - Enema Treatment	Simple MI Requiring Surgery	Complex MI Requiring Surgery	Reported Outcomes/ Complications/Mortality	Conclusions
- Shinar et al., 2020 [12] - Case Series and Meta-Analysis	Identifying prenatal predictors of neonatal surgery	24 patients with MI and CF, from 244 MI studied patients			Postoperative mortality rate of 8.1% and a survival rate of 100% in neonates not requiring surgery	Meconium pseudocysts, bowel dilation, and ascites are prenatal predictors of neonatal surgery in cases of meconium peritonitis
- Padoan et al., 2019 [13] - Retrospective, multicenter, observational study	Identifying the risk factors for poor 12-month clinical outcomes in MI-CF newborns	24/52 patients treated with enema—success rate 58% (14 cases)	- 38 patients with simple MI - 33 patients with complicated MI needed surgery - 40 subjects underwent intestinal resection - 41 patients needed a stoma		- 31 patients (37%) experienced negative outcomes; the risk factors were prenatally diagnosed intestinal obstruction and a need for intensive care and oxygen therapy - 13/71 patients (18%) had to undergo further abdominal surgery during the first month of life, for complications - Mortality rate 4.7%	High b-IRT levels, prenatally diagnosed intestinal obstruction, a severe post-surgical clinical picture and early liver disease are risk factors for negative outcomes. Breastfeeding may be protective.
- Caro-Domínguez et al., 2018 [14] - Retrospective comparative study	Role of postnatal radiographic and sonographic findings in predicting the need for surgery in neonates with MI	14 patients successfully treated with enema	- 23 patients required surgery (62%) - **Only 8% of patients had CF**		- diffuse peritoneal calcification as an isolated finding can be successfully treated non-operatively	Imaging findings that predicted the need for surgery were intestinal obstruction, ascites, volvulus, and pneumoperitoneum
- Long et al., 2021 [8] - Prospective population-cohort study	Outcome and factors associated with successful non-operative management	12/33 patients were treated with enema alone (36%)	- 20/33 patients were treated with enema and laparotomy (61%) - 1 patient with simple MI was primary operated (3%) - 9/21 (43%) had stoma formation	- 10/23 had enema and laparotomy - 13/23 had primary laparotomy - 15 (65%) had stoma formation	- When using an enema to decompress, infants with simple MI took 6 days to begin complete enteral feedings, whereas those who underwent a laparotomy after an enema took 15 days - Three contrast enemas (5%) were followed by complications: one drop in serum sodium and two intestinal perforations - Nine infants from 24 who had stomas (38%) had complications - Mortality rate was 4%	Compared to those who underwent a laparotomy, infants with simple MI who had successful enema decompression were more likely to have experienced recurrent enemas. Time to full feeding was shortened in cases when non-operative treatment was successful.

Table 1. *Cont.*

Author and Publication Year and Study Design	Purpose of the Study	Simple MI - Enema Treatment	Simple MI Requiring Surgery	Complex MI Requiring Surgery	Reported Outcomes/ Complications/Mortality	Conclusions
- Farrelly et al., 2014 [10] - Retrospective case note analysis	Outcomes of the surgical management for MI and DIOS in CF	19/30 patients with simple MI were treated with enema and only 5 responded	25 patients with simple MI and 29 with complicated MI were operated: - 39 (72%) had divided stomas, 7 (13%) were managed with enterotomy and washout, and 8 (15%) with resection and primary anastomosis		- time to closure for patients managed with stomas was 47 days (4–202) - significant difference in LOS between operative patients managed with and without stomas: 49 versus 23 days - Presentation with MI did not predispose to later development of DIOS *per se* - no postoperative deaths	Compared to therapy with stomas, retaining intestinal continuity at the initial laparotomy for MI appears to be safe, associated with shorter hospital stays, and does not increase the rate of unplanned re-laparotomy - patients who presented with MI had a predisposition to develop a more severe form of DIOS necessitating surgery
- Jessula et al., 2018 [15] - Retrospective cohort review of prospectively collected data	Identifying if specific genetic subtypes and the presence of echogenic bowel on prenatal US are associated with either MI or operative requirement in the neonatal period	7 patients with simple MI were treated conservatively and did not require any surgical intervention	- 3 patients with simple MI and 16 with complicated MI were operated - 2 patients had surgeries performed in another province - 6/19 patients had enterotomy + washout - 5/19 patients had resection and primary anastomosis - 6/19 patients had resection and ostomy - 4/17 patients had a jejunal atresia, 1 patient had duodenal atresia and 1 had gastroschisis		- 6 operated patients presented complications (2 perforations and 4 bowel obstructions) - median age at surgery was 2 days - Median NICU and hospital stays were 34.5 and 70 days while median time on TPN and time to ostomy reversal were 28.5 and 97 days, respectively	- Prematurity and LBW are risk factors for MI and need for surgery. Specific genotypes and echogenic bowel were not predictors of either. - Comparing patients managed with and without ostomies, median times on TPN, in NICU, and in hospital were not significantly different

Table 1. *Cont.*

Author and Publication Year and Study Design	Purpose of the Study	Simple MI - Enema Treatment	Simple MI Requiring Surgery	Complex MI Requiring Surgery	Reported Outcomes/ Complications/Mortality	Conclusions
- Boczar et al., 2015 [9] - Retrospective study	Evaluation of diagnostic and treatment procedures in children with MI	5/8 patients with simple MI received enemas, with no success	- 8 patients with simple MI received a Bishop–Koop stoma and - 2 patients with complicated MI received a stoma - 5 patients were operated on during the first day of life, 4 on the second day and 1 on the third day of life		- The mean hospital stay was 22.9 days - In 8 children the stoma was taken out at the mean age of 19.4 months, in one patient the stoma closed spontaneously	The Bishop–Koop stoma, permitting the passage through the whole gastrointestinal tract, is a safe option - There were no abnormalities related to the electrolyte balance, excessive fluid loss, or body weight deficiencies associated with the stoma.
- Askarpour et al., 2020 [16] - Retrospective analysis	Surgical outcomes of neonates with meconium ileus who underwent Santulli ileostomy were compared to cases submitted to loop ileostomy		- 53 patients with MI received an ostomy - 28 Santulli ileostomy - 23 loop ileostomy		- necrosis, anastomotic leak, adhesive intestinal obstruction did not differ between the groups - skin excoriation, ostomy prolapsed, and surgical site infection was significantly lower in the Santulli ileostomy group compared to the loop group - ileostomy output in the first week and in 4th week was significantly lower in Santulli group - hospitalization in the Santulli group was 12 ± 2.34 days and after loop ileostomy was 14.24 ± 1.47 day ($p < 0.001$)	The Santulli ileostomy procedure has advantages over loop ileostomy in terms of postoperative outcomes, providing the finest esthetic results with the least amount of problems.

MI—meconium ileus; CF—cystic fibrosis; b-IRT—blood immunoreactive trypsinogen; LOS—length of stay; LBW—lower birth weight; US—ultrasound.

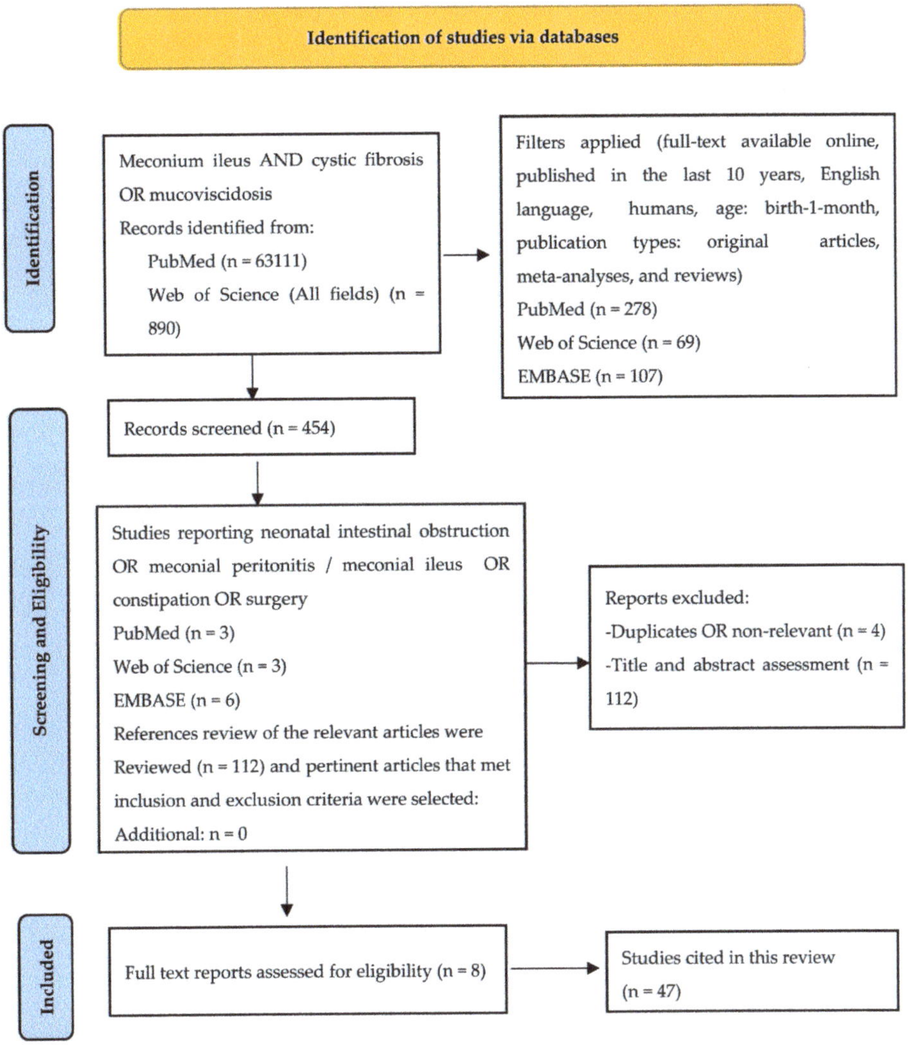

Figure 1. PRISMA flowchart. Notes: PRISMA figure adapted from Liberati A, et al. [11], Creative Commons.

3.1. *Prenatal Diagnosis and Fetal Risk Factors*

An intrauterine growth restriction and prenatal ultrasound findings including hyperechoic masses (signifying inspissated stool in the distal ileum), peritoneal calcifications, or non-visualization of the gallbladder may suggest CF in a high-risk fetus [2,17]. Fetal meconium is hypoechoic or isoechoic to surrounding abdominal structures in the second and third trimesters, whereas MI manifests as a hyperechoic mass with sonographic density higher than that of the liver or bone. If the prenatal ultrasound is abnormal, the parents' carrier status should be determined using a common mutation panel or entire CFTR gene sequencing. Adequate genetic counseling must be provided to address the risks of having a child with CF and its potential consequences if both parents are carriers of the disease. Then, the fetus should undergo ultrasound monitoring every six weeks and the delivery should be scheduled at a tertiary care facility with a multidisciplinary team including an experienced perinatologist, a pediatric surgeon, and a well-equipped neonatal intensive care unit (NICU). One will expect a premature birth and a reduced birth weight; the reduced birth weight of neonates with cystic fibrosis (CF) is mostly due to reduced intrauterine growth, which is only partially accounted for by shorter gestations [18].

In the last 10 years, we only found three original studies addressing the issue of prenatal ultrasound findings and the impact on postnatal management of neonates with MI and CF. In 2020, Shinar et al. analyzed a case series and performed a meta-analysis for identifying prenatal predictors of neonatal surgery; they identified 24 patients with MI and CF from 244 MI studied patients and found that meconium pseudocysts, bowel dilation, and ascites are prenatal predictors of neonatal surgery in cases of meconium peritonitis. Their postoperative mortality rate was 8.1% and the survival rate 100% for neonates not requiring surgery [12]. Padoan et al., in a retrospective, multicenter, observational study on 71 patients, also found that prenatally diagnosed intestinal obstruction is a risk factor for negative 12-month clinical outcomes in MI-CF newborns [13].

Jessula et al. in 2018 also performed a retrospective cohort review of prospectively collected data in order to identify if specific genetic subtypes and the presence of echogenic bowel on prenatal US are associated with either MI or operative requirement in the neonatal period. They identified seven patients with simple MI, who were treated conservatively and did not require any surgical intervention, three patients with simple MI, and sixteen with complicated MI who were operated. Prematurity and LBW were risk factors for MI and the need for surgery. Specific genotypes and echogenic bowel were not predictors of either [15].

3.2. Clinical Presentation and Diagnosis of Meconium Ileus

Increased sodium resorption through unregulated ENaCs is accompanied by water resorption and results in dehydrated mucus in the lungs and luminal contents of the small bowel, beginning from intrauterine life. Due to the deficiency in pancreatic enzymes and abnormal mucin production the meconium is thickened, protein-rich, and inspissated in the distal ileum, causing intrinsic obstruction and dilation of the small intestine upstream, until its perforation with meconium peritonitis. Approximately 15–20% of fetuses with cystic fibrosis manifest from birth with simple or complicated meconial ileus with meconium peritonitis. Although the clinical, ultrasound, and radiological appearance is different for simple versus complicated meconium ileus, the definitive diagnosis of cystic fibrosis is established based on genetic testing or biochemical alterations of the CFTR. In assessing the infant's clinical condition, a laboratory assessment that considers lactate, hemoglobin, white blood cell counts (WBC), and electrolytes is also needed [3,19].

The method for screening newborns for CF is usually predicated on two assessments of immunoreactive trypsinogen levels detected in a dried blood spot on the Guthrie card, the first test in the days 2–5 of life and the second being carried out within 30 days of birth [20]. This algorithm has a rather high false-positive result rate; also, the diagnosis is not ruled out in the event of a negative newborn screening result [Smith]. High b-IRT level was detected as a risk factor for negative 12-month clinical outcomes in MI-CF newborns in the study conducted by Padoan et al. in 2019 [13]. Sweat testing is performed to confirm or rule out cystic fibrosis if screening results are positive. In cases where the newborn is well-hydrated and not edematous, a sweat chloride test can be performed as soon as 48 h after delivery. This test is diagnostic at concentrations higher than 60 mmol/L and represents the gold standard biochemical analysis for CF. Nonetheless, many children diagnosed with MI require primary genetic testing because they are either too little, underweight, edematous, or too sick to undergo sweat testing right away.

CFTR functional testing and the identification of two mutations linked to cystic fibrosis are additional methods of diagnosis. A specific set of mutant probes can be used to evaluate one of the 40 most prevalent mutations seen in over 90% of mucoviscidosis patients. Anyway, this method is less sensitive than an expanded gene analysis, and is less likely to reveal polymorphisms and mutations of unknown significance [21].

3.2.1. Simple Meconium Ileus

Simple MI manifests from birth with the impossibility of eliminating meconium, bilious vomiting, and distended abdomen, with dilated intestinal loops visible on the abdominal wall (Figure 2).

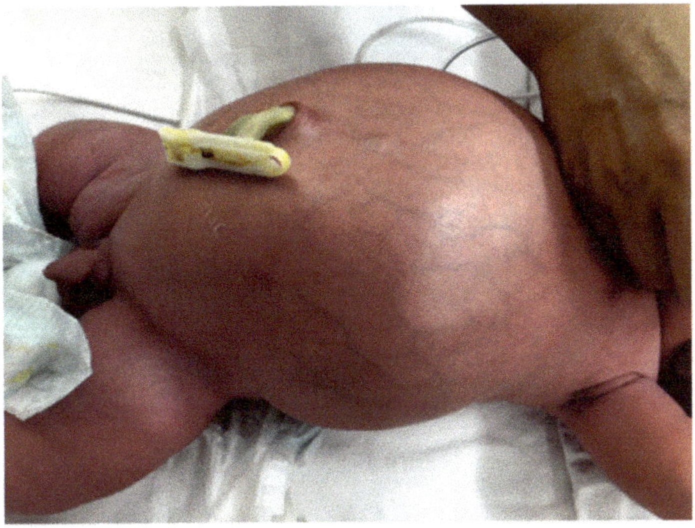

Figure 2. Clinical appearance of a patient with simple meconium ileus.

These clinical manifestations will raise the suspicion of cystic fibrosis and investigations will be continued with thoracoabdominal X-ray, ultrasound, genetic investigations, and sweat test. The ultrasound may show pseudo-thickening of the bowel walls because of thick and adhesive meconium. Stratified and dehydrated meconium causes the bowel lining to have increased echo intensity. Intestinal gases cannot be eliminated due to the high density of meconium and its adhesion to the intestinal walls, so that the abdomen becomes intensely weathered, occlusive, but in the absence of air–fluid levels. The abdominal radiograph has almost the same appearance in the supine and erect position with distended loops without air–fluid levels and a ground glass or 'soap-bubble' appearance (Neuhauser's sign) (Figure 3). Another typical occurrence on X-ray is inspissated pellets along the large intestine wall. If there is a total obstruction, there might not be any air in the rectum.

It could be acceptable to take blood and urine cultures and think about starting broad spectrum antibiotic medication if there is a fever or an elevated white blood cell count [22]. A nasogastric tube is implanted to facilitate the decompression of the stomach and proximal small bowel, to stop more bilious emesis and lower the risk of aspiration. Neonates with simple MI may achieve successful decompression after noninvasive management with Gastrografin or other contrast repeated enemas performed under fluoroscopic or ultrasound guidance, the success rates varying between 5% and 83% [2,8]. According to some authors, the percentage of babies who are treated without surgery has been declining over time [8,23]. In the last 10 years, we only found five studies reporting a total number of 133 cases of simple MI [8–10,13,15]; from them, 70 patients received at least one enema, with a success rate of 54% (38 patients responded to enemas and did not required any surgical intervention; that means a 28.5% rate of conservative management for simple MI).

The newborn needs to undergo fluid resuscitation (150 mL/kg/day minimum) via an intra-venous (IV) line prior to contrast because the hypertonicity of the enema might cause severe fluid changes, cardiovascular collapse, and even end-organ damage including necrotizing enterocolitis [3]. Up to 2–3 gentle enemas with hypertonic solution or acetylcysteine can be performed, under imaging control, with the visualization of the filling of the distal ileum, followed by the evacuation of meconium, as Noblett described since 1969 [24]. The perforation risk is between 2.7% and 23%; therefore, in order to react appropriately to complications like the necessity for urgent surgical intervention, the presence of an IV line is imperative [3]. In spite of this evidence, the agents that are currently used more frequently, at least in the United States, are Omnipaque (240–350 mOsm/kg water) and Cysto-contray II (400 mOsm/kg water), which are significantly less toxic and less hyperosmolar than Gastrografin [25]. Successful conservative management is associated with a shorter time to full feeds—6 (2–10) days in contrast with 15 days (9–19) in those with laparotomy [8]. In a recently published prospective study on 56 neonates with MI and CF, there was significant variation in the number of enemas per infant (1–4), as well as the concentration of the contrast agents. The mortality rate was 4% [8]. The UK and Ireland have highly diverse and non-standardized early management practices for newborns with MI [8]. Anyway, this was the only study reporting in detail the number and the type of hypertonic solution used for enema, and the results cannot be extrapolated due to the small number of cases (12 cases) [8]. After disimpaction of the terminal ileum with Gastrografin, Noblett used to recommend the administration of 5 mL of 10% N-Acetylcysteine every 6 h through the nasogastric tube, but that could cause chemical aspiration pneumonia. That is why some authors only recommend the continuation of enemas with saline solution, under serial radiological control [3,17].

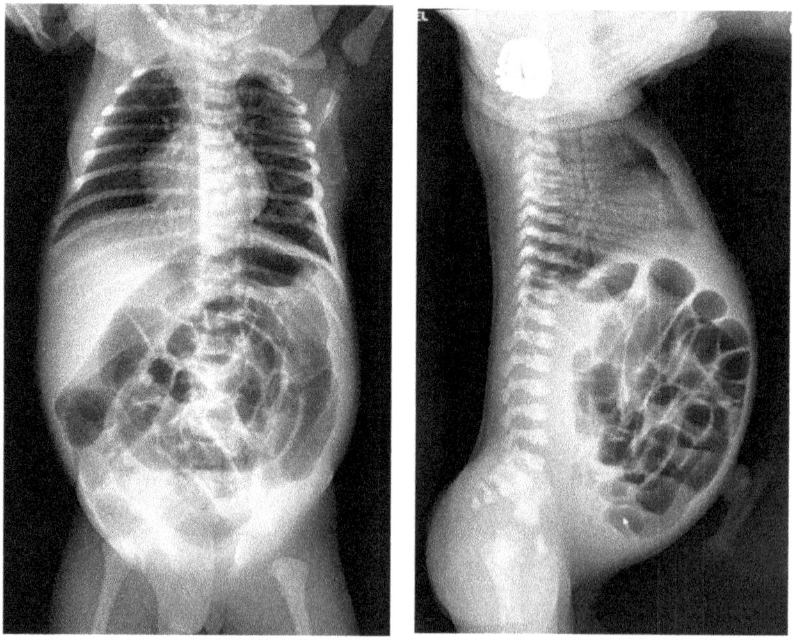

Figure 3. Abdominal X-ray showing dilated intestinal loops and a ground glass appearance; antero-posterior incidence and profile incidence.

If the enema maneuver fails or the patient's condition worsens, then surgical intervention will be performed through mini-laparotomy and resection of the impacted ileum with primary anastomosis or the creation of an ileostomy proximal to the impacted area with dehydrated meconium will be performed (Figures 4 and 5).

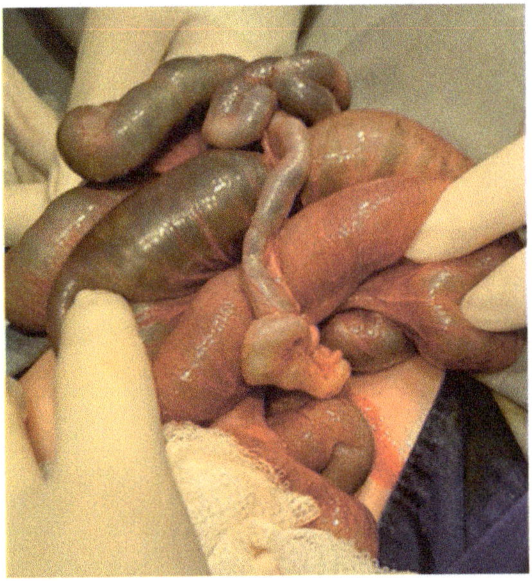

Figure 4. Intraoperative appearance of a meconium ileus showing a mesenteric defect, dilated intestinal loops and a meconium inspissated distal ileum.

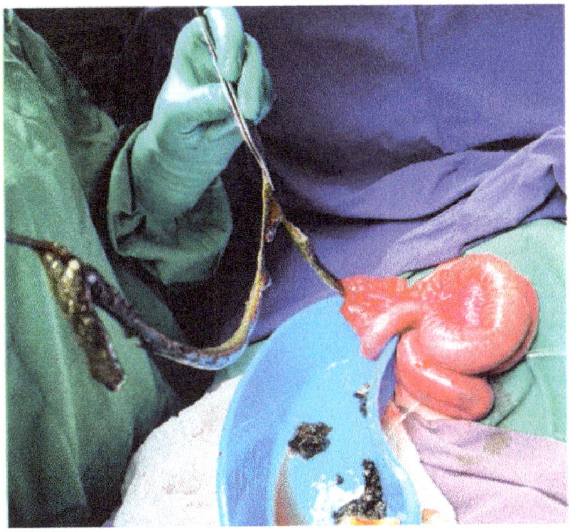

Figure 5. Intraoperative appearance of a dense, adherent meconium extracted from distal ileum.

The exact moment of the surgical intervention, the type of stoma, the postoperative management, or the optimal moment of closing the stoma varies depending on the case; there is no consensus in these respects. The Bishop–Koop distal stoma with a proximal end-to-side anastomosis, Santulli proximal stoma with a side-to-end distal anastomosis, or Mikulicz double barrel enterostomy are examples of traditional options for creating an ostomy [1,2,16]. Other therapeutic alternatives include enterotomy with evacuation of meconium and intraoperative saline or acetylcysteine irrigations, continued postoperatively through one of the mentioned stomas, or appendicostomy with saline irrigations intra and postoperatively [26]. Also, a minimal enterotomy with the insertion of a T-tube is sometimes recommended, the irrigations on the tube continuing postoperatively until a normal intestinal transit is obtained, at which point the T-tube is removed and the digestive fistula closes spontaneously. If the terminal ileum is blocked with meconium pellets that cannot be detached without significant damage, then resection of the respective area and primary anastomosis or ileostomy are recommended [26].

Boczar et al. in 2015 retrospectively studied eight patients with simple MI and two with complicated MI. Five from eight patients with simple MI received enemas with no success and all received a Bishop–Koop stoma. Their conclusion was that the Bishop–Koop stoma, permitting the passage through the whole gastrointestinal tract, is a safe option; there were no abnormalities related to the electrolyte balance, excessive fluid loss, or body weight deficiencies associated with the stoma [9].

3.2.2. Complicated Meconium Ileus

Intestinal atresia, prenatal volvulus with gangrene or perforation of the dilated intestinal loops which can lead to a meconium cyst, and meconium peritonitis are the characteristics of complicated meconium ileus [3,27]. The clinical presentation is influenced by the timing of the perforation. There is a chance that some meconium may be reabsorbed in the peritoneum prior to birth if perforation happens earlier in pregnancy, leaving only a few calcifications seen on ultrasound or abdominal X-ray after birth. A higher likelihood of meconium peritonitis or meconium cyst is observed if necrosis and perforation happen near to delivery. In a recent study, about 40% of all patients with MI had the complex form; of these, 13% (or one-third of all problematic cases) had intestinal atresia, and more than half of them also had intestinal volvulus. Given that between 8 and 11% of children with ileal atresia also have a CF diagnosis, these data lend support to the recent demand for a CF-oriented diagnostic work-up in any infant presenting with volvulus or jejunal/ileal atresia [13].

The clinical presentation is usually more spectacular than in the case of simple MI, with bilious vomiting, marked abdominal distension, abdominal wall edema, fever (Figure 6). Respiratory distress may also be caused by substantial abdominal distention. If the neonate is stable, a diagnostic contrast enema can help identify malrotation by pinpointing the cecum's location and identify a microcolon caused by proximal obstruction in the terminal ileum. If the patient's clinical condition is deteriorated, a simple abdominal X-ray (Figure 7) and an ultrasound are sufficient to guide operative management. Anyway, infants with complicated MI will always require surgery [8].

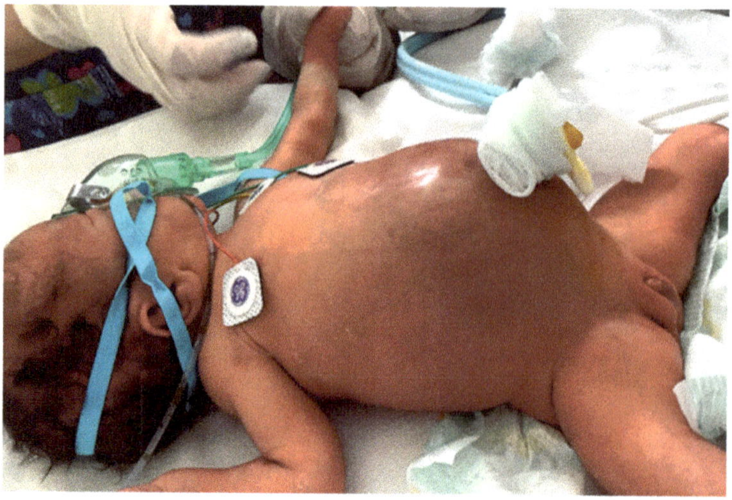

Figure 6. Clinical appearance of a patient with meconium peritonitis.

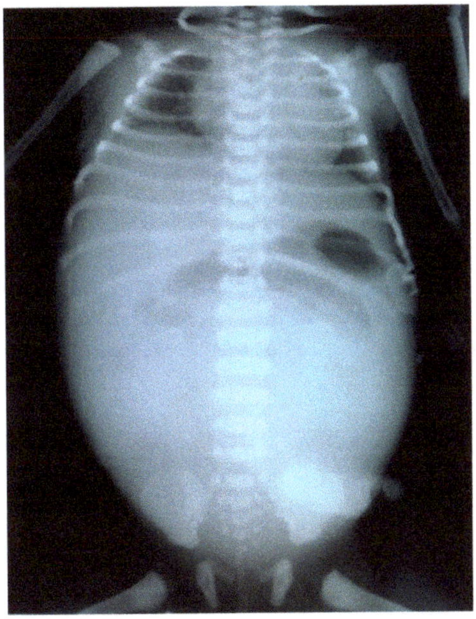

Figure 7. Abdominal X-ray showing dilated intestinal loops in the upper part of the abdomen and opacity due to meconium cyst in the rest of the abdomen.

Free intraperitoneal fluid with floating echogenic particles, single or numerous pseudocysts, collapsed bowel loops alternating with dilated intestinal loops, and hepatic or splenic calcifications can be seen on the postnatal ultrasound of a patient with complicated MI [28]. Caro-Domínguez et al. in 2018, in a retrospective comparative study, wanted to find out the role of postnatal radiographic and sonographic findings in predicting the need for surgery in neonates with MI. They demonstrated that diffuse peritoneal calcification as an isolated finding can be successfully treated non-operatively and imaging findings that predicted the need for surgery were intestinal obstruction, ascites, volvulus, and pneumoperitoneum [14].

Clinical presentation of a complicate MI may be a meconium pseudocyst with a fibrous wall with or without calcifications and the loops situated peripheral and usually posterior to the cyst. There are also possible thick vascular adhesions dotted with calcifications. Another form of presentation can be meconial ascites, which can become infected after birth [29]. These cases require surgical intervention to evacuate the ascites or pseudocyst, with the reduction of abdominal pressure. The membrane of the pseudocyst must be excised, this being sometimes difficult because it is very adherent to the intestinal loops (Figure 8). Once more, in order to remove the obstruction and provide continuous irrigation after surgery, an ostomy must usually be created. Padoan et al. demonstrated that a severe post-surgical clinical picture is a risk factor for negative 12-month clinical outcomes in MI-CF newborns; 18% of operated newborns had to undergo further abdominal surgery during the first month of life, for complications [13]. According to other reports, between 20% and 38% of patients with complicated MI will require reoperation for various complications [8,30].

Nevertheless, no comprehensive research has been conducted so far to determine the ideal surgical protocol for MI [17]. A proximal, distal, or Mikulicz double-barreled ileostomy; T-tube enterostomy; appendicostomy for irrigation and evacuation of impacted meconium; or resection of terminal ileon with primary anastomosis or with ileostomy may all be attempted. We found only three studies that reported the types of stomas performed and another study comparing the outcomes of patients depending on the surgical management [8,10,15,16].

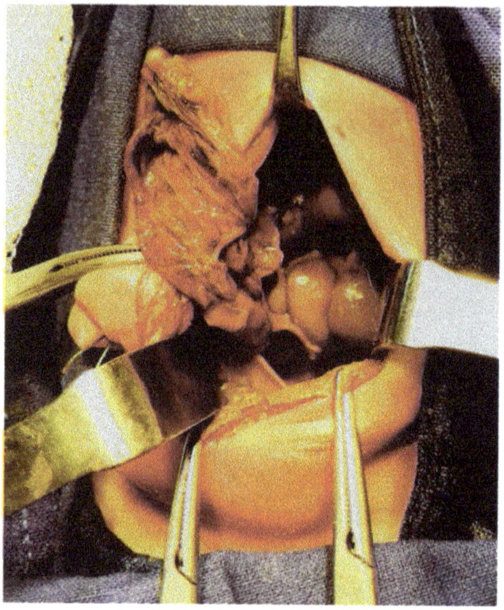

Figure 8. Intraoperative appearance of a meconium peritonitis with removal of the cystic membrane.

In the study conducted by Long et al., of the babies having laparotomies, 24 (56%) had a stoma formation; the type of stoma was known in 13 infants: 10 had Mikulicz double-barreled ileostomy, one newborn had a 'T-tube' ileostomy, and two had loop ileostomy. No infant was known to have a Bishop–Koop or a Santulli stoma. Nine infants from 24 who had stomas (38%) had complications and the mortality rate was 4%. Anyway, there was no comparation between the outcome of the patients depending on the type of stoma [8].

Askarpour et al. in 2020 performed a retrospective analysis to determine the surgical outcomes of neonates with meconium ileus who underwent Santulli ileostomy compared to cases submitted to loop ileostomy. They analyzed 28 Santulli ileostomy and 23 loop ileostomy cases and found that necrosis, anastomotic leak, and adhesive intestinal obstruction did not differ between the groups. Skin excoriation, ostomy prolapsed, and surgical site infection was significantly lower in the Santulli ileostomy group as compared to the loop group. Ileostomy output in the first week and fourth week was significantly lower in the Santulli group; also, hospitalization in the Santulli group was 12 ± 2.34 days and in the loop ileostomy group was 14.24 ± 1.47 day ($p < 0.001$). The Santulli ileostomy procedure has advantages over loop ileostomy in terms of postoperative outcomes, providing the finest esthetic results with the least amount of problems [16].

On the other hand, Farrelly et al. in 2014 analyzed 39 newborns with divided stomas, 7 with enterotomy and washout, and 8 with resection and primary anastomosis. They concluded that compared to therapy with stomas, retaining intestinal continuity at the initial laparotomy for MI appears to be safe, associated with shorter hospital stays, and does not increase the rate of unplanned re-laparotomy [10].

Jessula et al., comparing a small lot of patients managed with and without ostomies (six patients had enterotomy and washout, five patients had resection and primary anastomosis, and six patients had resection and ostomy), found that median times on TPN, in NICU, and in hospital were not significantly different [15].

Continuous fluid resuscitation is part of postoperative care, as well as oral feedings accompanied by vitamins and pancreatic enzyme supplementation once the dehydrated meconium was eliminated. Within 6 to 12 weeks, stomas should be closed to help prevent long-term issues with fluid, electrolyte, and nutritional losses. Due to their higher risk of newborn cholestasis, infants with MI also need to have their liver function checked every week. In addition, hyponatremia can occur in CF patients as a result of increased sweating and intestinal sodium loss [31]. The spot urine sodium to creatinine ratio, which has a goal of 17 to 52 mmol/mmol, is a more sensitive indicator of sodium status. This is especially true in infants who have had substantial bowel resection, whether or not they have an ileostomy, because of the excessive fluid and sodium loss [17].

3.3. Short- and Long-Term Prognosis

For patients with simple MI, successful conservative management is associated with a shorter time to full feeds, 6 days in contrast with 15 days in those with laparotomy, as demonstrated by Long et al. in 2021 in a prospective population-cohort study [8]. Farelly et al. reported a significant difference in LOS between operative patients managed with and without stomas: 49 versus 23 days [10].

When it comes to infants with complex MI, they frequently need TPN and lipids at first to sustain their growth. To reduce the incidence of cholestasis, the lipid selection should, if at all possible, favor an anti-inflammatory profile that includes fish oil and medium chain triglycerides (MCT). Proteins can be more easily digested using formulae based on amino acids or protein hydrolysates, whereas MCT are absorbed straight into portal circulation, avoiding the lymphatic system [32]. Breastmilk or conventional formulae can be offered as soon as the baby's gastrointestinal tolerance increases and they continue to heal from the initial insult of MI [13]. The combined pathophysiology of exposure to TPN and lipids, nothing *per os* condition encouraging biliary sludge, CFTR malfunction within biliary ducts, and intestinal obstruction are the primary causes of increased liver enzymes and cholestasis. When enteric feedings are introduced and advanced and ursodeoxycholic acid is used, the newborn cholestasis typically resolves entirely within three months. Although there has been evidence of a link between history of MI and CF-associated liver illness later in life, this link is still debatable because different research has produced conflicting results [6,33,34]. Supplementation of the diet with fat-soluble vitamin and pancreatic enzymes should also be carried out in children who start enteral nutrition with formula or breastmilk, starting with 2000–4000 lipase units per 120 mL of formula [35]. To maximize the effectiveness of pancreatic enzymes, acid-suppressing drugs such proton-pump inhibitors (PPIs) or histamine blockers are required to raise the pH of the gastric and proximal duodenal fluid [3].

An overall body sodium deficit may arise from excessive intestinal sodium losses when an ileostomy is present, contributing to metabolic acidosis and poor weight gain [2]. Thus, a supplementation of sodium may be given by increasing sodium in TPN or increasing sodium supplementation in enteral feeds. All these special dietary needs lead to prolonged hospitalization of patients with complex MI. In the study conducted by Jessula et al., median NICU and hospital stays were 34.5 and 70 days while median time on TPN and time to ostomy reversal were 28.5 and 97 days, respectively [15].

Patients with CF and MI have equivalent pulmonary function to those without MI at the ages of 15 and 25, but may have lower height and weight percentiles [2,36]. The relationship between the initial MI presentation and subsequent morbidity and mortality has been investigated in a number of retrospective or prospective studies [10,36,37]. There were no long-term differences between the groups in the retrospective studies that evaluated the nutritional status and pulmonary function of patients with CF and MI versus controls who were diagnosed due to other symptoms [10,36]. A nutritional deficiency was linked to worsening lung function in children and adolescents with cystic fibrosis, but not to morbidity in the prospective study conducted by Huaschild et al. [37].

Anyway, according to other studies on this issue, having MI will still put the patient at a major disadvantage even in this decade, with a significant higher mortality. These studies found growth retardation in patients with CF who present with MI and worse than ideal results in later life, particularly when it comes to a reduced forced expiratory volume in 1 s (FEV_1) [13,38]. Out of a total of 107 CF patients analyzed over a period of over 18 years, the

25 patients diagnosed with MI had the worst pubertal growth and adult height compared to patients diagnosed later, based on other symptoms [39]. In our study, the mortality rate varied between 0% and 8.1% for the neonates with MI and CF [8,10,12,13].

Regarding the long-term evolution of digestive disorders in patients with cystic fibrosis, MI has previously affected about 50% of distal intestinal obstruction syndrome patients (DIOS) [40]. DIOS is the meconium ileus equivalent, affecting 15 to 20% of children and adults with cystic fibrosis. Farelly et al. showed that presentation with MI did not predispose to later development of DIOS *per se*, but patients who presented with MI had a predisposition to develop a more severe form of DIOS necessitating surgery [10]. Other digestive complications of CF are rectal prolapse and fibrosing colonopathy, with episodes of intestinal occlusion due to stenosis [41] (Figure 9).

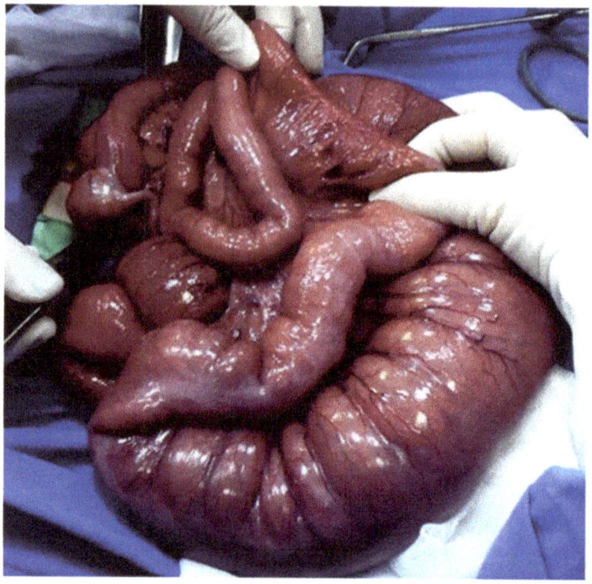

Figure 9. Intestinal stenosis with dilation of the ileon above in a patient with CF.

Patients diagnosed later, without MI, have the benefit of a less severe disease but the drawback of a delayed diagnosis. Patients with MI may have a more severe disease but benefit from an early diagnosis and treatment. That is why some authors even advise treating every MI patient as though they have CF until CF is ruled out in order to provide the best possible care, which includes starting pancreatic enzyme replacement therapy—a crucial step in the process [42].

4. Discussions

Cystic fibrosis, also called mucoviscidosis, is one of the most frequent autosomal recessive genetic disease among Caucasians, with an incidence of 1 in 2500 live births [1,41]. If in the previous decades the life expectancy of these patients was 30–40 years, thanks to the discoveries and innovations in the genetic, medical, and technological fields; more aggressive use of antibiotics; and intensive nutritional support, currently the life expectancy exceeds 50 years on average [43]. The first manifestation of this condition can be MI, and this form of neonatal occlusion can endanger the patient's life. Although these days approximately 80% of simple and severe MI cases have both early and late survival rates regularly documented [3,44], there is still no standardized protocol of diagnostic methods and no consensus on treatment methods. In 2014, Smyth et al. published the "European Cystic Fibrosis Society Standards of Care Best Practice guidelines", but the chapter "What is the best way to manage meconium ileus (MI) in patients with CF?" only has a few lines mentioning that both surgical and non-surgical management should be known to the surgical team; a complicated MI may need longer hospital stays, be more severe, and be more challenging to treat; it could be necessary to use a facility experienced in the dietary management of small bowel syndrome for postoperative care [45].

This is the only systematic review in the last 20 years regarding the diagnosis and treatment of meconium ileus in cystic fibrosis, trying to find the latest recommendations regarding the diagnosis and treatment of MI in CF. Although the diagnosis can be established prenatally, we only found three original studies addressing the issue of prenatal ultrasound findings and the impact on postnatal management of neonates with MI and CF [12,13,15], and no study about possible prenatal management. Treating moms with CFTR correctors and potentiators to act on aberrant CFTR in the fetus is one possible option to take into consideration. The natural course of MI may be altered by these drugs if they are begun at an early enough stage [3,46,47]. To stop the development of a microcolon or other problems, in utero surgical decompression of the occluded bowel or correction of MI would be another possible prenatal intervention.

Neonates with simple MI may achieve successful decompression after noninvasive management with Gastrografin, other contrast repeated enemas, or with acetylcysteine, but the percentage of babies who are treated without surgery has been declining over time. In the last 10 years, we only found 5 studies reporting the results after conservative treatment of MI, with a mean success rate of 28.5%. These results could be the result of contrast agent use, radiologist experience changes, or unwillingness to repeat enemas. Consequently, increased rates of surgical intervention are currently noted. There is a need for more precise guidelines regarding when to resort to surgical treatments, as there remains a considerable percentage of cases (up to 72%) in which the conservative therapy may not be effective. Surgeons should advise repeat enemas prior to laparotomy in patients who are stable. If the enema maneuver fails or the patient's condition worsens, then surgical intervention will be performed and a stoma created. Although many reviews discuss the benefits or disadvantages of various types of stomas or resection of the distal ileal loop and primary anastomosis, the only original study from the analyzed period recommends the Bishop–Koop stoma for simple meconium ileus that does not respond to enemas [9]. If simple MI responds to enemas, there is still no consensus on the method of continuing the treatment with acetylcysteine or on the moment when enemas are no longer necessary.

For complicated MI, although alternative techniques have been identified, the two basic categories of strategies are those that involve creating a stoma and those that preserve bowel continuity. Comparing patients managed with and without ostomies, median times on TPN, in NICU, and in hospital were not significantly different in the study conducted by Jessula et al. on 19 patients [15]. Instead, in their 2014 study on 54 patients, Farelly et al. concluded that compared to therapy with stomas, retaining intestinal continuity at the initial laparotomy for MI appears to be safe, associated with shorter hospital stays, and does not increase the rate of unplanned re-laparotomy [10]. They reported an increased incidence of complex MI (49%), without mentioning exactly what type of complex MI the patients had. However, in this way they justified the low rate of use of conservative therapeutic methods (Gastrografin enema successful in only 9%) [10]. Regarding the type of stoma, no conclusion can be drawn from the studies of the last 10 years; it seems anyway that Santulli or Bishop–Koop type stomas have superior results compared to loop stomas in patients with complicated MI [9,16]. For a correct comparison of the data and relevant conclusions, there should be uniformity and a standardization of the diagnosis and the treatment methods.

Study Limitations

Frequent to most systematic reviews on MI treatments, include the small number of original studies in the last 10 years and small number of analyzed patients (out of 566 publications verified, only 8 met the inclusion criteria). The conclusions reached may not be robust or generalizable due to the small dataset. Most studies were retrospectively conducted which also limits the generalization of the results and there may be a high risk of reporting bias. Conservative or surgical management is not standardized between studies and very little comparative data exist to determine which kind of surgery or stoma is ideal, which make it difficult to harmonize results. Neonates with MI and pediatric patients with CF had promising responses to treatment with CFTR correctors and potentiators to act on aberrant CFTR, but RCTs are needed to comprehensively understand their efficacy. Early diagnosis of CF and the initiation of appropriate, multidisciplinary management of MI may help mitigate the risk of developing irreversible digestive and pulmonary damage that will necessitate invasive surgical interventions in these patients.

5. Conclusions

Neonates with cystic fibrosis and meconium ileus are treated in very different ways and according to different national standards. This brings to light a major problem in the subject because it could be difficult to attain firm findings due to the diversity of practices. This study reveals a lack of strong data to support management decisions, unequivocally shows that the care of infants with MI is not standardized, and suggests a great need for international collaborative studies.

Anyway, until proven otherwise, each patient with MI should be treated as though they have CF and receive the proper care, as research has demonstrated that early detection and treatment by a multidisciplinary team improves these patients' short- and long-term prognosis. When feasible, non-operative management is probably ideal for the baby because it saves surgery and makes the transition to full enteral feedings easier. If laparotomy is needed, ileostomy formation is the most common approach. The prognosis for CF patients with MI is now similar to that of CF patients without MI thanks to the use of contrast enemas as a treatment for simple MI, improved surgical methods, and early adoption of nutritional support for complicated MI.

Author Contributions: Conceptualization, M.A.D., E.Ţ. and L.M.T.; methodology, G.G.; software, V.Ţ.; validation, V.Ţ., E.C. and L.I.B.; formal analysis, V.B.; investigation, D.E.M.; data curation, G.G.; writing—original draft preparation, E.Ţ. and E.M.; writing—review and editing, M.A.D. and I.C.R.; visualization, L.M.T.; supervision, E.Ţ. and V.Ţ. All authors equally contributed to the article. All authors have read and agreed to the published version of the manuscript.

Funding: This research received no external funding.

Institutional Review Board Statement: Not applicable.

Informed Consent Statement: The authors have obtained the consent of the parents to use images for medical and scientific purposes.

Data Availability Statement: Dataset available on request from the authors.

Conflicts of Interest: The authors declare no conflicts of interest.

References

1. Richards, M.; Waldhausen, J.H. Meconium Ileus. *Clin. Colon Rectal Surg.* **2018**, *31*, 121–126. [CrossRef] [PubMed]
2. Carlyle, B.E.; Borowitz, D.S.; Glick, P.L. A review of pathophysiology and management of fetuses and neonates with meconium ileus for the pediatric surgeon. *J. Pediatr. Surg.* **2012**, *47*, 772–781, Erratum in *J. Pediatr. Surg.* **2012**, *47*, 1633. [CrossRef] [PubMed]
3. Sathe, M.; Houwen, R. Meconium ileus in Cystic Fibrosis. *J. Cyst. Fibros.* **2017**, *16* (Suppl. 2), S32–S39. [CrossRef]
4. Sun, L.; Rommens, J.M.; Corvol, H.; Li, W.; Li, X.; Chiang, T.A.; Lin, F.; Dorfman, R.; Busson, P.-F.; Parekh, R.V.; et al. Multiple apical plasma membrane constituents are associated with susceptibility to meconium ileus in individuals with cystic fibrosis. *Nat. Genet.* **2012**, *44*, 562–569. [CrossRef] [PubMed]
5. Blackman, S.M.; Deering–Brose, R.; McWilliams, R.; Naughton, K.; Coleman, B.; Lai, T.; Algire, M.; Beck, S.; Hoover-Fong, J.; Hamosh, A.; et al. Relative contribution of genetic and nongenetic modifiers to intestinal obstruction in cystic fibrosis. *Gastroenterology* **2006**, *131*, 1030–1039. [CrossRef] [PubMed]
6. Butnariu, L.I.; Ţarcă, E.; Cojocaru, E.; Rusu, C.; Moisă, M.; Constantin, M.-M.L.; Gorduza, E.V.; Trandafir, L.M. Genetic Modifying Factors of Cystic Fibrosis Phenotype: A Challenge for Modern Medicine. *J. Clin. Med.* **2021**, *10*, 5821. [CrossRef] [PubMed]

7. Yule, A.; Sills, D.; Smith, S.; Spiller, R.; Smyth, A.R. Thinking outside the box: A review of gastrointestinal symptoms and complications in cystic fibrosis. *Expert Rev. Respir. Med.* **2023**, *17*, 547–561. [CrossRef] [PubMed]
8. Long, A.-M.; Jones, I.H.; Knight, M.; McNally, J.; Saeed, A.; Lopes, J.; Garrett-Cox, R.; Sherwood, W.; Besarovic, S.; Jones, C.; et al. Early management of meconium ileus in infants with cystic fibrosis: A prospective population cohort study. *J. Pediatr. Surg.* **2021**, *56*, 1287–1292. [CrossRef]
9. Boczar, M.; Sawicka, E.; Zybert, K. Meconium ileus in newborns with cystic fibrosis—Results of treatment in the group of patients operated on in the years 2000–2014. *Dev. Period Med.* **2015**, *19*, 32–40.
10. Farrelly, P.J.; Charlesworth, C.; Lee, S.; Southern, K.W.; Baillie, C.T. Gastrointestinal surgery in cystic fibrosis: A 20-year review. *J. Pediatr. Surg.* **2014**, *49*, 280–283. [CrossRef]
11. Liberati, A.; Altman, D.G.; Tetzlaff, J.; Mulrow, C.; Gøtzsche, P.C.; Ioannidis, J.P.; Clarke, M.; Devereaux, P.J.; Kleijnen, J.; Moher, D. The PRISMA statement for reporting systematic 426 reviews and meta-analyses of studies that evaluate healthcare interventions: Explanation and elaboration. In *BMJ*; 2009; 21, p. 339. Available online: https://www.ncbi.nlm.nih.gov/pmc/articles/PMC2714672/ (accessed on 15 March 2024).
12. Shinar, S.; Agrawal, S.; Ryu, M.; Van Mieghem, T.; Daneman, A.; Ryan, G.; Zani, A.; Chiu, P.; Chitayat, D. Fetal Meconium Peritonitis—Prenatal Findings and Postnatal Outcome: A Case Series, Systematic Review, and Meta-Analysis. Fetale Mekoniumperitonitis—Pränatale Befunde und postnatales Outcome: Eine Fallserie, systematische Übersicht und Metaanalyse. *Ultraschall Med. Eur. J. Ultrasound* **2022**, *43*, 194–203. [CrossRef] [PubMed]
13. Padoan, R.; Cirilli, N.; Falchetti, D.; Cesana, B.M.; Meconium Ileus Project Study Group. Risk factors for adverse outcome in infancy in meconium ileus cystic fibrosis infants: A multicentre Italian study. *J. Cyst. Fibros.* **2019**, *18*, 863–868. [CrossRef] [PubMed]
14. Caro-Domínguez, P.; Zani, A.; Chitayat, D.; Daneman, A. Meconium peritonitis: The role of postnatal radiographic and sonographic findings in predicting the need for surgery. *Pediatr. Radiol.* **2018**, *48*, 1755–1762. [CrossRef] [PubMed]
15. Jessula, S.; Hof, M.V.D.; Mateos-Corral, D.; Mills, J.; Davies, D.; Romao, R.L.P. Predictors for surgical intervention and surgical outcomes in neonates with cystic fibrosis. *J. Pediatr. Surg.* **2018**, *53*, 2150–2154. [CrossRef] [PubMed]
16. Askarpour, S.; Ayatipour, A.; Peyvasteh, M.; Javaherizadeh, H. A comparative study between Santulli ileostomy and loop ileostomy in neonates with meconium ileus. *Abcd-Arquivos Bras. Cir. Dig. Arch. Dig. Surg.* **2020**, *33*, e1485. [CrossRef] [PubMed]
17. Parikh, N.S.; Ibrahim, S.; Ahlawat, R. Meconium Ileus. In *StatPearls [Internet]*; StatPearls Publishing: Treasure Island, FL, USA, 2024; Updated 8 August 2023. Available online: https://www.ncbi.nlm.nih.gov/books/NBK537008/ (accessed on 17 March 2024).
18. Schlüter, D.K.; Griffiths, R.; Adam, A.; Akbari, A.; Heaven, M.L.; Paranjothy, S.; Andersen, A.-M.N.; Carr, S.B.; Pressler, T.; Diggle, P.J.; et al. Impact of cystic fibrosis on birthweight: A population based study of children in Denmark and Wales. *Thorax* **2019**, *74*, 447–454. [CrossRef]
19. Belu, A.; Trandafir, L.M.; Țarcă, E.; Cojocaru, E.; Frăsinariu, O.; Stârcea, M.; Moscalu, M.; Tiutiuca, R.C.; Luca, A.C.; Galaction, A. Variations in Biochemical Values under Stress in Children with SARS-CoV-2 Infection. *Diagnostics* **2022**, *12*, 1213. [CrossRef] [PubMed] [PubMed Central]
20. Athanazio, R.A.; Filho, L.V.R.F.d.S.; Vergara, A.A.; Ribeiro, A.F.; Riedi, C.A.; Procianoy, E.d.F.A.; Adde, F.V.; Reis, F.J.C.; Ribeiro, J.D.; Torres, L.A.; et al. Brazilian guidelines for the diagnosis and treatment of cystic fibrosis. *J. Bras. Pneumol.* **2017**, *43*, 219–245. [CrossRef] [PubMed] [PubMed Central]
21. O'Sullivan, B.P.; Freedman, S.D. Cystic fibrosis. *Lancet* **2009**, *373*, 1891–1904. [CrossRef]
22. Duceac, L.D.; Marcu, C.; Ichim, D.L.; Ciomaga, I.M.; Tarca, E.; Iordache, A.C.; Ciuhodaru, M.I.; Florescu, L.; Tutunaru, D.; Luca, A.C.; et al. Antibiotic Molecules Involved in Increasing Microbial Resistance. *Rev. Chim.* **2019**, *70*, 2622–2626. [CrossRef]
23. Copeland, D.R.; Peter, S.D.S.; Sharp, S.W.; Islam, S.; Cuenca, A.; Tolleson, J.S.; Dassinger, M.S.; Little, D.C.; Jackson, R.J.; Kokoska, E.R.; et al. Diminishing role of contrast enema in simple meconium ileus. *J. Pediatr. Surg.* **2009**, *44*, 2130–2132. [CrossRef] [PubMed]
24. Noblett, H.R. Treatment of uncomplicated meconium ileus by gastrografin enema: A preliminary report. *J. Pediatr. Surg.* **1969**, *4*, 190–197. [CrossRef] [PubMed]
25. Burke, M.S.; Ragi, J.M.; Karamanoukian, H.L.; Kotter, M.; Brisseau, G.F.; Borowitz, D.S.; Ryan, M.E.; Irish, M.S.; Glick, P.L. New strategies in nonoperative management of meconium ileus. *J. Pediatr. Surg.* **2002**, *37*, 760–764. [CrossRef] [PubMed]
26. Pandey, A.; Singh, A.K.; Rawat, J.; Singh, S.; Wakhlu, A.; Kureel, S.N. Management Strategy of Meconium Ileus-Outcome Analysis. *J. Indian Assoc. Pediatr. Surg.* **2019**, *24*, 120–123. [CrossRef] [PubMed] [PubMed Central]
27. Best, E.J.; O'brien, C.M.; Carseldine, W.; Deshpande, A.; Glover, R.; Park, F. Fetal Midgut Volvulus with Meconium Peritonitis Detected on Prenatal Ultrasound. *Case Rep. Obstet. Gynecol.* **2018**, *2018*, 5312179. [CrossRef] [PubMed] [PubMed Central]
28. Veyrac, C.; Baud, C.; Prodhomme, O.; Saguintaah, M.; Couture, A. US assessment of neonatal bowel (necrotizing enterocolitis excluded). *Pediatr. Radiol.* **2012**, *42* (Suppl. 1), 107–114. [CrossRef]
29. Khan, S.A.; Khare, M.; Dagash, H.; Kairamkonda, V. Meconium pseudocyst presenting as massive ascites in a new-born. *Radiol. Case Rep.* **2018**, *14*, 235–237. [CrossRef] [PubMed] [PubMed Central]
30. Steven, L.C.; Gavel, G.; Young, D.; Carachi, R. Immunoreactive trypsin levels in neonates with meconium ileus. *Pediatr. Surg. Int.* **2006**, *22*, 236–239. [CrossRef]

31. Allouzi, S.; Rihawi, B.; Allouzi, J.; Allouzi, M.I.; Abdulrahman, N.; Abdullah, M. A unique presentation of hyponatremia and seizures in a 2-month-old child with cystic fibrosis: A case report. *Ann. Med. Surg.* **2023**, *85*, 4150–4152. [CrossRef] [PubMed] [PubMed Central]
32. Trandafir, L.M.; Frăsinariu, O.E.; Țarcă, E.; Butnariu, L.I.; Constantin, M.M.L.; Moscalu, M.; Temneanu, O.R.; Popescu, A.S.M.; Popescu, M.G.M.; Stârcea, I.M.; et al. Can Bioactive Food Substances Contribute to Cystic Fibrosis-Related Cardiovascular Disease Prevention? *Nutrients* **2023**, *15*, 314. [CrossRef] [PubMed]
33. Leeuwen, L.; Magoffin, A.K.; Fitzgerald, D.A.; Cipolli, M.; Gaskin, K.J. Cholestasis and meconium ileus in infants with cystic fibrosis and their clinical outcomes. *Arch. Dis. Child.* **2014**, *99*, 443–447. [CrossRef] [PubMed]
34. Fiorotto, R.; Strazzabosco, M. Pathophysiology of Cystic Fibrosis Liver Disease: A Channelopathy Leading to Alterations in Innate Immunity and in Microbiota. *Cell. Mol. Gastroenterol. Hepatol.* **2019**, *8*, 197–207. [CrossRef] [PubMed]
35. Zheng, Y.; Mostamand, S. Nutrition in children with exocrine pancreatic insufficiency. *Front. Pediatr.* **2023**, *11*, 943649. [CrossRef] [PubMed] [PubMed Central]
36. Sanders, D.B.; Slaven, J.E.; Maguiness, K.; Chmiel, J.F.; Ren, C.L. Early-Life Height Attainment in Cystic Fibrosis Is Associated with Pulmonary Function at Age 6 Years. *Ann. Am. Thorac. Soc.* **2021**, *18*, 1335–1342. [CrossRef] [PubMed]
37. Hauschild, D.B.; Rosa, A.F.; Ventura, J.C.; Barbosa, E.; Moreira, E.A.M.; Ludwig Neto, N.; Moreno, Y.M.F. Association of nutritional status with lung function and morbidity in children and adolescents with cystic fibrosis: A 36-month cohort study. *Rev. Paul Pediatr.* **2018**, *36*, 8. [CrossRef] [PubMed] [PubMed Central]
38. Tan, S.M.J.; Coffey, M.J.; Ooi, C.Y. Differences in clinical outcomes of paediatric cystic fibrosis patients with and without meconium ileus. *J. Cyst. Fibros.* **2019**, *18*, 857–862. [CrossRef] [PubMed]
39. Zhang, Z.; Lindstrom, M.J.; Farrell, P.M.; Lai, H.J.; with the Wisconsin Cystic Fibrosis Neonatal Screening Group. Pubertal Height Growth and Adult Height in Cystic Fibrosis After Newborn Screening. *Pediatrics* **2016**, *137*, e20152907. [CrossRef] [PubMed]
40. Kelly, T.; Buxbaum, J. Gastrointestinal Manifestations of Cystic Fibrosis. *Dig. Dis. Sci.* **2015**, *60*, 1903–1913. [CrossRef]
41. Tobias, J.; Tillotson, M.; Maloney, L.; Fialkowski, E. Meconium Ileus, Distal Intestinal Obstruction Syndrome, and Other Gastrointestinal Pathology in the Cystic Fibrosis Patient. *Surg. Clin. N. Am.* **2022**, *102*, 873–882. [CrossRef]
42. Sathe, M.; Houwen, R. Is meconium ileus associated with worse outcomes in cystic fibrosis? *J. Cyst. Fibros.* **2019**, *18*, 746. [CrossRef] [PubMed]
43. van der Doef, H.P.J.; Kokke, F.T.M.; van der Ent, C.K.; Houwen, R.H.J. Intestinal obstruction syndromes in cystic fibrosis: Meconium ileus, distal intestinal obstruction syndrome, and constipation. *Curr. Gastroenterol. Rep.* **2011**, *13*, 265–270. [CrossRef] [PubMed]
44. Grosse, S.D.; Rosenfeld, M.; Devine, O.J.; Lai, H.J.; Farrell, P.M. Potential impact of newborn screening for cystic fibrosis on child survival: A systematic review and analysis. *J. Pediatr.* **2006**, *149*, 362–366. [CrossRef] [PubMed]
45. Smyth, A.R.; Bell, S.C.; Bojcin, S.; Bryon, M.; Duff, A.; Flume, P.; Kashirskaya, N.; Munck, A.; Ratjen, F.; Schwarzenberg, S.J.; et al. European Cystic Fibrosis Society Standards of Care: Best Practice guidelines. *J. Cyst. Fibros.* **2014**, *13*, S23–S42. [CrossRef]
46. Solomon, G.M.; Marshall, S.G.; Ramsey, B.W.; Rowe, S.M. Breakthrough therapies: Cystic fibrosis (CF) potentiators and correctors. *Pediatr. Pulmonol.* **2015**, *50*, S3–S13. [CrossRef] [PubMed] [PubMed Central]
47. Skilton, M.; Krishan, A.; Patel, S.; Sinha, I.P.; Southern, K.W. Potentiators (specific therapies for class III and IV mutations) for cystic fibrosis. *Cochrane Database Syst. Rev.* **2019**, *2019*, CD009841. [CrossRef]

diagnostics MDPI

Article

Assessing Differential Transfusion Requirements for Children with Congenital Malformations vs. Pediatric Acute Abdomen Emergencies

Alin Ionescu [1,2], Alexandra Mihăilescu [3], Adela Chiriță-Emandi [3], Nitesh Munagala [4], Vlad Laurențiu David [5], Raluca Dumache [6], Dorel Săndesc [7], Ovidiu Bedreag [7], Roxana Folescu [8,*], Felix Bratosin [9], Paula Irina Barata [10,11], Dan-Mihai Cristescu [2,12] and Mihai Alexandru Săndesc [13]

1 Center for Preventive Medicine, "Victor Babeș" University of Medicine and Pharmacy, 300041 Timișoara, Romania; ionescu.alin@umft.ro
2 Doctoral School, "Victor Babeș" University of Medicine and Pharmacy, 300041 Timisoara, Romania; dancristescu93@gmail.com
3 Centre of Genomic Medicine, Genetics Discipline, "Victor Babeș" University of Medicine and Pharmacy, 300041 Timisoara, Romania; alexandra.mihailescu@umft.ro (A.M.); adela.chirita@umft.ro (A.C.-E.)
4 Guntur Medical College Affiliated with Dr. NTR University of Health Sciences, Vijayawada 520008, India; munagalanitesh@gmail.com
5 Department of Pediatric Surgery and Orthopedics, "Victor Babeș" University of Medicine and Pharmacy, 300041 Timisoara, Romania; david.vlad@umft.ro
6 Center for Ethics in Human Genetic Identifications, "Victor Babeș" University of Medicine and Pharmacy, 300041 Timisoara, Romania; raluca.dumache@umft.ro
7 Research Center CCATITM, "Victor Babeș" University of Medicine and Pharmacy, 300041 Timisoara, Romania; sandesc.dorel@umft.ro (D.S.); bedreag.ovidiu@umft.ro (O.B.)
8 Discipline of Family Medicine, "Victor Babeș" University of Medicine and Pharmacy, 300041 Timisoara, Romania
9 Department of Infectious Disease, "Victor Babeș" University of Medicine and Pharmacy, 300041 Timisoara, Romania; felix.bratosin@umft.ro
10 Center for Research and Innovation in Precision Medicine of Respiratory Diseases, "Victor Babeș" University of Medicine and Pharmacy, 300041 Timisoara, Romania; barata.paula@student.uvvg.ro
11 Department of Physiology, Faculty of Medicine, "Vasile Goldis" Western University of Arad, 310025 Arad, Romania
12 Research Centre of Timisoara Institute of Cardiovascular Diseases, "Victor Babes" University of Medicine and Pharmacy, 300041 Timisoara, Romania
13 Research Center Professor Doctor Teodor Șora, "Victor Babeș" University of Medicine and Pharmacy, 300041 Timisoara, Romania; sandesc.mihai@umft.ro
* Correspondence: folescu.roxana@umft.ro

Abstract: Background and Objectives: This retrospective study aimed to evaluate the efficacy of preoperative blood transfusions in correcting anemia for pediatric patients with congenital malformations (CMs) versus those with acute abdomen (AA) conditions. The study hypothesized that the response to transfusions might vary significantly between these groups due to the differences in the underlying pathology and clinical status. Methods: The study included 107 pediatric patients admitted to Timisoara 'Louis Turcanu' Emergency Hospital for Children between January 2015 and May 2023, who required blood transfusions for preoperative anemia. Hemoglobin (HGB), hematocrit (HCT), and red blood cell counts (RBC) were assessed at admission, 48 h post-transfusion, and at discharge. Statistical analyses, including Student's *t*-test, Pearson correlation, and chi-square tests, were utilized to compare outcomes between the groups. The study population was divided into 53 children with CM and 54 with AA. Results: Initial analyses showed that children with CM had statistically significantly higher baseline HGB (8.54 ± 1.00 g/dL vs. 7.87 ± 1.02 g/dL, $p = 0.001$) and HCT ($26.07 \pm 3.98\%$ vs. $23.95 \pm 2.90\%$, $p = 0.002$) compared to those with AA. Post-transfusion, children with CM exhibited a greater increase in HGB, with the highest increases noted in patients with central nervous system defects (mean increase of 3.67 g/dL, $p = 0.038$). In contrast, the increases in HGB for children with AA were less pronounced, with the highest being 2.03 g/dL in those with peritonitis ($p = 0.078$). Conclusions: No significant gender differences were noted in response to transfusion. Children with congenital malformations respond more effectively to preoperative blood transfusions compared to those with acute abdomen conditions. These findings suggest that differential transfusion strategies may be required based on the underlying medical condition to optimize the management of preoperative anemia in pediatric patients. Tailoring transfusion approaches according to specific patient needs and conditions could enhance clinical outcomes and resource utilization in pediatric surgical settings.

Keywords: anemia; blood transfusion; congenital malformations; pediatric patients; children

1. Introduction

Anemia is a significant and modifiable risk factor associated with elevated perioperative morbidity and mortality. It is estimated that a quarter of the world's population is affected by anemia, with around 40% of children under five being diagnosed with anemia in 2023 [1,2].

It is essential to identify and, if possible, promptly correct the etiology of anemia, as it varies significantly among different age groups. In neonates, anemia is often due to hemorrhage and hemolysis (e.g., isoimmune hemolysis or glucose-6-phosphate dehydrogenase deficiency), rather than decreased production [3]. Additionally, congenital anomalies and conditions associated with blood loss, such as surgical procedures, can contribute to anemia in this age group. For example, a newborn who undergoes surgery is expected to develop anemia subsequently due to perioperative blood loss. In the pediatric population beyond the neonatal period, common causes of anemia include iron deficiency, infections, hemoglobinopathies, and other chronic conditions [1]. Iron deficiency remains one of the most critical causes of anemia in children worldwide. Gedfie et al. [4], in a systematic review, reported a global prevalence of iron-deficiency anemia of 16.42%, while the prevalence of iron deficiency reached 17.95% in children under 5 years of age. Moreover, they highlighted considerable variability among different geographic regions. Similar findings were reported by Nazari et al. [5], who found prevalences of 18.2% for iron-deficiency anemia and 27.7% for iron deficiency in Iranian children under 6 years of age. Certain causes of anemia, such as sickle cell disease and leishmaniasis, are significantly more prevalent in specific geographic areas. Therefore, geographic and age-related factors should be carefully considered, and a thorough history should be obtained [6,7].].

Regardless of the etiology, when a blood transfusion is necessary, blood requirements should be thoroughly calculated to avoid hypervolemia and other transfusion reactions. Thus, age, clinical status, and comorbidities, as well as weight and increment in hemoglobin, should all be considered before making clinical decisions [8,9].

Transfusion-associated circulatory overload (TACO) is a serious transfusion complication associated with increased morbidity and mortality [10]. It is characterized by pulmonary edema and congestive heart failure due to increased hydrostatic blood pressure from volume overload following blood transfusion [11]. However, overload and pulmonary edema are not common complications in children when transfused with the correct volumes at appropriate rates. The data regarding the prevalence of TACO in pediatric patients are inconsistent, partly due to varying definitions and patient populations studied. For instance, De Cloedt L et al. [12] reported incidence rates ranging from 1.5% to 76%, depending on the criteria used to define TACO and whether a 10% or 20% threshold increase in blood volume was considered. The wide range reflects differences in patient groups, including those with and without comorbidities that predispose them to circulatory overload. In children without comorbidities, the incidence of transfusion complications, including TACO, is significantly lower when transfusions are administered with careful attention to volume and rate. Therefore, adherence to appropriate transfusion protocols is essential to minimize the risk of TACO and other transfusion-related complications in pediatric patients.

The efficient treatment of anemia is crucial in patients scheduled for surgery since the condition has been associated with an increased risk of postoperative complications, longer hospitalization, and a higher mortality rate. In a study published by Faraoni et al. [13], preoperative anemia was associated with higher in-hospital mortality (OR 2.17) in children undergoing noncardiac surgery. Likewise, Scott et al. [14], in a meta-analysis of children aged between 28 days and 12 years, reported a 24% decrease in death risk for each 1g/dL increase in hemoglobin.

Depending on age categories, anemia can arise from various origins, such as congenital anomalies, conditions that predispose individuals to blood loss, surgical interventions, and chronic disease [15–18]. For instance, newborns undergoing surgical procedures often face a high risk of developing anemia due to intraoperative or postoperative blood loss. Moreover, the mechanisms responsible for the complications linked to anemia are related to the pathophysiological response to hypoxia. To illustrate, in the case of cerebrovascular events, the hyperkinetic state associated with anemia determines the hyperexpression of different adhesion molecules in endothelial cells, consequently increasing the risk of thrombi [19]. In addition, impaired oxygen delivery to organs reduces the tolerance to ischemia and hemorrhage. In bacterial infections, many pathways seem to act synergically (e.g., enhanced erythropoietic drive, hemolysis, immune dysfunction) [20].

The aim of the current study was to evaluate the differences in the efficacy of preoperative blood transfusions in correcting anemia between children with congenital malformations (CMs) and those with acute abdomen (AA). We hypothesized that children with CMs—chronic conditions allowing for planned transfusions—would exhibit better correction of anemia compared to children with AA, where the acute nature of the condition limits the time for preoperative optimization. By comparing these two groups, we aimed to determine whether the ability to plan transfusions impacts their effectiveness, despite the predictability suggested by the chronic versus acute distinction.

2. Materials and Methods

2.1. Participant Selection

The current study followed the PICO statement (Population, Intervention, Comparison, Outcome). Population: Pediatric patients admitted to the Timisoara 'Louis Turcanu' Emergency Hospital for Children requiring preoperative blood transfusions to correct anemia. Intervention: Blood transfusion to manage preoperative anemia in children with congenital malformations (CM). Comparison: Pediatric patients with acute abdomen (AA) conditions requiring similar preoperative blood transfusions. Outcome: Efficacy of blood transfusions in increasing hemoglobin levels, evaluated through hemoglobin (HGB), hematocrit (HCT), and red blood cell counts (RBC) assessed at admission, 48 h post-transfusion, and at discharge.

This retrospective study included 107 surgical pediatric patients admitted to Timisoara 'Louis Turcanu' Emergency Hospital for Children, who received preoperative blood transfusion between January 2015 and May 2023.

Inclusion criteria were represented by the requirement of blood transfusion for preoperative anemia correction.

Exclusion criteria were represented by the presence of associated malignancies and primary hematological disorders. Patients that had both diverticulitis and congenital diverticulum were also excluded from the current study.

We evaluated three consecutive hemograms for each participant: at admission (baseline), at 48 h' post-transfusion, and upon discharge from the hospital.

Anemia was defined by the hemoglobin values, according to the definition of the World Health Organization (WHO): 12–59 months of age lower than 11.0 g/dL, 5–11 years of age <11.5 g/dL, 12–14 years <12.0 g/dL, female 15–17 years of age <12.0 g/dL, and male 15–17 years of age <13.0 g/dL.

The study was approved by the Ethics Committee of the "Victor Babes" University of Medicine and Pharmacy Timișoara (68/01.10.2018 rev 2024), Romania, and conducted in accordance with the Declaration of Helsinki.

2.2. Laboratory Variables

A Sysmex XN-550 Hematology Analyzer (Kobe, Hyogo, Japan) was used for in vitro diagnostic use in determining whole blood diagnostic parameters. The method used fluorescence flow cytometry, flow cytometry, DC impedance method with hydrodynamic focusing, and cyanide-free SLS method. Parameters analyzed included: white blood cells (WBCs), red blood cells (RBCs), hemoglobin (HGB), hematocrit (HCT), mean corpuscular volume (MCV), mean corpuscular hemoglobin (MCH), mean corpuscular hemoglobin concentration (MCHC), platelet count (PLT), red cell distribution width (RDW), red cell distribution width–standard deviation (RDW-SD), red cell distribution width–coefficient of variation (RDW-CV), platelet distribution width (PDW), mean platelet volume (MPV), platelet–large cell ratio (P-LCR), platelets (PCTs), neutrophils (NEUTs), lymphocytes (LYMPHs), monocytes (MONOs), eosinophils (EOs), basophils (BASOs), NEUT%, LYMPH%, MONO%, EO%, BASO%, and immature granulocyte (IG). However, our analysis focused on RBC, HGB, and HCT, as markers of anemia.

2.3. Transfusions

Blood transfusions were initiated based on the WHO guidelines for hemoglobin concentrations that indicate severe anemia, with a general recommendation of 7 g/dL, which necessitates immediate correction to mitigate the risk of hypoxia and other complications. In cases of CM, transfusions were planned based on the anticipated blood loss during upcoming surgeries, considering the patient's overall health and ability to tolerate anemia. Conversely, for AA, transfusions were often emergent, driven by acute blood losses and the need to stabilize the patient's condition rapidly. Consistent with contemporary pediatric care standards, the protocol aimed to minimize blood transfusions. This was achieved by employing restrictive transfusion strategies, where transfusions were only given when necessary and in the smallest effective volumes to reduce risks of transfusion-related complications. In the initial transfusion, patients were closely monitored through serial hemograms measured at admission, 48 h post-transfusion, and at discharge. Adjustments to the transfusion plan were made based on these ongoing assessments to ensure optimal patient outcomes without excessive blood administration.

2.4. Statistical Analysis

Data analysis was performed using the statistical software IBM SPSS Statistics 25 (SPSS Inc. Chicago, IL, USA). The Kolmogorov–Smirnov test was used to determine the normality of data. The Student's *t*-test was used to compare continuous variables between the two groups, and Pearson correlation coefficient was used to assess associations between certain variables. Chi-square test was used to assess the differences in sex distribution between CM and AA groups. Age was accounted for by including it as a covariate in multivariate regression models evaluating the efficacy of blood transfusions. Additionally, we conducted subgroup analyses within specific age brackets to further assess the impact of age on transfusion outcomes. By adjusting for age, we aimed to ensure that any observed differences in transfusion efficacy between the CM and AA groups were attributable to the clinical conditions rather than age disparities between the groups. Continuous variables were compared using the Student's *t*-test for normally distributed data or the Mann–Whitney U test for non-normally distributed data, while categorical variables were compared using the chi-square test. A p-value of <0.05 was considered statistically significant.

3. Results

Demographics

The patients were aged between 1 day to 17 years. The cohort was divided into two subgroups according to their diagnosis: 53 participants with congenital malformations (diaphragmic hernia, esophageal atresia, gastroschisis, Hirschsprung disease, spina bifida, and congenital hydronephrosis) and 54 participants with anemia that were diagnosed with acute abdomen (acute appendicitis, peritonitis, diverticulitis, intestinal obstruction, and trauma-related blood loss). A more detailed overview of the patients is presented in Table 1.

Table 1. Patients' diagnostics identified in the study cohort.

Group	Gender	Diagnosis	Count	Total
CM	F	Gastrointestinal tract malformation	12	15
		Central nervous system defect	2	
		Cleft palate	1	
	M	Gastrointestinal tract malformation	27	38
		Urinary tract malformation	5	
		Diaphragmatic hernia	2	
		Cleft palate	1	
		Central nervous system defect	2	
		Pulmonary sequestration	1	
AA	F	Gastrointestinal tract hemorrhage	2	22
		Intraperitoneal bleeding	2	
		Appendicitis	5	
		Peritonitis	5	
		Intestinal obstruction	7	
		Necrotizing enterocolitis	1	
	M	Gastrointestinal tract hemorrhage	2	32
		Intraperitoneal bleeding	10	
		Appendicitis	3	
		Peritonitis	6	
		Intestinal obstruction	9	
		Necrotizing enterocolitis	2	

The mean age of the subjects included in this study was 29.86 ± 56.67 months, while gender distribution showed predominantly males 70/107 (65%). The mean values of age, hospitalization period, and sex distribution are shown in Table 2. While males are predominant in both groups, their weighting is significantly higher in the Congenital Malformation group (71.70%) in comparison to the Acute Abdomen group (59.26%). Additionally, there is a statistically significant difference regarding age ($p < 0.001$) with patients from the CM group being younger than those from the acute abdomen group.

Table 2. Cohort demographics (gender distribution, age, hospitalization period).

Variables	All N = 107	Female N = 37	Male N = 70	*p*-Value	CM N = 53	AA N = 54	*p*-Value
Gender F/M N, (%)/N, (%)	37 (34.58%)/ 70 (65.42%)	37	70	-	15 (28.30%)/ 38 (71.70%)	22 (40.74%)/ 32 (59.26%)	<0.001 *
Age in months	29.86 ± 56.67	41.06 ± 66.35	23.93 ± 50.32	0.175 **	16.94 ± 23.94	52.34 ± 69.42	<0.001 **
Hospitalization days (mean, ± SD)	17.02 ± 12.94	15.11 ± 7.47	18.03 ± 15.00	0.182 **	15.08 ± 7.99	18.93 ± 16.27	0.123 **

* Chi-Square Test; ** *t* test.

Data analysis revealed statistically significant lower values of the baseline level of hemoglobin ($p = 0.001$) and hematocrit ($p = 0.002$) in the AA versus the CM group. In a likewise manner, differences in the aforementioned parameters were observed at the 48 h follow-up ($p = 0.001$ and $p = 0.005$, accordingly). These findings are presented in Table 3. The variation in hemoglobin levels at admission, at the 48 h follow-up and at discharge with regard to diagnosis and gender is presented in Figures 1–3. When the cohort was divided by gender into two groups, males (N = 70) and females (N = 37), the data analysis did not find any statistically significant differences regarding both demographic data and blood parameters (Tables 2 and 3). At discharge, 57% of all subjects had anemia, with no differences between AA and CM groups.

Table 3. Blood parameter comparison between groups.

Variables	All N = 107	Female N = 37	Male N = 70	*p*-Value	Congenital Malformation N = 53	Acute Abdomen N = 54	*p*-Value
Baseline evaluation							
RBC ($\times 10^6$/mm^3)	2.89 ± 0.42	2.82 ± 0.49	2.92 ± 0.36	0.307 **	2.89 ± 0.42	2.88 ± 0.40	0.927 **
HGB (g/dL)	8.21 ±1.07	8.11 ± 1.25	8.25 ± 0.95	0.560 **	8.54 ± 1.00	7.87 ± 1.02	0.001 **
HCT (%)	25.01 ±3.62	24.66 ± 4.45	25.19 ± 3.11	0.521 **	26.07 ± 3.98	23.95 ± 2.90	0.002 **
Evaluation at 48 h following the transfusion							
RBC ($\times 10^6$/mm^3)	4.05 ±0.66	3.95 ± 0.77	4.09 ± 0.59	0.340 **	4.09 ± 0.56	4.00 ± 0.74	0.451 **
HGB (g/dL)	11.77 ± 1.88	11.62 ± 2.27	11.85 ± 1.64	0.596 **	12.35 ± 1.49	11.20 ± 2.05	0.001 **
HCT (%)	34.26 ± 4.96	33.74 ± 6.14	34.52 ± 4.23	0.491 **	35.60 ± 4.13	32.94 ± 5.37	0.005 **
Evaluation at discharge							
RBC ($\times 10^6$/mm^3)	3.99 ± 0.69	3.87 ± 0.73	4.05 ± 0.66	0.204 **	3.90 ± 0.59	4.07 ± 0.77	0.204 **
HGB (g/dL)	11.30 ± 1.55	11.04 ± 1.78	11.43 ± 1.40	0.256 **	11.43 ± 1.33	11.16 ± 1.72	0.359 **
HCT (%)	33.49 ± 4.32	32.86 ± 5.10	33.81 ± 3.84	0.325 **	33.47 ± 3.89	33.49 ± 4.73	0.984 **
Anemia at discharge	61(57%)	24 (64.8%)	37(52.8%)	0.794 *	30 (56.6%)	31 (57.4%)	0.898 *

RBC: red blood cell; HGB: hemoglobin; HCT: hematocrit; * Chi-Square Test; ** *t* test.

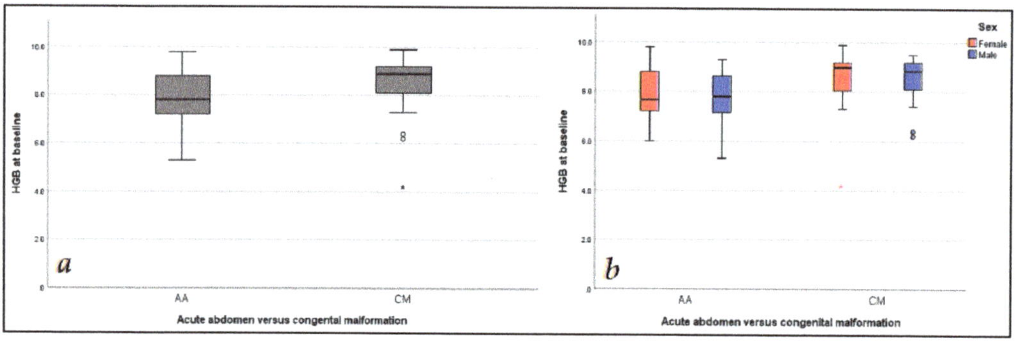

Figure 1. Hemoglobin level values: (**a**) baseline hemoglobin level AA vs. CM groups; (**b**) baseline hemoglobin level comparison according to gender and diagnosis.

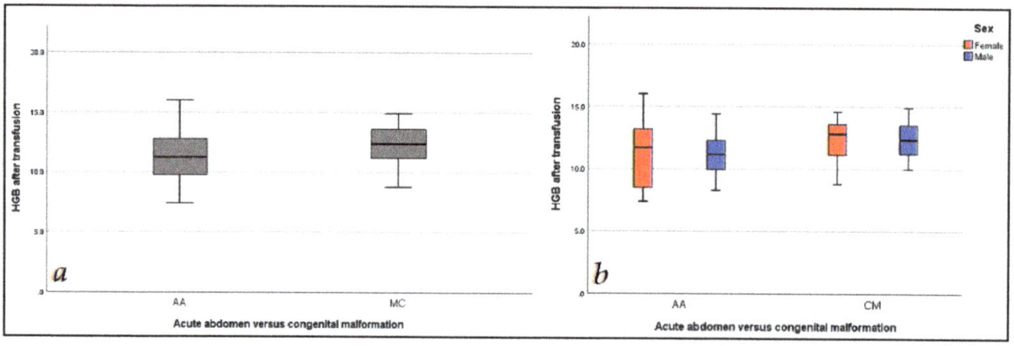

Figure 2. Hemoglobin level values: (**a**) hemoglobin at the 48 h follow-up AA vs. CM groups; (**b**) hemoglobin at the 48 h follow-up level comparison according to gender and diagnosis.

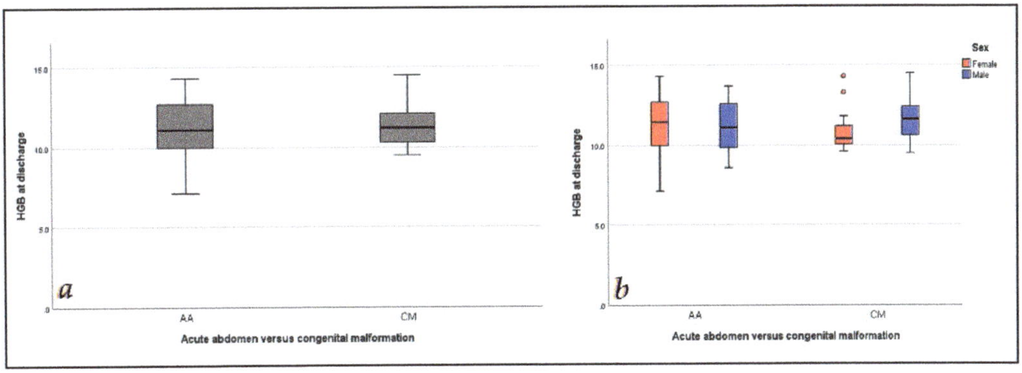

Figure 3. Hemoglobin levels values: (**a**) hemoglobin level at discharge level comparison between AA and CM groups; (**b**) hemoglobin level at discharge regarding gender and diagnosis.

The data analyzed from Table 4 indicated statistically significant differences in blood parameters between the CM and AA groups, stratified by age. For each age category, the CM group consistently demonstrated higher levels of RBC, HGB, and HCT compared to the AA group. Notably, in the youngest cohort (0–12 months), CM patients exhibited a mean HGB level of 8.67 g/dL, significantly higher than the 7.78 g/dL observed in AA patients, with a *p*-value of 0.001, suggesting a robust difference in the initial hemoglobin status between these groups. The statistical tests employed, including *t*-tests for comparing means and chi-square tests for comparing proportions, consistently showed these differences across all age categories. Similarly, the anemia rates at discharge were lower in the CM group across all ages, with *p*-values consistently below 0.05, indicating a statistically significant better outcome in anemia management for the CM group compared to the AA group.

Table 4. Blood parameter comparison between age-specific subgroups of CM and AA.

Age Groups	Subgroup	N	RBC ($\times$ 106/mm^3)	HGB (g/dL)	HCT (%)	Anemia at Discharge
0–12 months	CM	16	2.86 ± 0.41	8.67 ± 1.02	25.94 ± 3.87	58%
	AA	18	2.81 ± 0.38	7.78 ± 1.09	23.87 ± 2.92	63%
12–24 months	CM	14	2.93 ± 0.45	8.74 ± 0.98	26.19 ± 4.01	54%
	AA	15	2.88 ± 0.42	7.95 ± 1.12	24.05 ± 3.08	59%
>24 months	CM	23	2.92 ± 0.44	8.50 ± 1.05	25.76 ± 3.98	57%
	AA	21	2.85 ± 0.39	8.02 ± 1.15	24.22 ± 2.85	60%

The data presented in Table 5 show a negative correlation between the baseline level of hemoglobin and age. The strength of the association varies between groups: weak in the AA group (r = −0.378, *p* = 0.005), strong in the CM group (r = −0.611), and moderate at the cohort level (r = −0.469). In addition, a positive correlation between the level of hemoglobin before and after blood transfusion was found in the CM group (r = 0.423, *p* = 0.002) and at the cohort level (r = 0.392).

Table 5. Pearson correlation analysis.

Variables	All n = 107		Acute Abdomen n = 54		Congenital Malformation n = 53	
	Pearson Correlation	p-Value	Pearson Correlation	p- Value	Pearson Correlation	p-Value
HGB baseline × age (months)	−0.469	<0.001	−0.378	0.005	−0.611	<0.001
HGB baseline × HBG after transfusion	0.392	<0.001	0.226	0.052	0.423	0.002

In the multivariate analysis of factors affecting hemoglobin correction post-transfusion in pediatric patients, significant differences were observed between children with congenital malformations (CMs) and those with acute abdomen (AA) conditions. Patients in the AA group demonstrated a statistically significant decrease in hemoglobin correction compared to the CM group, with a coefficient of −0.87 (p = 0.004). This finding suggests that children with acute abdomen may have less effective anemia correction through transfusion, which could be due to factors such as ongoing blood loss or a more severe initial state of anemia. Additionally, the analysis indicated that age negatively influenced hemoglobin correction, with each additional month of age reducing hemoglobin levels by 0.02 g/dL (p = 0.037), highlighting a lesser efficacy of transfusion in older children within the studied cohort.

The study also explored the roles of gender and other variables in transfusion outcomes. Females tended to have higher increases in hemoglobin levels post-transfusion compared to males, although this difference did not reach statistical significance (coefficient = 0.54, p = 0.112). Conversely, higher baseline hemoglobin levels significantly predicted better post-transfusion outcomes, with an increase of 0.49 g/dL for each unit increase in initial hemoglobin (p < 0.001). Additionally, a longer hospitalization was associated with better hemoglobin recovery, with each additional day linked to an increase of 0.07 g/dL in hemoglobin levels (p = 0.028). These results underscore the complexity of factors influencing the efficacy of blood transfusions in pediatric surgical patients, suggesting that individual patient characteristics and clinical settings play critical roles in determining transfusion requirements and outcomes (Table 6).

Table 6. Multivariate analysis of factors affecting hemoglobin correction post-transfusion.

Variable	Coefficient	Standard Error	p-Value
Group (Reference: CM)		12	
Acute Abdomen (AA)	−0.87	0.28	0.004
Age (Months)	−0.02	0.01	0.037
Gender (Reference: Male)			
Female	0.54	0.33	0.112
Baseline Hemoglobin (g/dL)	0.49	0.09	<0.001
Hospitalization Days	0.07	0.03	0.028

In the subgroup analysis of hemoglobin correction post-transfusion, children diagnosed with congenital malformations (CMs) generally exhibited higher mean increases in hemoglobin levels compared to those with acute abdomen (AA) emergencies. Specifically, central nervous system defects within the CM category showed the most significant improvement in hemoglobin levels, with a mean increase of 3.67 g/dL (p = 0.038). This statistically significant finding indicates a robust response to transfusion in this subgroup. In contrast, gastrointestinal tract malformations and diaphragmatic hernias also showed increases, 3.24 g/dL and 2.98 g/dL respectively, but the changes were not statistically significant (p = 0.052 and p = 0.112, respectively), suggesting variable efficacy of transfusions within different types of congenital malformations.

On the other hand, children in the AA group had lower mean increases in hemoglobin levels following transfusion, with none reaching statistical significance. The highest increase was observed in children with peritonitis, who showed a mean increase of 2.03 g/dL

($p = 0.078$), followed by intestinal obstruction and appendicitis with increases of 1.89 g/dL ($p = 0.093$) and 1.76 g/dL ($p = 0.101$), respectively. These results suggest that children with AA conditions may have a less effective response to transfusions, possibly due to ongoing blood loss or the acute nature of their conditions. This differential response underscores the need for tailored transfusion strategies based on the specific underlying condition and severity of anemia at presentation, as presented in Table 7.

Table 7. Subgroup analysis of hemoglobin correction by specific condition.

Diagnosis Category	Mean Hemoglobin Increase (g/dL)	*p*-Value
Congenital Malformations		
Gastrointestinal Tract Malformation	3.24	0.052
Central Nervous System Defect	3.67	0.038
Diaphragmatic Hernia	2.98	0.112
Acute Abdomen		
Appendicitis	1.76	0.101
Intestinal Obstruction	1.89	0.093
Peritonitis	2.03	0.078

4. Discussion

Our study evaluated the efficacy of preoperative blood transfusions in correcting anemia among pediatric patients with congenital malformations (CMs) and those with acute abdomen (AA), providing new insights into how the chronic nature of CMs and the acute presentation of AA impact transfusion outcomes. In CM patients, scheduled transfusions led to a significant increase in hemoglobin levels 48 h post-transfusion, with a mean increase of 3.81 g/dL (from 8.54 ± 1.00 g/dL to 12.35 ± 1.49 g/dL, $p < 0.001$). Conversely, in the AA group, although the urgency limits preoperative optimization, transfusions still resulted in a meaningful hemoglobin increase of 3.33 g/dL (from 7.87 ± 1.02 g/dL to 11.20 ± 2.05 g/dL, $p < 0.001$), albeit to a lesser extent than in CM patients. The magnitude of hemoglobin correction was significantly greater in the CM group compared to the AA group (coefficient = −0.87, $p = 0.004$), highlighting challenges in managing anemia in acute settings. Within-group analyses identified that in CM patients, factors like baseline anemia severity and comorbidities affected transfusion outcomes, while in AA patients, factors such as the extent of acute blood loss and hemodynamic instability played significant roles. These findings suggest that optimizing transfusion timing in CM patients enhances anemia-correction efficacy, whereas in AA patients, the acute nature of their condition may limit the effectiveness of transfusions despite timely intervention.

Anemia is a relatively common finding in patients undergoing surgery, detected during the initial assessment or postoperative care. Preoperative anemia can be found in approximately 30–40% of the patients undergoing major surgery, while the prevalence of postoperative anemia reaches up to 90% [21]. Perioperative anemia has been assessed as an independent risk factor for perioperative morbidity and mortality by numerous studies. Anemia has been associated with poor clinical outcomes, prolonged hospitalization, increased need for ICU care, higher mortality, and an increased rate of complications [22–24]. Careful surveillance and timely identification of at-risk patients enable adequate preoperative treatment, such as iron supplementation (for non-critical patients qualifying for procedures) or blood transfusions (requiring emergency surgery). Nonetheless, the appropriate treatment will be chosen considering the etiology, clinical status, age, weight, particularities, and bleeding risks associated with the surgical procedure required.

The sex distribution in our study was uneven, with a significantly higher number of male subjects in both the AA and CM groups. However, the proportion of males was significantly bigger in the CM group (70.70%) compared to the AA group (59.26%) (chi-square test $p < 0.001$). Numerous studies presented in the literature highlighted the role gender plays as a risk factor for congenital malformations. For instance, Tennant et al. [25], in a study on 12.795 cases of congenital anomalies, reported that males accounted for

54.9% of cases. Moreover, when compared to female fetuses, pregnancies with male fetuses were associated with a higher risk of congenital anomalies (RR, male vs. female = 1.15). Sokal et al. [26], in a population-based study that included 794.169 children (born between 1990 and 2009), reported that the overall risk for congenital anomalies was 26% higher in male versus female subjects (PR [M:F] 1.26). Likewise, Shaw et al. [27] reported that the prevalence of birth defects was 22% higher among males. Lary et al. [28] examined the records for 1968 through 1995 from the Metropolitan Atlanta Congenital Defects Program in order to assess the sex-specific prevalence of different congenital disabilities. Their findings suggest that females have a higher prevalence of nervous and endocrine system anomalies, while males are at a higher risk for all the other birth defects. For example, gastrointestinal tract defects and urinary tract anomalies were 55% and 67%, respectively, more prevalent among male subjects.

Our results indicated a negative correlation between age and hemoglobin baseline levels in both groups, especially in the CM group, showing that younger age is correlated with higher blood count values. Several reasons could explain this phenomenon. Firstly, the differences in the etiology of anemia might provide a plausible explanation since the acute abdomen can be associated with a significantly higher or faster blood loss. Secondly, there is a physiological difference in red blood cell count and erythrocyte morphology in neonates compared to adults. For instance, the volume of red blood cells is 21% larger, and the diameter is 13% bigger in neonates compared to adults [29]. Younger age (neonatal presentation) was more prevalent in the congenital malformation group, as they were observed immediately after birth. To illustrate, Bower et al. [30] analyzed the Western Australian Birth Defects Registry data. They reported that in 18.7% of cases, the birth defects were diagnosed prenatally, while a further 47.8% were diagnosed by the age of 1 month. Zhu et al. [31] reported a diagnosis rate at birth of 29.7%. Hemoglobin levels at baseline positively correlated with the values after transfusion, further showing that milder anemia is easier to correct with blood transfusions.

There were statistically significant differences regarding the prevalence of anemia at discharge between the AA and CM groups or between male and female groups. This is probably because all children were treated following similar guidelines and treatment protocols and benefited from identical healthcare standards.

The novelty of our study lies in the detailed examination of transfusion efficacy within specific pediatric surgical populations and the identification of factors that influence outcomes in each group. While it is generally understood that scheduled transfusions are preferable when time permits, our study quantifies this advantage and underscores the importance of individualized transfusion strategies. Our findings suggest that in CM patients, proactive anemia management should be a priority to optimize surgical outcomes. In AA patients, despite the limitations imposed by the acute nature of their condition, efforts should be made to correct anemia as effectively as possible, perhaps by exploring rapid-acting interventions or protocols tailored to emergency settings.

The limitations of the current study consist in the relatively small number of subjects (107), as well as the lack of data regarding additional parameters like serum iron level, ferritin, serum folate and cobalamin levels, etc., that could prove useful in identifying additional predictors for blood-transfusion requirements. One should also take into account the possibility that patients with congenital malformations might experience difficulties in absorbing nutrients, which can result in malnutrition and anemia. Moreover, ongoing blood loss or a more severe initial state of anemia may be influenced by various confounding factors, such as the differences in blood transfusion principles among surgeons. Future studies that use larger cohorts, with either pediatric or adult participants, from more areas of the world are welcomed additions to this theme, mainly if they include further knowledge of patient blood-management strategies that can reduce the need for transfusion in anemia patients undergoing surgeries.

5. Conclusions

In this study, the children suffering from acute abdomen presented more severe anemia before the transfusion, compared to those with congenital malformations. In addition, the anemia was more difficult to correct in the acute abdomen group, suggesting that careful surveillance is needed for this group. No statistically significant differences regarding blood parameters were observed between genders, suggesting that gender does not influence the efficacy of blood transfusion at this age.

Author Contributions: Conceptualization, A.I., N.M. and A.M.; methodology, A.I., N.M. and A.M.; software, A.I., N.M. and A.M.; validation, A.C.-E. and V.L.D.; formal analysis, A.C.-E. and V.L.D.; investigation, A.C.-E. and V.L.D.; resources, R.D. and D.S.; data curation, R.D. and D.S.; writing—original draft preparation, R.D., A.I. and D.S.; writing—review and editing, O.B., R.F., P.I.B., D.-M.C., F.B. and M.A.S.; visualization, O.B., R.F., P.I.B., D.-M.C., F.B. and M.A.S.; supervision, O.B., R.F., P.I.B., D.-M.C., F.B. and M.A.S.; project administration, O.B., R.F., P.I.B., D.-M.C., F.B. and M.A.S. All authors have read and agreed to the published version of the manuscript.

Funding: This research received no external funding.

Institutional Review Board Statement: The study was conducted in accordance with the Declaration of Helsinki and approved by the Ethics Committee of "Victor Babes" University of Medicine and Pharmacy from Timisoara (68/01.10.2018 rev 2024).

Informed Consent Statement: Informed consent was obtained from all subjects involved in the study.

Data Availability Statement: The data will be available on request from the corresponding author. The data are not publicly available due to privacy.

Acknowledgments: We would like to acknowledge Victor Babes University of Medicine and Pharmacy Timisoara for their support in covering the costs of publication for this research paper.

Conflicts of Interest: The authors declare no conflicts of interest.

References

1. Martinez-Torres, V.; Torres, N.; Davis, J.A.; Corrales-Medina, F.F. Anemia and Associated Risk Factors in Pediatric Patients. *Pediatr. Health Med. Ther.* **2023**, *14*, 267–280. [CrossRef] [PubMed] [PubMed Central]
2. Chaparro, C.M.; Suchdev, P.S. Anemia Epidemiology, Pathophysiology, and Etiology in Low- and Middle-income Countries. *Ann. N. Y. Acad. Sci.* **2019**, *1450*, 15–31. [CrossRef] [PubMed]
3. Lokeshwar, M.R.; Dalal, R.; Manglani, M.; Shah, N. Anemia in Newborn. *Indian J. Pediatr.* **1998**, *65*, 651–661. [CrossRef] [PubMed]
4. Gedfie, S.; Getawa, S.; Melku, M. Prevalence and Associated Factors of Iron Deficiency and Iron Deficiency Anemia Among Under-5 Children: A Systematic Review and Meta-Analysis. *Glob. Pediatr. Health* **2022**, *9*, 2333794X2211108. [CrossRef]
5. Nazari, M.; Mohammadnejad, E.; Dalvand, S.; Ghanei Gheshlagh, R. Prevalence of Iron Deficiency Anemia in Iranian Children under 6 Years of Age: A Systematic Review and Meta-Analysis. *J. Blood Med.* **2019**, *10*, 111–117. [CrossRef]
6. Kato, G.J.; Piel, F.B.; Reid, C.D.; Gaston, M.H.; Ohene-Frempong, K.; Krishnamurti, L.; Smith, W.R.; Panepinto, J.A.; Weatherall, D.J.; Costa, F.F.; et al. Sickle Cell Disease. *Nat. Rev. Dis. Primers* **2018**, *4*, 18010. [CrossRef]
7. Varma, N.; Naseem, S. Hematologic Changes in Visceral Leishmaniasis/Kala Azar. *Indian J. Hematol. Blood Transfus.* **2010**, *26*, 78–82. [CrossRef]
8. Hamouda, M.A.; Al Barbry, D.H.; El Mahdy, A.M. Importance of Preoperative Full Blood Count in Pediatric Patients Undergoing Surgeries. *Benha J. Appl. Sci.* **2019**, *4*, 17–21. [CrossRef]
9. Davies, P.; Robertson, S.; Hegde, S.; Greenwood, R.; Massey, E.; Davis, P. Calculating the Required Transfusion Volume in Children. *Transfusion* **2007**, *47*, 212–216. [CrossRef]
10. Yanagisawa, R.; Fujihara, I.; Komori, K.; Abe, S.; Ono, T.; Sakashita, K.; Nakamura, T. Transfusion-Associated Circulatory Overload in a Pediatric Patient with Neuroblastoma. *Transfus. Apher. Sci.* **2017**, *56*, 445–447. [CrossRef]
11. Piccin, A.; Cronin, M.; Brady, R.; Sweeney, J.; Marcheselli, L.; Lawlor, E. Transfusion-associated Circulatory Overload in Ireland: A Review of Cases Reported to the National Haemovigilance Office 2000 to 2010. *Transfusion* **2015**, *55*, 1223–1230. [CrossRef] [PubMed]
12. De Cloedt, L.; Emeriaud, G.; Lefebvre, É.; Kleiber, N.; Robitaille, N.; Jarlot, C.; Lacroix, J.; Gauvin, F. Transfusion-associated Circulatory Overload in a Pediatric Intensive Care Unit: Different Incidences with Different Diagnostic Criteria. *Transfusion* **2018**, *58*, 1037–1044. [CrossRef] [PubMed]
13. Faraoni, D.; DiNardo, J.A.; Goobie, S.M. Relationship Between Preoperative Anemia and In-Hospital Mortality in Children Undergoing Noncardiac Surgery. *Anesth. Analg.* **2016**, *123*, 1582–1587. [CrossRef] [PubMed]

14. Scott, S.; Chen-Edinboro, L.; Caulfield, L.; Murray-Kolb, L. The Impact of Anemia on Child Mortality: An Updated Review. *Nutrients* **2014**, *6*, 5915–5932. [CrossRef]
15. Skorupski, C.P.; Cheung, M.C.; Lin, Y. Preoperative anemia in major elective surgery. *Can. Med. Assoc. J.* **2023**, *195*, E551. [CrossRef]
16. Lăzărescu, A.E.; Văduva, A.O.; Hogea, G.B.; Croicu, C.; Pătraşcu, J.M., Jr.; Petrescu, P.H.; Andor, B.C.; Muntean, M.D.; Pătraşcu, J.M. Comparing PRP and bone marrow aspirate effects on cartilage defects associated with partial meniscectomy: A confocal microscopy study on an animal model. *Rom. J. Morphol. Embryol.* **2021**, *62*, 263–268. [CrossRef]
17. Feier, C.V.I.; Muntean, C.; Faur, A.M.; Gaborean, V.; Petrache, I.A.; Cozma, G.V. Exploring Inflammatory Parameters in Lung Cancer Patients: A Retrospective Analysis. *J. Pers. Med.* **2024**, *14*, 552. [CrossRef]
18. Loghin, A.; Preda, O.; Bacârea, V.; Moldovan, C.; Porav-Hodade, D.; Dema, A.; Berger, N.; Borda, A. Predictive preoperatory variables of the prostate tumor volume. *Rom. J. Morphol. Embryol.* **2011**, *52* (Suppl. 1), 363–368.
19. Kaiafa, G.; Savopoulos, C.; Kanellos, I.; Mylonas, K.S.; Tsikalakis, G.; Tegos, T.; Kakaletsis, N.; Hatzitolios, A.I. Anemia and Stroke: Where Do We Stand? *Acta Neurol. Scand.* **2017**, *135*, 596–602. [CrossRef]
20. Abuga, K.M.; Muriuki, J.M.; Williams, T.N.; Atkinson, S.H. How Severe Anaemia Might Influence the Risk of Invasive Bacterial Infections in African Children. *Int. J. Mol. Sci.* **2020**, *21*, 6976. [CrossRef]
21. Gómez-Ramirez, S.; Jericó, C.; Muñoz, M. Perioperative Anemia: Prevalence, Consequences and Pathophysiology. *Transfus. Apher. Sci.* **2019**, *58*, 369–374. [CrossRef] [PubMed]
22. Gelebo, K.G.; Neme, D.; Destaw, B.; Aweke, Z.; Kasa, S.M. The Effect of Preoperative Anemia on Perioperative Outcomes among Patients Undergoing Emergency Surgery: A Multicenter Prospective Cohort Study. *Heliyon* **2023**, *9*, e17804. [CrossRef] [PubMed]
23. Pan, K.; Pang, S.; Robinson, M.; Goede, D.; Meenrajan, S. A Review of Perioperative Anemia: A Modifiable and Not so Benign Risk Factor. *J. Fam. Med. Prim. Care* **2022**, *11*, 5004. [CrossRef] [PubMed]
24. Baron, D.M.; Hochrieser, H.; Posch, M.; Metnitz, B.; Rhodes, A.; Moreno, R.P.; Pearse, R.M.; Metnitz, P. Preoperative Anaemia Is Associated with Poor Clinical Outcome in Non-Cardiac Surgery Patients. *Br. J. Anaesth.* **2014**, *113*, 416–423. [CrossRef]
25. Tennant, P.W.G.; Samarasekera, S.D.; Pless-Mulloli, T.; Rankin, J. Sex Differences in the Prevalence of Congenital Anomalies: A Population-Based Study. *Birth Defects Res. Part A Clin. Mol. Teratol.* **2011**, *91*, 894–901. [CrossRef]
26. Sokal, R.; Tata, L.J.; Fleming, K.M. Sex Prevalence of Major Congenital Anomalies in the United Kingdom: A National Population-based Study and International Comparison Meta-analysis. *Birth Defects Res. Part A Clin. Mol. Teratol.* **2014**, *100*, 79–91. [CrossRef]
27. Shaw, G.M.; Carmichael, S.L.; Kaidarova, Z.; Harris, J.A. Differential Risks to Males and Females for Congenital Malformations among 2.5 Million California Births, 1989–1997. *Birth Defects Res. Part A Clin. Mol. Teratol.* **2003**, *67*, 953–958. [CrossRef]
28. Lary, J.M.; Paulozzi, L.J. Sex Differences in the Prevalence of Human Birth Defects: A Population-based Study. *Teratology* **2001**, *64*, 237–251. [CrossRef]
29. Linderkamp, O.; Wu, P.Y.K.; Meiselman, H.J. Geometry of Neonatal and Adult Red Blood Cells. *Pediatr. Res.* **1983**, *17*, 250–253. [CrossRef]
30. Bower, C.; Rudy, E.; Callaghan, A.; Quick, J.; Nassar, N. Age at Diagnosis of Birth Defects. *Birth Defects Res. Part A Clin. Mol. Teratol.* **2010**, *88*, 251–255. [CrossRef]
31. Zhu, J.L.; Madsen, K.M.; Vestergaard, M.; Olesen, A.V.; Basso, O.; Olsen, J. Paternal Age and Congenital Malformations. *Hum. Reprod.* **2005**, *20*, 3173–3177. [CrossRef]

diagnostics

MDPI

Article

Manometric Evaluation of the Sphincter Complex in Anterior Anus and Mild Anorectal Malformations—An Important Diagnostic Tool

Jonathan Hencke *, Raphael Staubach and Steffan Loff

Department of Pediatric Surgery, Olgahospital, Klinikum Stuttgart, Kriegsbergstrasse 62, 70174 Stuttgart, Germany
* Correspondence: j.hencke@klinikum-stuttgart.de

Abstract: Background: Distinguishing between the anatomical variant of an anterior anus and mild forms of imperforate anus with rectoperineal fistula often requires inspection, calibration, and, in uncertain cases, electrical stimulation (ES) under general anesthesia. Anorectal manometry (AM), despite its ability to assess sphincter configuration and function, is rarely reported as a diagnostic tool. This study evaluated the utility of AM in such cases. **Methods:** A retrospective analysis of AM and clinical data from 38 patients (35 female, 3 male) with suspected anterior anus was conducted from October 2009 to September 2021. Water-perfused catheter probes with eight radial channels were used to perform pull-through maneuvers. Sphincter locations were identified through vector reconstruction, and pressure ratios of the anterior part to the circumference were recorded. Results were compared to clinical data, including ES findings. Statistical significance was assessed using Mann–Whitney U and Chi-Square tests. **Results:** Following AM, ES was unnecessary in 25 patients. Of the remaining patients, 83% showed abnormal sphincter configurations on ES, and seven underwent anoplasty. Patients with abnormal sphincter complexes demonstrated significantly lower mean anterior pressures (61.2 mmHg vs. 136.4 mmHg, U = 336.5, $p = 0.001$) and a trend toward lower anterior-to-circumferential pressure ratios (mean 0.42 vs. 0.85, U = 613, $p = 0.270$). Constipation was also more frequent in this group ($X^2(1,N = 38) = 4.1$, $p = 0.044$). Average anterior pressures < 75 mmHg and ratios < 0.7 indicated an anus outside the sphincter complex (sensitivity 80%, specificity 90%). **Conclusions:** AM proves valuable for evaluating ambiguous anterior anus cases, potentially reducing reliance on ES under general anesthesia. 3D high-resolution AM may further increase diagnostic accuracy.

Keywords: anterior anus; anorectal malformation; anorectal manometry; sphincter complex

1. Introduction

In some children, caregivers observe an anteriorized anal opening, often raising concerns about a possible anorectal malformation (ARM). An anus located closer to the genitalia than normal, while still having an average diameter, an adequate perineal body, and surrounded by sphincter muscles, is presently understood as an anatomical variant [1]. Various terms for this are used: 'anterior anus' (AA), 'ectopic anus' or, 'ventral anal ectopy', with, 'anterior anus' being the preferred definition. It must be distinguished from an imperforate anus with a rectoperineal fistula and anal canal stenosis, both considered pathological in contrast [1]. On the one hand, there is a need to identify mild forms of

ARM that are sometimes missed but could lead to severe sequelae, especially constipation [2]. On the other hand, it is crucial to avoid misdiagnosing a normally functioning anus and subjecting children to unnecessary surgery. Recently, the ARM-Net Consortium published a comprehensive position paper with clear definitions [1] aiming to standardize the evaluation and treatment of children with an anteriorized anal opening. According to their guidelines, children are categorized as 'normal anus' (normal position, normal diameter, surrounded by sphincter muscle), 'anterior anus' (anterior position, normal diameter, surrounded by sphincter muscle), 'congenital anal stenosis' (normal or anterior position, reduced diameter, surrounded by sphincter muscle), and 'perineal fistula' (anterior position, possibly abnormal diameter, not surrounded by sphincter muscle). For differentiation, the authors suggest a systematic approach involving inspection, measuring the position using the ano-perineal index (API), determination of the caliber with Hegar dilators, and elicitation of the anocutaneous reflex to observe sphincter contraction. The API was first proposed by Reisner et al. in 1984 [3] and has become the standard measurement of anal position. It is measured as the ratio of the distance between the scrotum/fourchette and anus and divided by the distance between the scrotum/fourchette and coccyx [3]. An API < 0.34 in girls and <0.46 in boys is considered an anteriorly displaced anus. In uncertain cases concerning the musculature, electrical stimulation (ES) under general anesthesia is the suggested method. Several alternative methods to assess the sphincter have been proposed in the literature. Transperineal sonography [4], endosonography [5], and magnetic resonance imaging [6] have been used with some success.

Manometric evaluation of the sphincter in AA is seldom documented, with only a handful of studies having investigated whether the sphincter muscle surrounds the anal canal [7,8]. In postoperative evaluation of ARMs, however, this is commonly employed to demonstrate sphincter integrity and the ability of the patient to squeeze sufficiently [9]. In our department, we have utilized anorectal manometry (AM) in various investigations, including AA, and thus, we wish to impart our experience in this regard.

2. Materials and Methods

We conducted a retrospective analysis of all patients undergoing AM for suspected AA between October 2009 and September 2021. Each patient received an enema prior to the exam and no sedative was administered. All patients underwent AM with identical equipment: a water-perfused eight-channel manometric catheter with radially placed channels, an outer diameter of 14 Fr, and without a balloon; an electric manometric water pump type PIP-4-8 SS (both Mui Scientific Inc., Mississauga, ON, Canada) with manometric sensors type DPT-6000 (CODAN pvp Critical Care GmbH, Forstinning, Germany) connected to a polygraph (Medtronic, Copenhagen, Denmark) and a computer. Recording and evaluation were performed with the Gastrotrac program (Alpine Biomedical Corp., Fountain Valley, CA, USA). To capture sphincter pressures, the catheter was positioned in the rectum and gradually pulled through the anal canal (at a rate of 1 cm per second) to record the circumferential pressures from the interior towards the exterior of the anal canal. This maneuver was repeated several times. Computerized vector reconstruction subsequently produced a three-dimensional image of the pressures and enabled identification of the high-pressure zone and the sphincter complex, respectively. For this retrospective study, a maximum of six pull-through maneuvers per patient were analyzed and the level with the highest pressure most closely resembling the sphincter complex was examined (Figure 1). All circumferential pressures at this level were recorded; the mean of both the circumference and the three anterior pressures (channels 1, 2, 8; Figure 1) were calculated along with the ratio between these means. As most patients underwent several pull-through maneuvers, we took the minimal, maximal, and mean value of these three measurements (circumferential and anterior pressure, as well as their ratio) in every patient.

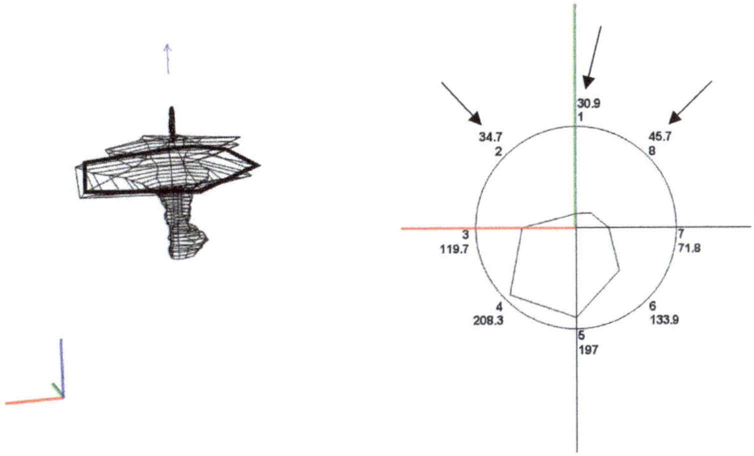

Figure 1. Vector reconstruction of a pull-through maneuver (**left**) with the corresponding transection (**right**); channels 1, 2, and 8 (arrows) are defined as 'anterior'.

Furthermore, we reviewed clinical data from the respective patients, including age, gender, clinical description of AA, whether calibration with Hegar dilators was performed and up to which size, utilization of ES and its result, instances of surgical correction, initial mention of constipation, and any mention of constipation or stool incontinence at follow-up. After data collection, the patients' information was anonymized for the purpose of analysis. The patients were categorized into two groups: Group A, comprising cases with an abnormal sphincter during ES or a recommendation for ES that was not performed; Group B with a normal sphincter during ES or cases where ES was deemed unnecessary after AM. Statistical analyses were conducted with Microsoft Excel (Version 16.95.1) for means, medians, and other descriptive statistics; the rest were performed with online statistical calculators: sensitivity and specificity calculator from medcalc.org; Mann–Whitney U test and Chi-Square test from soscistatistics.com. Statistical significance was defined as $p < 0.05$. Ethical approval for the retrospective use of patient data without individual consent was obtained from the Institutional Ethics Committee of the University of Heidelberg, Mannheim Medical Faculty, protocol code 2022-821.

3. Results

We identified 38 patients undergoing AM due to clinical suspicion of AA, with the vast majority (35 patients) being female. The age at the initial examination ranged from 35 days to 4 years, with a mean of 8.1 months; the majority (34 patients) were examined in their first year of life. In three cases, AM was repeated at a later stage (ranging from two weeks to twelve months later), either due to inconclusive results at the initial assessment or excessive agitation hindering reliable measurements. Details on constipation, however, were available for all patients, with nine individuals presenting symptoms of constipation at the time of AM.

Regrettably, clinical reports lacked standardization. Descriptions of the anatomy were available for 20 patients, with most cases reporting a small, narrow perineum and measured the perineal length; occasionally, the anal crease, a perineal groove, or the presence of an anal dimple were described. Hegar size was noted in 21 patients; sometimes, the calibration was halted without reaching the maximum possible caliber despite the expected Hegar size being higher. Only one case exhibited a clearly stenotic anal canal with an 8–9 mm diameter. The average diameter across cases was 11.05 mm. The ano-perineal index (API) was not documented for any patient.

The number of pull-through maneuvers per exam ranged from one to ten with an average of 4.5. After AM, further evaluation with ES under general anesthesia was deemed unnecessary in 24 patients. Among the remaining cases, 12 underwent ES with 10 patients (83%) exhibiting an abnormal sphincter complex. In two cases, ES was recommended but not executed (and no surgical intervention occurred). The reports of ES frequently depicted the center of the sphincter complex as being dorsal to the anal opening and noted a complete absence of sphincter muscle on the anterior aspect of the anus. Conversely, the two patients with a normal sphincter during ES either displayed an anus completely encircled by the sphincter or only a slightly weaker anterior part. Group A (abnormal sphincter verified in ES or recommended ES) consisted of 12 patients, while Group B consisted of 26 patients.

We conducted a comparison of circumferential pressures, anterior pressures, and their respective ratio between the two groups; the results are presented in Table 1 and visualized in Figures 2–4. Analysis revealed a trend towards lower circumferential pressures as demonstrated in Figure 2. While there was an obvious tendency for lower anterior pressures (Figure 3) and lower ratio of anterior-to-circumferential pressures to be exhibited in Group A (Figure 4), it was only statistically significant for lower anterior pressures ($U = 336.5$, $p = 0.001$).

Table 1. Comparison of circumferential and anterior pressures and their ratio between Group A and B.

		Abnormal Sphincter/Group A (12 pat.), Mean Values	**Normal Sphincter/Group B (26 pat.), Mean Values**	**Mann–Whitney U (U=)**	***p*=**
Circumferential pressures	Mean	107.6 mmHg	144.3 mmHg	629.5	0.33
	Min	87.7 mmHg	121.6 mmHg	506.5	0.10
	Max	131.1 mmHg	170.3 mmHg	484.5	0.08
Anterior pressures in mmHg	Mean	61.2 mmHg	136.4 mmHg	336.5	0.001
	Min	43 mmHg	113.6 mmHg	384.5	0.03
	Max	83.1 mmHg	162 mmHg	475.5	0.06
Ratio anterior: circumferential pressures	Mean	0.52	0.93	633	0.35
	Min	0.42	0.86	613	0.27
	Max	0.65	1.02	603	0.23

As illustrated in Figure 5, there are two outliers, with one of them having a stenotic anal opening. Notably, the majority of cases with an abnormal sphincter were clustered within the area of anterior pressures under 75 mmHg and ratios under 0.7. When establishing these values as a combined cut-off threshold, we reached a sensitivity of 80% (95% CI 44–98%) and a specificity of 90% (95% CI 74–98%) for an abnormal sphincter.

We compared constipation rates between Group A and B, revealing that 45% of Group A patients were reported as constipated at the time of AM while 15% of Group B had a diagnosis of constipation ($X^2(1,N = 38) = 4.1$, $p = 0.04$). Seven patients underwent anoplasty after ES. All patients undergoing surgery presented for follow-up visits, with the most recent visit at a mean age of 5.3 years, range 1.1–12.1 years. Of all remaining patients without surgery, 17 were followed up at a mean age of 4.2 years, range 6 months–13.3 years. No documentation on follow-up visits was found in our hospital records for 14 patients. Two patients undergoing anoplasty were reported as constipated at follow-up, while five were mentioned to be without constipation; when compared with preoperative constipation rates, three experienced an improvement in constipation, two were already without constipation before the procedure, one remained constipated, and one developed constipation after surgery. Most other patients not undergoing anoplasty were without constipation at the time of AM and follow-up (14/17, 82%), with one showcasing improvement at follow-up while one remained constipated; however, the follow-up period in this case was very short (1 month). One patient developed severe constipation, and it is noteworthy that AM had indicated the suspicion of an abnormal sphincter in this patient (mean anterior pressure 73 mmHg and ratio 0.66). Although ES was recommended, the parents opted for further treatment in a different hospital, where bowel management was initiated and a sigmoid resection due to constipation took place; the patient presented her case to a different department of our hospital several years later.

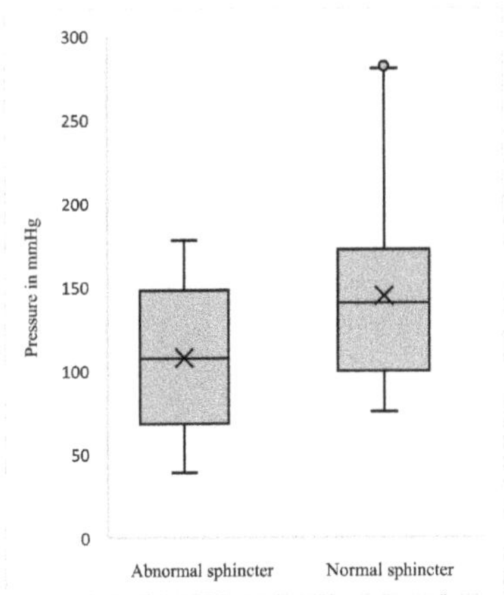

Figure 2. Boxplot of mean circumferential pressures.

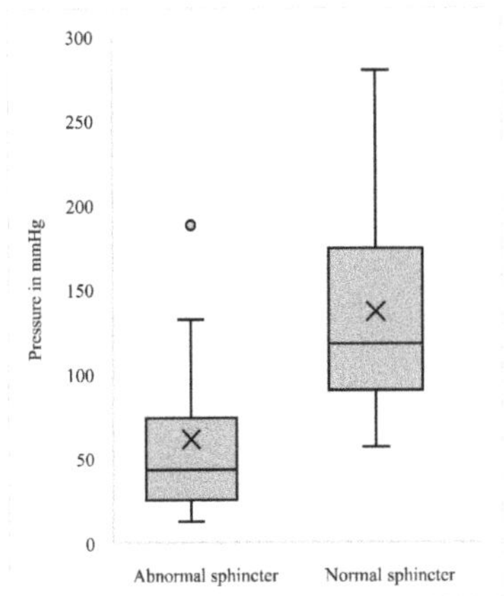

Figure 3. Boxplot of mean anterior pressures.

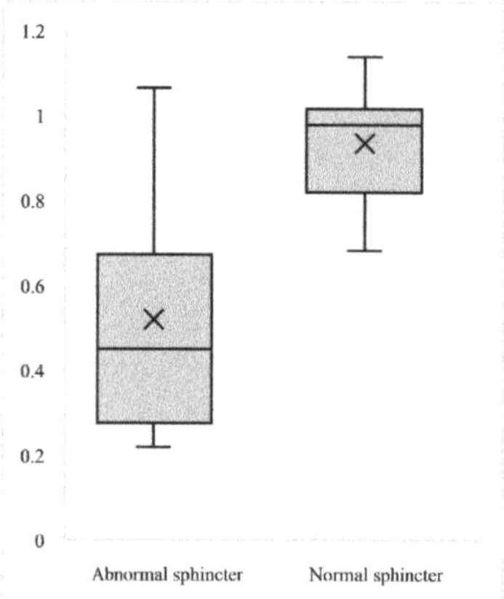

Figure 4. Boxplot of mean ratio anterior-to-circumferential pressures.

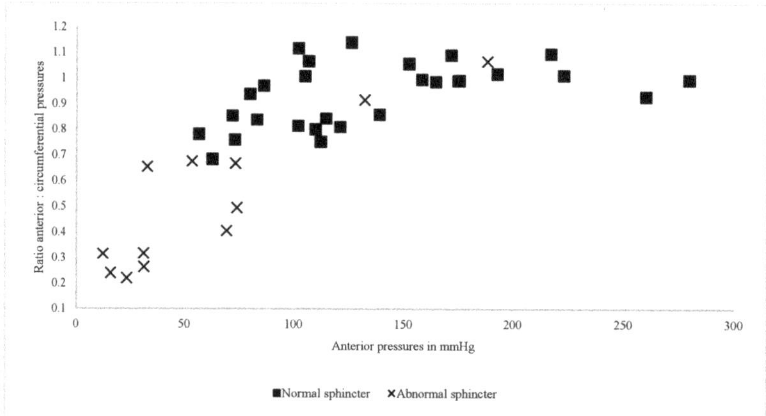

Figure 5. Scatter plot comparing mean anterior pressures and their ratio to circumferential pressures between patients.

4. Discussion

Our results demonstrated a good overlap between findings from clinical, manometric, and electric stimulation data for identifying ARM and AA. This supports the use of AM to evaluate the anal canal in ambiguous cases. Both the statistical significance for lower anterior pressures and the trend towards lower ratios between anterior and circumferential pressures support the presumed findings. The sensitivity and specificity, although not perfect, further bolsters the employment of AM as a promising diagnostic adjunct. Furthermore, the clinical data, with low rates of constipation in Group B (assumed to have a normal sphincter), reinforce the categorization into the groups.

Given the incidence of AA and clinically unremarkable ARM in the general population, our study represents a relatively good number of subjects; however, this was only possible in the form of a retrospective study, which unfortunately lacked standardization and showed inconsistent follow-ups. Especially the missing clinical information on API, Hegar size and description of the severity of constipation or bowel function at presentation or at follow-up in the whole study population would have strengthened the results. There are different definitions and classifications (e.g., Rome IV) of constipation, but we had to rely on the mere mention of constipation in the patient's record due to incomplete records.

Another aspect is an error inherent in AM itself: As most of the children were in their first year of life, no command to squeeze could be given. However, the pull-through maneuvers of the water-perfused catheter usually cause enough anal stimulation to elicit contraction of the sphincter, especially in younger children. The pull-through maneuvers were accomplished by estimating the correct speed (1 cm/s) with the markings on the catheter and a sound at 1 s intervals, but this manual technique is, of course prone, to error. In the same way, not all children were at rest, which might have caused measurement artifacts. Other centers routinely use sedation for AM in children, while we have good experience of reliable measurements without any sedation, especially in the first year of life. The selective utilization of ES only in clinically very suspicious patients and those with conspicuous AM results also undermines the validity of our results. However, this could not be mitigated given the retrospective nature of this study. This study is not free from different sources of bias: there is certainly some selection bias as some patients may have had an almost normal anal position which may not be classified as an AA when measuring the API. AM, the reported incidence of constipation and especially ES can also be prone to considerate observer bias without standardized protocols.

A few studies from various time periods have employed anorectal manometry in AA, with most involving different definitions and techniques, which hampers direct comparison of results: the first study by Kerremans et al. from 1974 utilized microballoons to measure resting pressure and presence of the recto-anal inhibitory reflex (RAIR) [10]; the second study by Schuster et al. from 2000 used the same equipment as our study, focusing on anal canal length and vector volume, as well as sphincter muscle asymmetry in a similar way as in our study [7]; Ruttenstock et al. from 2013 also used water-perfused catheters to evaluate anal canal length, resting pressure, and RAIR in pre- and post-operative cases of ARM [11]. The most recent study from 2023 employed three-dimensional high-resolution AM (3D-HRAM) [8]. However, it is worth noting that all these studies differ in their definition of AA and mild ARM. The older studies used the term 'ectopic anus', with most patients suffering from constipation and having undergone some form of anoplasty. Kerremans et al. already acknowledged the possibility of a functionally normal AA without constipation, thus not requiring surgery [10]. The study by Schuster et al. compared children with 'ectopic anus' and pre-existing severe constipation to normal children [7]. Some of these children with 'ectopic anus' might be more accurately categorized as ARM with a non-stenotic perineal fistula according to contemporary definitions. The correct measurement of anal canal length and the respective vector volumetry, as in the study by Schuster et al. [7], may depend on a very precise and consistent pull of the catheter in manual pull-through maneuvers; therefore, these parameters were not measured in our study.

The most recent study using 3D-HRAM warrants a special mention: although the study did not adhere to the ARM-Net's definitions of AA, it demonstrated a significant concordance between 3D-HRAM findings and ES results, comparing children with mild ARM with constipated children and those with Hirschsprung' disease [8]. The study reported 100% sensitivity and specificity, as ES consistently confirmed the predictions made with 3D-HRAM, particularly if the sphincter was interrupted anteriorly. Since 2022, we transitioned our AM equipment to a solid-state catheter, enabling the application of 3D-HRAM. This should provide an improved image and eliminate the errors caused by the pull-through maneuvers. It is worth noting that normal pressure values should not simply be transferred from studies with water-perfused catheters to the use of solid-state catheters; usually pressures are higher with solid-state sensors [12]. So far, we have examined ten patients with suspected AA with this system with promising results; examples of the recordings and 3D reconstructions are shown in Figure 6a–d. 3D-HRAM provides an excellent image of sphincter function, a feat that is difficult to reproduce with other methods.

ES, in comparison, would require video recording to offer a similar objectivity. Since most of our recent patients did not present stenosis or constipation and only a minority showed a slightly weaker anterior sphincter section, only one is planned to be further examined by ES and undergo surgery if ES confirms an anal location clearly outside the sphincter complex.

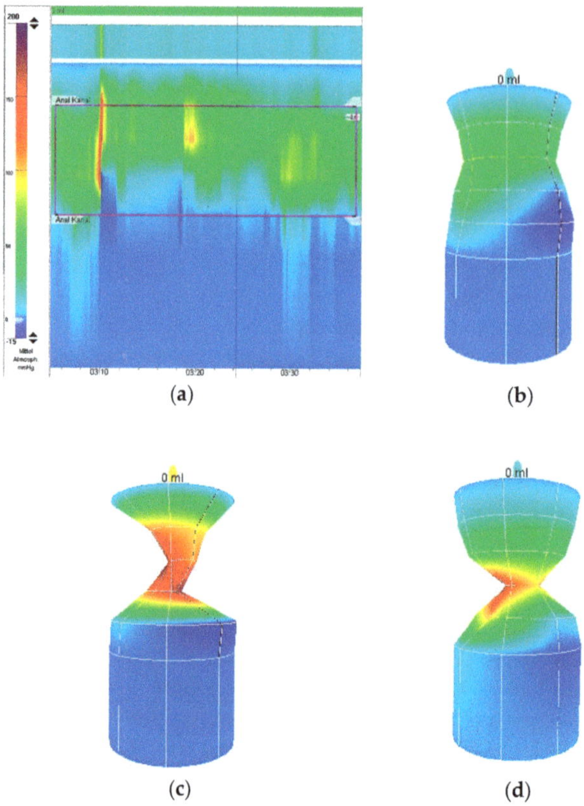

Figure 6. (**a**) 3D-HRAM recording of resting pressure with an occasional squeeze pressure during sneezing; (**b**) 3D reconstruction of AA at rest with circular sphincter complex; (**c**) 3D reconstruction of anal squeeze in the same patient; (**d**) slight anterior weakness during squeeze in a different patient.

Adherence to definitions, as advocated by recent guidelines, will help standardize studies, diagnostics, and treatment. Although further studies are necessary, consistent protocols and the increased use of 3D-HRAM are likely to improve diagnostic accuracy. In our current practice, we aim to gather comprehensive data: API, anal caliber, detailed description of outer anal appearance, and clinical symptoms. We encourage our colleagues in the field of pediatric colorectal surgery to adopt this approach and utilize AM, especially 3D-HRAM, if available, for sphincter assessment in order to decrease the need for general anesthesia in ES. Moreover, AM can be readily performed in an outpatient clinic, alleviating concerns for parents who may be apprehensive about their infant receiving general anesthesia; this aspect is also relevant in cases of limited operating room time availability.

The need for surgical treatment in AA and especially in mild ARM remains an ongoing debate. The altered recto-anal angle in AA may impede defecation by creating a rectal 'cul-de-sac' and lead to constipation [10]. In the past, constipated cases of AA have been corrected surgically [7,13], while newer studies with relatively large cohorts and long-term follow-up, extending into adolescence and adulthood, have shown that this is mostly unnecessary [14,15]. While constipation was reported up to three times more often in AA than in controls, it remained a minority occurrence (10–36%) and could always be treated conservatively. Additionally, none showed stool incontinence or a higher rate of urinary tract infections. Even stenotic cases could successfully be managed with serial dilations [14]. Hence, surgical correction of the anal position in AA is now considered outdated. Mild forms of ARM with perineal fistula may also sometimes be treated by dilations alone, as some studies show that preserving as much of the anal canal as possible is associated with improved outcomes [11,16]. This should also be incorporated into the surgical approach [17]. Overall, we have to acknowledge that mild types of ARM exist on a spectrum like all other ARM; the transition to AA may not always be clear-cut and some may require a formal surgical correction by anterior or posterior sagittal anorectoplasty more than others.

The establishment of clear definitions (AA vs. ARM with perineal fistula) is a necessary first step. Further research and, for example, a scoring system consisting of anatomic and clinical information are needed to evaluate which ARM patients benefit most from conservative as opposed to surgical treatment.

Author Contributions: Conceptualization, J.H. and S.L.; methodology, J.H.; formal analysis, J.H.; investigation, J.H.; data curation, J.H.; writing—original draft preparation, J.H.; writing—review and editing, J.H., R.S., and S.L.; visualization, J.H.; supervision, S.L. All authors have read and agreed to the published version of the manuscript.

Funding: This research received no external funding.

Institutional Review Board Statement: The study was conducted in accordance with the Declaration of Helsinki and approved by the Institutional Ethics Committee of the University of Heidelberg, Mannheim Medical Faculty (protocol code 2022-821 protocol code, 26 April 2022).

Informed Consent Statement: Patient consent was waived since no identification through data is possible due to anonymization and institutional data protection. Waiving of patient consent was approved by the Institutional Ethics Committee.

Data Availability Statement: Due to institutional data protection regulations, the data of this study are not publicly available and will only be shared upon reasonable request.

Conflicts of Interest: The authors declare no conflicts of interest.

Abbreviations

The following abbreviations are used in this manuscript:

ARM	Anorectal malformation
AA	Anterior anus
API	Ano-perineal index
ES	Electrical stimulation
AM	Anorectal manometry
RAIR	Recto-anal inhibitory reflex
3D-HRAM	Three-dimensional high-resolution anorectal manometry

References

1. Amerstorfer, E.E.; Schmiedeke, E.; Samuk, I.; Sloots, C.E.J.; van Rooij, I.A.L.M.; Jenetzky, E.; Midrio, P. Clinical Differentiation between a Normal Anus, Anterior Anus, Congenital Anal Stenosis, and Perineal Fistula: Definitions and Consequences—The ARM-Net Consortium Consensus. *Children* **2022**, *9*, 831. [CrossRef] [PubMed]
2. Eltayeb, A.A. Delayed presentation of anorectal malformations: The possible associated morbidity and mortality. *Pediatr. Surg. Int.* **2010**, *26*, 801–806. [CrossRef] [PubMed]

3. Reisner, S.H.; Sivan, Y.; Nitzan, M.; Merlob, P. Determination of Anterior Displacement of the Anus in Newborn Infants and Children. *Pediatrics* **1984**, *73*, 216–217. [CrossRef] [PubMed]
4. Haber, H.P.; Warmann, S.W.; Fuchs, J. Transperineal sonography of the anal sphincter complex in neonates and infants: Differentiation of anteriorly displaced anus from low-type imperforate anus with perineal fistula. *Ultraschall. Med.* **2008**, *29*, 383–387. [CrossRef] [PubMed]
5. Keshtgar, A.S.; Athanasakos, E.; Clayden, G.S.; Ward, H.C. Evaluation of outcome of anorectal anomaly in childhood: The role of anorectal manometry and endosonography. *Pediatr. Surg. Int.* **2008**, *24*, 885–892. [CrossRef] [PubMed]
6. Thambidorai, C.R.; Raghu, R.; Zulfiqar, A. Magnetic resonance imaging in anterior ectopic anus. *Pediatr. Surg. Int.* **2008**, *24*, 161–165. [CrossRef] [PubMed]
7. Schuster, T.; Joppich, I.; Schneider, K.; Jobst, G. A computerised vector manometry study of the so-called ectopic anus. *Pediatr. Surg. Int.* **2000**, *16*, 8–14. [CrossRef] [PubMed]
8. den Hollander, V.E.C.; Gerritsen, S.; van Dijk, T.H.; Trzpis, M.; Broens, P.M.A. Diagnosing Mild Forms of Anorectal Malformation With Anorectal Manometry: A Prospective Study. *Am. J. Gastroenterol.* **2023**, *118*, 546–552. [CrossRef] [PubMed]
9. Evans-Barns, H.M.E.; Tien, M.Y.; Trajanovska, M.; Safe, M.; Hutson, J.M.; Dinning, P.G.; King, S.K. Post-Operative Anorectal Manometry in Children following Anorectal Malformation Repair: A Systematic Review. *J. Clin. Med.* **2023**, *12*, 2543. [CrossRef] [PubMed]
10. Kerremans, R.P.J.; Penninckx, F.M.A.; Beckers, J.P.V. Functional Evaluation of Ectopic Anus and Its Surgical Consequences. *Am. J. Dis. Child.* **1974**, *128*, 811–814. [CrossRef] [PubMed]
11. Ruttenstock, E.M.; Zani, A.; Huber-Zeyringer, A.; Höllwarth, M.E. Pre- and Postoperative Rectal Manometric Assessment of Patients with Anorectal Malformations: Should We Preserve the Fistula? *Dis. Colon. Rectum.* **2013**, *56*, 499–504. [CrossRef] [PubMed]
12. Vitton, V.; Ben Hadj Amor, W.; Baumstarck, K.; Grimaud, J.C.; Bouvier, M. Water-perfused manometry vs three-dimensional high-resolution manometry: A comparative study on a large patient population with anorectal disorders. *Color. Dis.* **2013**, *15*, 726–731. [CrossRef] [PubMed]
13. Hendren, W.H. Constipation caused by anterior location of the anus and its surgical correction. *J. Pediatr. Surg.* **1978**, *13*, 505–512. [CrossRef] [PubMed]
14. Kyrklund, K.; Pakarinen, M.P.; Taskinen, S.; Rintala, R.J. Bowel function and lower urinary tract symptoms in females with anterior anus treated conservatively: Controlled outcomes into adulthood. *J. Pediatr. Surg.* **2015**, *50*, 1168–1173. [CrossRef] [PubMed]
15. Duci, M.; Fascetti-Leon, F.; Bogana, G.; Gamba, P.; Midrio, P. Conservative management of anterior located anus: A medium-long term follow up. *J. Pediatr. Surg.* **2021**, *56*, 2277–2280. [CrossRef] [PubMed]
16. Pakarinen, M.P.; Rintala, R.J. Management and outcome of low anorectal malformations. *Pediatr. Surg. Int.* **2010**, *26*, 1057–1063. [CrossRef] [PubMed]
17. Pakarinen, M.P.; Goyal, A.; Koivusalo, A.; Baillie, C.; Turnock, R.; Rintala, R.J. Functional outcome in correction of perineal fistula in boys with anoplasty versus posterior sagittal anorectoplasty. *Pediatr. Surg. Int.* **2006**, *22*, 961–965. [CrossRef] [PubMed]

diagnostics

MDPI

Article

Functional Independence of Taiwanese Children with Silver–Russell Syndrome

Hung-Hsiang Fang [1,2], Chung-Lin Lee [1,3,4,5,6], Chih-Kuang Chuang [7,8], Huei-Ching Chiu [1], Ya-Hui Chang [1,4], Yuan-Rong Tu [7], Yun-Ting Lo [4], Jun-Yi Wu [4], Yen-Yin Chou [9], Chung-Hsing Wang [10], Shio-Jean Lin [11], Shao-Yin Chu [12], Chen Yang [13], Tsung-Ying Ou [14], Hsiang-Yu Lin [1,4,5,6,7,15,*] and Shuan-Pei Lin [1,4,5,7,16,*]

1 Department of Pediatrics, MacKay Memorial Hospital, Taipei 104, Taiwan; spty871029@hotmail.com (H.-H.F.); clampcage@gmail.com (C.-L.L.); g880a01@mmh.org.tw (H.-C.C.); wish1001026@gmail.com (Y.-H.C.)
2 Department of Pediatrics, Tri-Service General Hospital, National Defense Medical Center, Taipei 114, Taiwan
3 Institute of Clinical Medicine, National Yang-Ming Chiao-Tung University, Taipei 112, Taiwan
4 International Rare Disease Center, MacKay Memorial Hospital, Taipei 104, Taiwan; andy11tw.e347@mmh.org.tw (Y.-T.L.); wl01723138@gmail.com (J.-Y.W.)
5 Department of Medicine, MacKay Medical College, New Taipei City 252, Taiwan
6 MacKay Junior College of Medicine, Nursing and Management, Taipei 112, Taiwan
7 Department of Medical Research, MacKay Memorial Hospital, Taipei 104, Taiwan; mmhcck@gmail.com (C.-K.C.); likemaruko@hotmail.com (Y.-R.T.)
8 College of Medicine, Fu-Jen Catholic University, Taipei 242, Taiwan
9 Department of Pediatrics, National Cheng Kung University Hospital, College of Medicine, National Cheng Kung University, Tainan 704, Taiwan; yenyin@mail.ncku.edu.tw
10 Division of Medical Genetics, Pediatric Endocrinology and Metabolism, China Medical University Children's Hospital, China Medical University, Taichung 404, Taiwan; a22340961@yahoo.com.tw
11 Department of Pediatrics, Genetic Counseling Center, Chi Mei Medical Center, Tainan 710, Taiwan; shiojean@gmail.com
12 Department of Pediatrics, Buddhist Tzu-Chi General Hospital, Hualien 970, Taiwan; hushaoyin@gmail.com
13 Department of Pediatrics, Taipei Medical University Hospital, Taipei 110, Taiwan; yeungsann@yahoo.com.tw
14 Department of Pediatrics, Dalin Tzu Chi Hospital, Buddhist Tzu Chi Medical Foundation, Chiayi 622, Taiwan; sleep12358@gmail.com
15 Department of Medical Research, China Medical University Hospital, China Medical University, Taichung 404, Taiwan
16 Department of Infant and Child Care, National Taipei University of Nursing and Health Sciences, Taipei 112, Taiwan
* Correspondence: lxc46199@ms37.hinet.net (H.-Y.L.); 4535lin@gmail.com (S.-P.L.); Tel.: +886-2-2543-3535 (H.-Y.L. & S.-P.L.); Fax: +886-2-2543-3642 (H.-Y.L. & S.-P.L.)

Abstract: Background: Silver–Russell syndrome (SRS) is a genetic disorder characterized by prenatal and postnatal growth retardation. Affected individuals commonly present with low birth weight, intrauterine growth restriction, postnatal short stature, hemihypotrophy, characteristic facial features, and body asymmetry. **Methods:** This study includes 24 Taiwanese children with SRS aged 2 years to 13 years and 3 months who were recruited at MacKay Memorial Hospital and other Taiwan hospitals between January 2013 and December 2024. Functional independence was assessed using the Functional Independence Measure for Children (WeeFIM) to evaluate self-care, mobility, and cognition domains. **Results:** The mean total WeeFIM score was 106.9 $\pm$ 23.2 (range: 54–126), with mean self-care, mobility, and cognition scores of 44.4 $\pm$ 13.8 (maximum 56), 32.4 $\pm$ 5.1 (maximum 35), and 30.2 $\pm$ 6.0 (maximum 35), respectively. The results of the restricted cubic spline analysis reveal a clear positive linear correlation before school age (approximately 72 months), followed by a plateau (p for nonlinearity < 0.05). Traceable molecular data were available for thirteen participants, of whom nine (69%) had loss of methylation at chromosome 11p15 (11p15LOM), and four (31%) had maternal uniparental disomy of chromosome 7 (upd(7)mat). Of the 24 children, 46% required assistance with bathing, which was strongly correlated with self-care ability and body height. In contrast, most of the children had independence in mobility tasks such as walking and stair climbing. However,

https://doi.org/10.3390/diagnostics15091109

some required support in cognitive tasks, including problem-solving, comprehension, and expression. Overall, the included children reached a functional plateau later than the normative population, with the greatest delays in self-care and mobility domains. **Conclusions:** This study highlights that Taiwanese children with SRS require support in self-care and cognitive tasks. Functional independence in self-care and mobility domains was positively associated with body height. The WeeFIM questionnaire effectively identified strengths and limitations, emphasizing the need for individualized support in daily activities.

Keywords: independent living; Silver–Russell syndrome; Taiwan; WeeFIM

1. Introduction

Silver–Russell syndrome (SRS; OMIM #180860) is a rare imprinting disorder characterized by prenatal and postnatal growth retardation [1,2]. The condition was first described by Silver et al. in 1953 [3] and Russell et al. in 1954 [4], who reported children with low birth weight, intrauterine growth restriction, postnatal short stature, hemihypotrophy, characteristic facial features, and body asymmetry. The estimated incidence of SRS ranges from 1:30,000 to 1:100,000, and nearly all individuals with SRS are born small for their gestational age [5].

The clinical diagnosis of SRS currently relies on the Netchine–Harbison clinical scoring system, which has been shown to have high sensitivity and strong negative predictive value [5–9]. The Netchine–Harbison system includes six criteria: small for gestational age (birth weight and/or birth length), postnatal growth failure, relative macrocephaly at birth, protruding forehead, body asymmetry, and feeding difficulties and/or low body mass index. A diagnosis of SRS can also be established through molecular testing, with the most common genetic findings including loss of methylation at chromosome 11p15 (11p15LOM) and maternal uniparental disomy of chromosome 7 (upd(7)mat) [10,11]. In rare cases, copy number variants and monogenic pathogenic variants in imprinted (*CDKN1C*, *IGF2*) and non-imprinted (*PLAG1*, *HMGA2*) genes have been demonstrated to contribute to the etiology [2,10,12,13].

As growth retardation can result from genetic, maternal, or environmental factors, comprehensive phenotypic profiling and timely molecular analysis are essential to diagnose SRS. Patients with imprinting center 1 hypomethylation are more likely to exhibit classical SRS features such as asymmetry, fifth-finger clinodactyly, and congenital anomalies compared to those with upd(7)mat [1,12].

The Functional Independence Measure for Children (WeeFIM) questionnaire is a practical tool for assessing functional outcomes [14,15], and it has been adapted for use in Chinese children [16]. Recognizing the need to assess the impact of SRS on functional independence, this study aims to quantify functional performance in Taiwanese children with SRS using the WeeFIM questionnaire, identify associated factors, and characterize functional limitations and impacts on daily caregiving.

2. Methods

2.1. Study Population

Twenty-four children with SRS aged from 2 years to 13 years and 3 months and their parents were recruited at MacKay Memorial Hospital and other Taiwan hospitals between January 2013 and December 2024. The parents and children completed the WeeFIM questionnaire at the clinic. The WeeFIM questionnaire was completed jointly by the child and their parent or legal guardian, with guidance and clarification provided by clinicians during outpatient clinic visits. This study was approved by the Institutional Review Board of MacKay Memorial Hospital (Reference number: 21MMHIS109e, approval date: 1 October 2021). All participants provided assent, while their parents or legal guardians signed a parental consent form.

Patient profiles and medical interventions were documented, and clinical features including molecular type, body height, early intervention history, and age at questionnaire completion were recorded. The diagnosis of SRS was confirmed either through molecular testing or clinical assessment. Early intervention history was obtained from parental reports or medical records. For patients with multiple questionnaire records, only the first completed questionnaire was selected.

2.2. WeeFIM Questionnaire

The WeeFIM questionnaire was designed for primary caregivers to directly assess their child's functional abilities and developmental disabilities [14,17]. The Chinese version of the WeeFIM questionnaire was used in this study to assess the functional independence of the enrolled children [16,18]. It was designed for children aged from 6 months to 7 years and can be used for individuals up to 21 years of age with developmental disabilities [19–23].

The WeeFIM questionnaire consists of 18 items categorized into three functional domains: self-care, mobility, and cognition. The self-care domain includes eight items: eating, grooming, bathing, upper-body dressing, lower-body dressing, toileting, bladder management, and bowel management. The mobility domain includes five items: chair transfer, toilet transfer, tub transfer, walking, and stair climbing. The cognition domain consists of five items: comprehension, expression, social interaction, problem-solving, and memory.

Each item is rated on a seven-point ordinal scale that reflects the level of assistance required for task completion, with higher scores corresponding to greater functional independence. A score of 1 indicates total assistance, where the participant is able to perform less than 25% of the task, while a score of 2 represents maximal assistance, with the participant able to complete 25–49% of the task. Moderate assistance (score of 3) indicates that the participant can perform 50–74% of the task, and minimal assistance (score of 4) denotes that the participant can perform at least 75% of the task. A score of 5 indicates that supervision, setup, or standby assistance is required, while a score of 6 represents modified independence, meaning that the participant can complete the task with an assistive device or with some safety or efficiency concerns. A score of 7 represents complete independence, indicating that the participant can complete the task safely and timely without the need of assistance or assistive devices [24].

The WeeFIM questionnaire has been widely used to assess functional abilities in children with developmental disorders, and it provides a standardized measure of self-care, mobility, and cognitive functioning. Scores ranging from 1 to 5 indicate dependence, requiring assistance for daily activities, whereas scores of 6 and 7 signify independence with no external support. The self-care, mobility, and cognition domain scores range from 8 to 56, 5 to 35, and 5 to 35, respectively, with a total WeeFIM score ranging from 18 to 126 [25].

2.3. Statistical Analysis

Descriptive statistics were used, and the results are presented as the median (interquartile range, IQR) and mean (standard deviation, SD), unless otherwise stated. All participants were under 16 years old. Due to the limited age range, the 24 enrolled children were stratified into three age groups (0–5, 6–10, and 11–15 years) for functional performance evaluation. The patients' WeeFIM scores were compared to normative Chinese children [16]. The differences in continuous variables (e.g., age, height, WeeFIM scores) among groups were analyzed using one-way analysis of variance (ANOVA), with Bonferroni correction applied for pairwise comparisons. Consistent with similar studies [26,27], the relationship between age, height, and WeeFIM scores was analyzed using linear regression, with age and height modeled as restricted cubic splines (RCS) with knots placed at the 10th, 50th, and 95th percentiles. RCS modeling was performed using R software, version 4.4.3 (R Foundation for Statistical Computing, Vienna, Austria), and the "rms" package version 7.0–0 (Frank E. Harrell Jr). All other statistical analyses were conducted using IBM SPSS Statistics software version 25.0 (IBM Corp., Armonk, NY, USA). A 2-sided p value of <0.05 was considered statistically significant.

3. Results

A total of 24 children (12 male and 12 female) with SRS were included in this study. Their age ranged from 2 years to 13 years and 3 months, with a median age at enrollment of 5 years and 8 months. The diagnosis of SRS was confirmed either by molecular studies or using clinical assessment [5]. Traceable molecular data were available for thirteen participants, of whom nine (69%) had 11p15LOM, and four (31%) had upd(7)mat. Data on height were available for 16 participants, and 8 children had a history of receiving early intervention.

The total WeeFIM score of the enrolled children ranged from 54 to 126 (median 117). Table 1 summarizes the total, mean, median, and IQR scores for each domain in the three age groups. The mean total WeeFIM score in the overall cohort was 106.9 $\pm$ 23.2 (range: 54–126), and the mean self-care, mobility, and cognition scores were 44.4 $\pm$ 13.8 (maximum 56), 32.4 $\pm$ 5.1 (maximum 35), and 30.2 $\pm$ 6.0 (maximum 35), respectively. The median IQR scores for the self-care, mobility, and cognition domains were 50.5 (36.5–55.5), 35.0 (33.5–35.0), and 32.0 (27.0–35.0), respectively. When grouped by age, significant differences were observed between groups in the self-care domain and total WeeFIM scores. The box plot in Figure 1A illustrates the distribution of scores across the self-care, mobility, and cognition domains, as well as total WeeFIM scores. The 16 children with recorded height data were divided into three groups based on height, from shortest to tallest. However, no significant differences were found between the height groups in self-care, mobility, or cognition domains, or in total WeeFIM score (Table 2). Figure 1B presents a box plot illustrating the distribution of self-care, mobility, cognition, and total WeeFIM scores among the participants grouped by height.

Based on the WeeFIM profiles of the participants stratified by age and height (Figure 2A,B), the lowest performance was in the bathing task. Table 3 summarizes the WeeFIM scores for the children requiring assistance or supervision versus those who were independent across the three domains. In the self-care domain, from 17% to 46% of the participants had scores ranging from 1 to 4, indicating varying levels of assistance required for different self-care tasks. Notably, 46% of the participants needed assistance with bathing. In contrast, most children demonstrated independence in mobility tasks, with 96% walking independently and 92% able to climb stairs without assistance. Despite their mobility independence, some children required support in problem-solving (33%), comprehension (21%), and expression (21%), highlighting cognitive challenges in daily functioning. To compare the functional development of the included children with the general population, Table 4 presents the age at which the 50th percentile of the included children attained level 6 on the WeeFIM scale. The attainment order differed slightly from the normative functional independence profile for Chinese children [16].

Table 1. WeeFIM scores of the children with Silver–Russell syndrome grouped by age.

Variable	Total (2.0–15.9 Years)	Group 1 (2.0–5.9 Years)	Group 2 (6.0–10.9 Years)	Group 3 (11.0–15.9 Years)	*p* Value
Number of children	24	14	6	4	
Age, year					
Mean ± standard deviation	6.7 ± 3.3	4.3 ± 1.2	8.6 ± 1.0 [a]	12.3 ± 0.7 [ab]	<0.001
Range	2.0–13.3	2.0–5.9	7.3–9.6	11.9–13.3	
Self-care score					0.009
Mean ± standard deviation	44.4 ± 13.8	37.5 ± 14.5	54.3 ± 2.0 [a]	53.5 ± 3.8	
Median [25th percentile, 75th percentiles]	50.5 [36.5, 55.5]	38.5 [26.0, 50.0]	55.0 [53.0, 56.0]	55.0 [51.0, 56.0]	
Mobility score					0.098
Mean ± standard deviation	32.4 ± 5.1	30.5 ± 6.1	35.0 ± 0	35.0 ± 0	
Median [25th percentile, 75th percentiles]	35.0 [33.5, 35.0]	34.0 [26.0, 35.0]	35.0 [35.0, 35.0]	35.0 [35.0, 35.0]	
Cognition score					0.337
Mean ± standard deviation	30.2 ± 6.0	28.9 ± 5.5	33.3 ± 2.7	29.8 ± 10.5	
Median [25th percentile, 75th percentiles]	32.0 [27.0, 35.0]	30.5 [23.0, 34.0]	35.0 [31.0, 35.0]	35.0 [24.5, 35.0]	
Total score					0.034
Mean ± standard deviation	106.9 ± 23.2	96.9 ± 25.3	122.7 ± 3.6	118.3 ± 14.2	
Median [25th percentile, 75th percentiles]	117.0 [98.5, 125.5]	102.0 [76.0, 117.0]	123.0 [121.0, 126.0]	125.0 [110.5, 126.0]	

Abbreviation: WeeFIM, functional independence measure for children; "a" and "b" denote significant differences compared to the 2.0–5.9 years and 6.0–10.9 years age groups, respectively, following Bonferroni correction.

Table 2. WeeFIM scores of children with Silver–Russell syndrome grouped by height.

Variable	Total (71.6–135.5 cm)	Group 1 (71.6–88.0 cm)	Group 2 (88.1–120.3 cm)	Group 3 (120.4–135.5 cm)	*p* Value
Number of children	16	5	6	5	
Height, cm					
Mean ± standard deviation	103.9 ± 19.2	83.0 ± 6.7	103.0 ± 11.0 [a]	125.8 ± 5.8 [ab]	<0.001
Range	71.6–135.5	71.6–88.0	88.9–120.3	121.3–135.5	
Self-care score					0.109
Mean ± standard deviation	44.0 ± 13.0	36.0 ± 15.0	43.0 ± 14.0	53.0 ± 3.0	
Median [25th percentile, 75th percentiles]	49.0 [31.0, 55.0]	35.0 [21.0, 48.0]	47.0 [27.0, 56.0]	54.0 [53.0, 55.0]	
Mobility score					0.221
Mean ± standard deviation	32.0 ± 5.0	29.0 ± 7.0	32.0 ± 4.0	35.0 ± 0	
Median [25th percentile, 75th percentiles]	35.0 [31.0, 35.0]	34.0 [23.0, 35.0]	35.0 [28.0, 35.0]	35.0 [35.0, 35.0]	
Cognition score					0.863
Mean ± standard deviation	29.0 ± 7.0	28.0 ± 7.0	30.0 ± 6.0	30.0 ± 9.0	
Median [25th percentile, 75th percentiles]	32.0 [24.0, 35.0]	31.0 [22.0, 33.0]	33.0 [25.0, 35.0]	35.0 [29.0, 35.0]	
Total score					0.250
Mean ± standard deviation	106.0 ± 23.0	93.0 ± 29.0	106.0 ± 23.0	118.0 ± 12.0	
Median [25th percentile, 75th percentiles]	116.0 [88.0, 125.0]	100.0 [63.0, 117.0]	114.0 [78.0, 126.0]	124.0 [117.0, 125.0]	

Abbreviation: WeeFIM, functional independence measure for children; "a" and "b" denote significant differences compared to the 71.6–88.0 cm and 88.1–120.3 cm height groups, respectively, following Bonferroni correction.

Table 3. Scores of individual WeeFIM tasks grouped into help, supervision, and no help categories in the children with Silver–Russell syndrome.

Task	Requiring Help (1–4 Points)		Requiring Supervision (5 Points)		Requiring No Help (6–7 Points)	
	n	%	*n*	%	*n*	%
Self-care						
Eating	5	21	5	21	14	58
Grooming	9	38	2	8	13	54
Bathing	11	46	0	0	13	54
Dressing upper	8	33	1	4	15	63
Dressing lower	6	25	2	8	16	67
Toileting	8	33	0	0	16	67
Bladder	4	17	1	4	19	79
Bowel	5	21	0	0	19	79
Mobility						
Chair transfer	1	4	4	17	19	79
Toilet transfer	2	8	3	13	19	79
Tub transfer	4	17	1	4	19	79
Walking	0	0	1	4	23	96
Stairs	2	8	0	0	22	92
Cognition						
Comprehension	5	21	0	0	19	79
Expression	5	21	0	0	19	79
Social interaction	3	13	4	17	17	71
Problem-solving	8	33	2	8	14	58
Memory	3	13	2	8	19	79

Abbreviation: WeeFIM, functional independence measure for children.

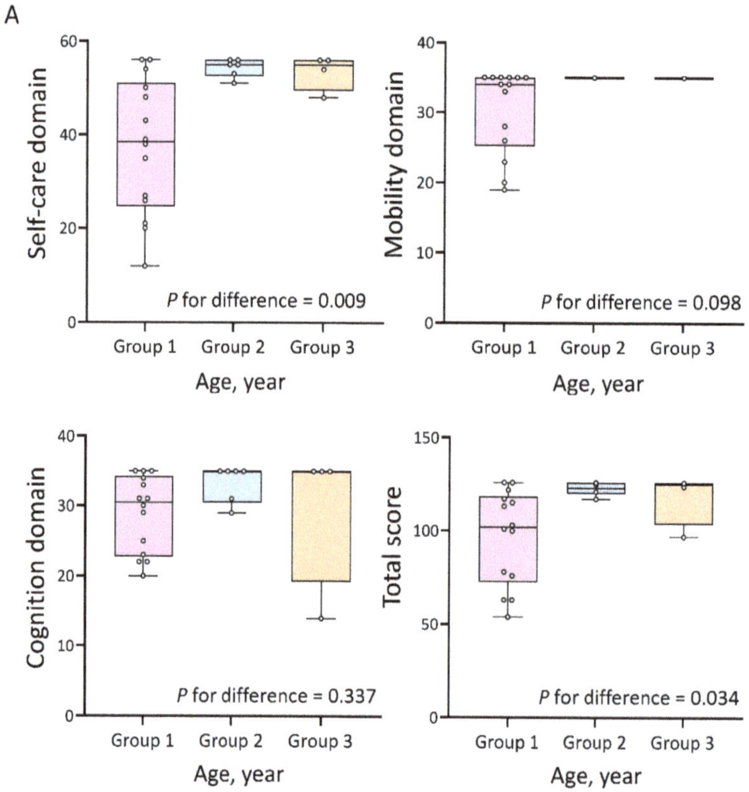

Figure 1. *Cont.*

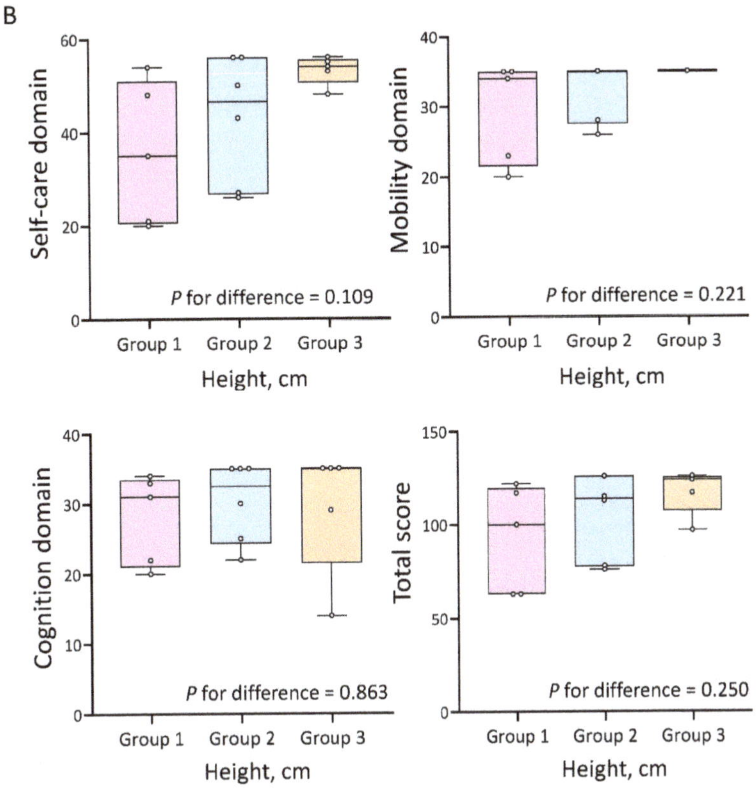

Figure 1. (**A**) Box plot illustrating the median and quartiles of total WeeFIM scores and domain-specific scores across three age groups: 2.0–5.9 yrs, 6.0–10.9 yrs, and 11.0–15.9 yrs. (**B**) Box plot illustrating the median and quartiles of total WeeFIM scores and domain-specific scores across three height-based groups: 71.6–88.0 cm, 88.1–120.3 cm, and 120.4–135.5 cm.

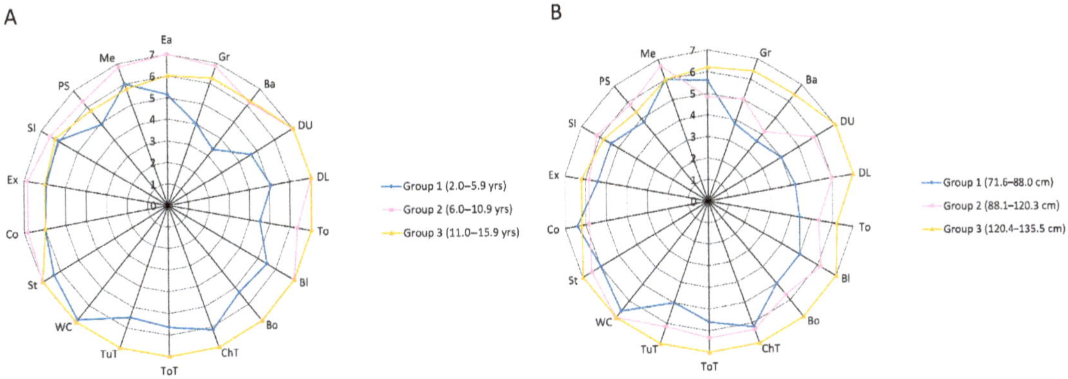

Figure 2. (**A**) WeeFIM profiles of the study participants stratified by three age groups; (**B**) WeeFIM profiles of the study participants stratified by three height-based groups. Ba = bathing; Bl = bladder; Bo = bowel; ChT = bed/chair/wheelchair transfer; Co = comprehension; DL = dressing (lower); DU = dressing (upper); Ea = eating; Ex = expression; Gr = grooming; Me = memory; PS = problem-solving; SI = social interaction; St = stairs; To = toileting; ToT = toilet transfer; TuT = tub/shower transfer; WC = walk/wheelchair.

Table 4. Order of 50th percentiles for attaining level 6 for children with Silver–Russell syndrome.

Order of Achievement	Items	25th Percentile (Months)	50th Percentile (Months)	75th Percentile (Months)
1	Walking	48.6	70.0	113.9
2	Stairs	52.2	70.2	113.9
3	Comprehension	52.2	70.5	113.9
4	Expression	52.2	70.5	113.9
5	Social interaction	52.2	70.5	108.5
6	Memory	52.2	70.5	113.9
7	Bladder	60.0	87.5	115.6
8	Bowel	60.0	87.5	115.6
9	Chair transfer	60.0	87.5	115.6
10	Toilet transfer	60.0	87.5	115.6
11	Tub transfer	60.0	87.5	115.6
12	Eating	63.1	88.7	113.9
13	Toileting	61.6	88.7	128.1
14	Problem-solving	60.0	88.7	113.9
15	Dressing lower	66.1	96.0	129.0
16	Grooming	70.0	102.0	115.6
17	Bathing	63.1	102.0	115.6
18	Dressing upper	63.1	102.0	142.3

We utilize restricted cubic splines in Figure 3 to visualize the relationships between age, height, and WeeFIM scores. The results show that the relationship between age and WeeFIM scores was generally nonlinear, except for the cognition domain, where the nonlinearity significance was 0.082. A clear positive linear correlation was observed before school age (approximately 72 months), after which the scores plateaued at varying ages depending on the specific WeeFIM domains (Figure 3A). By contrast, the relationship between height and WeeFIM scores was generally linear, except for the cognition domain (p for linearity = 0.608) (Figure 3B).

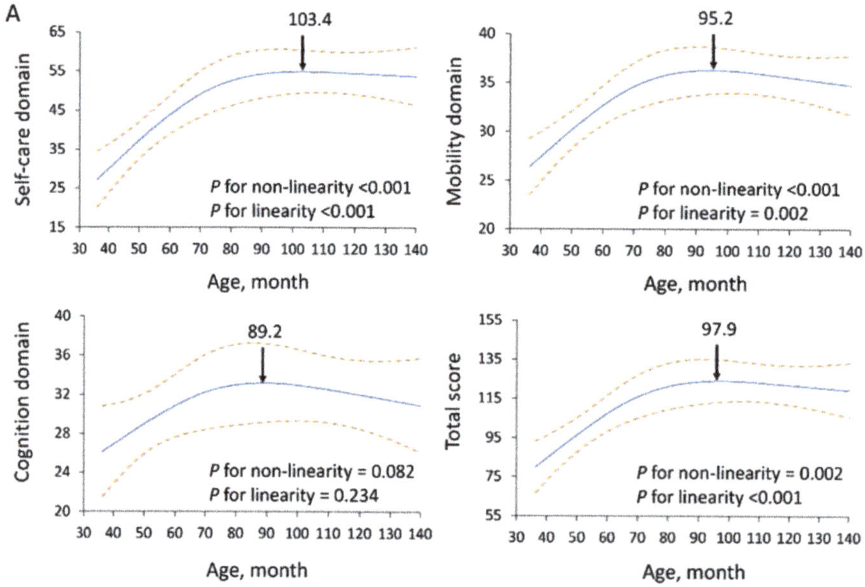

Figure 3. *Cont.*

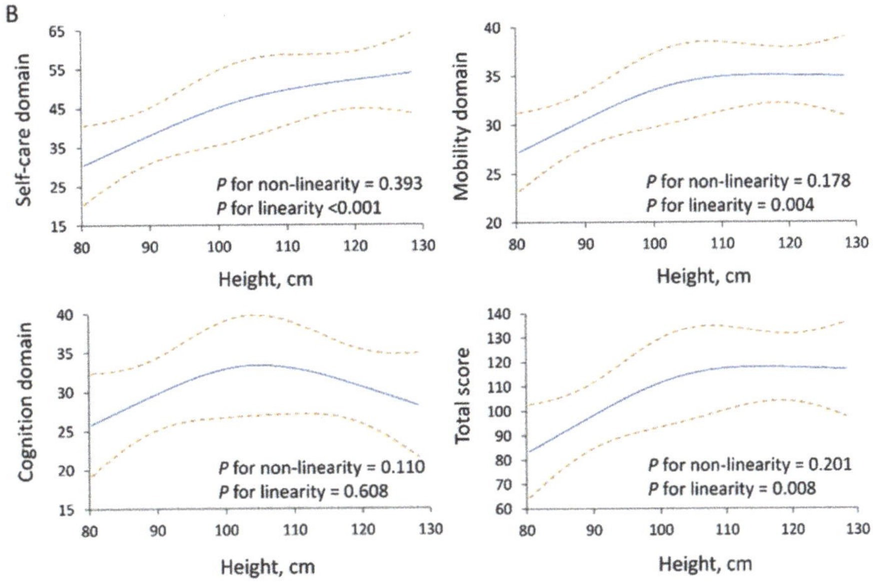

Figure 3. (**A**) Linear and nonlinear relationships of age-related trends in self-care, mobility, cognition, and total WeeFIM scores. (**B**) Linear and nonlinear relationships of height-related trends in self-care, mobility, cognition, and total WeeFIM scores. The solid blue line represents the predicted mean score based on a restricted cubic spline regression model and the dashed orange lines represent the 95% confidence intervals of the predicted scores.

The results also show no significant differences in the mean total WeeFIM score between those with the 11p15LOM (105.3 ± 25.5) and upd(7)mat (109.3 ± 11.3) type and the corresponding self-care (42.9 ± 14.4 and 47.8 ± 6.3), mobility (31.6 ± 5.6 and 34.5 ± 1.0), and cognition (30.9 ± 6.0 and 27.0 ± 8.8) scores. Sex-specific WeeFIM scores have not previously been reported, and our results show no significant differences in the total score between boys (103.9 ± 21.7) and girls (109.9 ± 25.2) and the corresponding self-care (42.3 ± 12.5 and 46.4 ± 15.2), mobility (32.4 ± 4.3 and 32.3 ± 6.0), and cognition (29.2 ± 7.3 and 31.2 ± 4.6) scores.

4. Discussion

In this study, we used the WeeFIM questionnaire to assess disabilities in self-care, mobility, and cognition domains and characterize the range of functional performance across these domains in children with SRS aged from 2 years to 13 years and 3 months. Overall, 79% of the children were independent in mobility, compared with 58% in cognition and 54% in self-care. These results are consistent with a previous study [28]. Among the children across the different age and height groups, the lowest WeeFIM subscores were observed in bathing (Figure 2A,B), and bathing performance was strongly correlated with self-care ability and body height.

The WeeFIM total score, self-care, and mobility domains were positively correlated with age ($p < 0.05$). Among the age groups, significant differences were observed in the self-care and total WeeFIM scores. The increasing trends plateaued at 103.4 months (normative population: 72 months) in the self-care domain, 95.2 months (54 months) in the mobility domain, 89.2 months (80 months) in the cognition domain, and 97.9 months (72 months) in the total WeeFIM score (Figure 3A). The children with SRS reached a functional plateau later than the normative population [16] in all three domains and the total WeeFIM score, with the most pronounced delays observed in the self-care and mobility domains.

RCS regression was performed to explore nonlinearity, followed by a two-piecewise linear regression model to determine turning points. The RCS analysis indicated nonlinear relationships between age and self-care (p for nonlinearity < 0.001; Figure 3A), mobility (p for nonlinearity < 0.001; Figure 3A), and total WeeFIM scores (p for nonlinearity = 0.002; Figure 3A). However, the relationship between age and cognition scores was linear (p for nonlinearity = 0.082; Figure 3A). To further validate these findings, simple linear regression was performed. Significant linear associations were observed in the self-care, mobility, and total WeeFIM scores ($p < 0.05$), whereas the cognition domain did not reach statistical significance ($p = 0.234$). Overall, there were progressive increases in self-care, mobility, cognition, and total WeeFIM scores with age, which plateaued upon reaching functional maturity. RCS analysis did not indicate a nonlinear relationship between height and self-care ($p = 0.393$; Figure 3B), mobility ($p = 0.178$; Figure 3B), cognition ($p = 0.110$; Figure 3B), or total WeeFIM score ($p = 0.201$; Figure 3B). To further assess linearity, simple linear regression was performed. Significant linear associations were identified in self-care, mobility, and total WeeFIM scores ($p < 0.05$), whereas the cognition domain did not reach significance ($p = 0.608$). Functional scores showed a positive association with height, except in the cognition domain. The children with SRS followed a different sequence in attaining functional performance, and specific tasks such as bathing and upper-body dressing took longer to achieve level 6 compared to the general population.

This study has several limitations. Firstly, due to the rarity of SRS, the sample size was small, which may limit the generalizability of the findings. Secondly, the participants were relatively young, potentially affecting the assessment of functional milestones in older individuals. In addition, as the original version of the WeeFIM questionnaire was not developed in Chinese, the translation may have introduced subtle nuances that were not fully recognized. To ensure accuracy and cultural relevance, further validation of the translated version is necessary. Thirdly, the records of the children were missing some data on height, molecular type, early intervention history, and developmental delays. To better understand the impact of these factors on motor and cognitive functioning in children with SRS, larger and more comprehensive studies are required.

5. Conclusions

The WeeFIM questionnaire responses reveal that the children with SRS had greater independence in mobility compared to self-care and cognitive functions. Our findings highlight that Taiwanese children with SRS require additional support in self-care and cognitive tasks. We also found that functional independence in self-care and mobility domains was positively associated with body height. These findings provide valuable insights for clinicians in identifying the functional strengths and challenges of children with SRS, facilitating the development of individualized support strategies to enhance daily living and overall quality of life.

Author Contributions: H.-H.F. performed acquisition, statistical analysis, interpretation of data, and drafting of the manuscript. S.-P.L. and H.-Y.L. participated in design of the study, interpretation of the data, and helped to draft the manuscript. C.-L.L., C.-K.C., H.-C.C., Y.-H.C., Y.-R.T., Y.-T.L., J.-Y.W., Y.-Y.C., C.-H.W., S.-J.L., S.-Y.C., C.Y. and T.-Y.O. were responsible for patient screening and revised the manuscript. All authors have read and agreed to the published version of the manuscript.

Funding: This research was supported by multiple grants from two major institutions. MacKay Memorial Hospital provided funding through grants MMH-E-114-13, MMH-MM-113-13, MMH-E-113-13, MMH-MM-112-14, and MMH-E-112-13. Additional support was received from the Ministry of Science and Technology, Executive Yuan, Taiwan through several research grants: NSTC-113-

2314-B-195-003, NSTC-113-2314-B-195-004, NSTC-113-2314-B-715-002, NSTC-113-2314-B-195-021, NSTC-113-2811-B-195-001, NSTC-112-2314-B-195-014-MY3, NSTC-112-2811-B-195-001, NSTC-112-2314-B-195-003, NSTC-111-2314-B-195-017, NSTC-111-2811-B-195-002, NSTC-111-2811-B-195-001, NSTC-110-2314-B-195-014, NSTC-110-2314-B-195-010-MY3, and NSTC-110-2314-B-195-029.

Institutional Review Board Statement: This study was conducted according to the guidelines of the Declaration of Helsinki. It was approved by the MacKay Memorial Hospital Institutional Review Board (Reference number: 21MMHIS109e, approval date: 1 October 2021) and was permitted to be published.

Informed Consent Statement: All participants provided assent, while their parents or legal guardians signed a parental consent form.

Data Availability Statement: All data are present within the article.

Acknowledgments: The successful completion of this research would not have been possible without the exceptional dedication and expertise of our clinical staff and research laboratory personnel. Their tireless commitment to excellence in both patient care and laboratory procedures was invaluable to this study.

Conflicts of Interest: The authors confirm that there are no competing interests or conflicts of interest, financial or non-financial, that could have influenced this study.

Abbreviations

SRS: Silver–Russell syndrome; 11p15LOM: loss of methylation at chromosome 11p15; upd(7)mat: maternal uniparental disomy of chromosome 7; WeeFIM: Functional Independence Measure for Children; IQR: interquartile range; SD: standard deviation; RCS: restricted cubic spline.

References

1. Binder, G.; Begemann, M.; Eggermann, T.; Kannenberg, K. Silver-Russell syndrome. *Best. Pract. Res. Clin. Endocrinol. Metab.* **2011**, *25*, 153–160. [CrossRef] [PubMed]
2. Saal, H.M.; Harbison, M.D.; Netchine, I. Silver-Russell Syndrome. In *GeneReviews®*; Adam, M.P., Feldman, J., Mirzaa, G.M., Pagon, R.A., Wallace, S.E., Amemiya, A., Eds.; University of Washington: Seattle, WA, USA, 1993.
3. Silver, H.K.; Kiyasu, W.; George, J.; Deamer, W.C. Syndrome of congenital hemihypertrophy, shortness of stature, and elevated urinary gonadotropins. *Pediatrics* **1953**, *12*, 368–376. [CrossRef] [PubMed]
4. Russell, A. A syndrome of intra-uterine dwarfism recognizable at birth with cranio-facial dysostosis, disproportionately short arms, and other anomalies (5 examples). *Proc. R. Soc. Med.* **1954**, *47*, 1040–1044.
5. Wakeling, E.L.; Brioude, F.; Lokulo-Sodipe, O.; O'Connell, S.M.; Salem, J.; Bliek, J.; Canton, A.P.M.; Chrzanowska, K.H.; Davies, J.H.; Dias, R.P.; et al. Diagnosis and management of Silver-Russell syndrome: First international consensus statement. *Nat. Rev. Endocrinol.* **2017**, *13*, 105–124. [CrossRef]
6. Azzi, S.; Salem, J.; Thibaud, N.; Chantot-Bastaraud, S.; Lieber, E.; Netchine, I.; Harbison, M.D. A prospective study validating a clinical scoring system and demonstrating phenotypical-genotypical correlations in Silver-Russell syndrome. *J. Med. Genet.* **2015**, *52*, 446–453. [CrossRef]
7. Netchine, I.; Rossignol, S.; Dufourg, M.-N.; Azzi, S.; Rousseau, A.; Perin, L.; Houang, M.; Steunou, V.; Esteva, B.; Thibaud, N.; et al. 11p15 imprinting center region 1 loss of methylation is a common and specific cause of typical Russell-Silver syndrome: Clinical scoring system and epigenetic-phenotypic correlations. *J. Clin. Endocrinol. Metab.* **2007**, *92*, 3148–3154. [CrossRef]
8. Dias, R.P.; Nightingale, P.; Hardy, C.; Kirby, G.; Tee, L.; Price, S.; MacDonald, F.; Barrett, T.G.; Maher, E.R. Comparison of the clinical scoring systems in Silver-Russell syndrome and development of modified diagnostic criteria to guide molecular genetic testing. *J. Med. Genet.* **2013**, *50*, 635–639. [CrossRef]
9. Lin, H.-Y.; Lee, C.-L.; Tu, Y.-R.; Chang, Y.-H.; Niu, D.-M.; Chang, C.-Y.; Chiu, P.C.; Chou, Y.-Y.; Hsiao, H.-P.; Tsai, M.-C.; et al. Quantitative DNA Methylation Analysis and Epigenotype-Phenotype Correlations in Taiwanese Patients with Silver-Russell Syndrome. *Int. J. Med. Sci.* **2024**, *21*, 8–18. [CrossRef]
10. Kurup, U.; Lim, D.B.N.; Palau, H.; Maharaj, A.V.; Ishida, M.; Davies, J.H.; Storr, H.L. Approach to the Patient With Suspected Silver-Russell Syndrome. *J. Clin. Endocrinol. Metab.* **2024**, *109*, e1889–e1901. [CrossRef]

11. Schonherr, N.; Meyer, E.; Eggermann, K.; Ranke, M.B.; Wollmann, H.A.; Eggermann, T. (Epi)mutations in 11p15 significantly contribute to Silver-Russell syndrome: But are they generally involved in growth retardation? *Eur. J. Med. Genet.* **2006**, *49*, 414–418. [CrossRef]
12. Lin, H.Y.; Lee, C.L.; Fran, S.; Tu, R.Y.; Chang, Y.H.; Niu, D.M.; Chang, C.Y.; Chiu, P.C.; Chou, Y.Y.; Hsiao, H.P.; et al. Epigenotype, Genotype, and Phenotype Analysis of Taiwanese Patients with Silver-Russell Syndrome. *J. Pers. Med.* **2021**, *11*, 1197. [CrossRef]
13. Singh, A.; Pajni, K.; Panigrahi, I.; Khetarpal, P. Clinical and Molecular Heterogeneity of Silver-Russell Syndrome and Therapeutic Challenges: A Systematic Review. *Curr. Pediatr. Rev.* **2023**, *19*, 157–168.
14. Ottenbacher, K.J.; Msall, M.E.; Lyon, N.; Duffy, L.C.; Granger, C.V.; Braun, S. Measuring developmental and functional status in children with disabilities. *Dev. Med. Child. Neurol.* **1999**, *41*, 186–194. [CrossRef]
15. Liu, M.; Toikawa, H.; Seki, M.; Domen, K.; Chino, N. Functional Independence Measure for Children (WeeFIM): A preliminary study in nondisabled Japanese children. *Am. J. Phys. Med. Rehabil.* **1998**, *77*, 36–44. [CrossRef]
16. Wong, V.; Wong, S.; Chan, K.; Wong, W. Functional Independence Measure (WeeFIM) for Chinese children: Hong Kong Cohort. *Pediatrics* **2002**, *109*, E36. [CrossRef]
17. Ottenbacher, K.J.; Msall, M.E.; Lyon, N.; Duffy, L.C.; Ziviani, J.; Granger, C.V.; Braun, S.; Feidler, R.C. The WeeFIM instrument: Its utility in detecting change in children with developmental disabilities. *Arch. Phys. Med. Rehabil.* **2000**, *81*, 1317–1326. [CrossRef]
18. Wong, S.S.; Wong, V.C. Functional Independence Measure for Children: A comparison of Chinese and Japanese children. *Neurorehabil Neural Repair.* **2007**, *21*, 91–96. [CrossRef]
19. Wong, V.; Chung, B.; Hui, S.; Fong, A.; Lau, C.; Law, B.; Lo, K.; Shum, T.; Wong, R. Cerebral palsy: Correlation of risk factors and functional performance using the Functional Independence Measure for Children (WeeFIM). *J. Child. Neurol.* **2004**, *19*, 887–893. [CrossRef]
20. Lee, C.; Lin, H.; Chuang, C.; Chiu, H.; Tu, R.; Huang, Y.; Hwu, W.; Tsai, F.; Chiu, P.; Niu, D.; et al. Functional independence of Taiwanese patients with mucopolysaccharidoses. *Mol. Genet. Genom. Med.* **2019**, *7*, e790. [CrossRef]
21. Lee, C.; Lin, H.; Tsai, L.; Chiu, H.; Tu, R.; Huang, Y.; Chien, Y.; Lee, N.; Niu, D.; Chao, M.; et al. Functional independence of Taiwanese children with Prader-Willi syndrome. *Am. J. Med. Genet. A* **2018**, *176*, 1309–1314. [CrossRef]
22. Lin, H.; Chuang, C.; Chen, Y.; Tu, R.; Chen, M.; Niu, D.; Lin, S. Functional independence of Taiwanese children with Down syndrome. *Dev. Med. Child. Neurol.* **2016**, *58*, 502–507. [CrossRef]
23. Syu, Y.-M.; Lee, C.-L.; Chuang, C.-K.; Chiu, H.-C.; Chang, Y.-H.; Lin, H.-Y.; Lin, S.-P. Functional Independence of Taiwanese Children with Osteogenesis Imperfecta. *J. Pers. Med.* **2022**, *12*, 1205. [CrossRef]
24. Sperle, P.A.; Ottenbacher, K.J.; Braun, S.L.; Lane, S.J.; Nochajski, S. Equivalence reliability of the functional independence measure for children (WeeFIM) administration methods. *Am. J. Occup. Ther.* **1997**, *51*, 35–41. [CrossRef]
25. Lin, H.-Y.; Lin, S.-P.; Lin, H.-Y.; Hsu, C.-H.; Chang, J.-H.; Kao, H.-A.; Hung, H.-Y.; Peng, C.-C.; Lee, H.-C.; Chen, M.-R.; et al. Functional independence of Taiwanese children with VACTERL association. *Am J Med Genet A* **2012**, *158*, 3101–3105. [CrossRef]
26. Chen, Q.; Hu, P.; Hou, X.; Sun, Y.; Jiao, M.; Peng, L.; Dai, Z.; Yin, X.; Liu, R.; Li, Y.; et al. Association between triglyceride-glucose related indices and mortality among individuals with non-alcoholic fatty liver disease or metabolic dysfunction-associated steatotic liver disease. *Cardiovasc. Diabetol.* **2024**, *23*, 232. [CrossRef]
27. Chen, Z.; Qiu, X.; Wang, Q.; Wu, J.; Li, M.; Niu, W. Serum vitamin D and obesity among US adolescents, NHANES 2011-2018. *Front. Pediatr.* **2024**, *12*, 1334139. [CrossRef]
28. Burgevin, M.; Lacroix, A.; Ollivier, F.; Bourdet, K.; Coutant, R.; Donadille, B.; Faivre, L.; Manouvrier-Hanu, S.; Petit, F.; Thauvin-Robinet, C.; et al. Executive functioning in adolescents and adults with Silver-Russell syndrome. *PLoS ONE* **2023**, *18*, e0279745. [CrossRef]

diagnostics

MDPI

Article

Incidental Calcifications of Carotid and Vertebral Arteries: Frequency and Associations in Pediatric Population

Turkhun Cetin [1], Gokce Cinar [2], Berna Ucan [2], Fulya Memis [3], Baris Irgul [1,*] and Sonay Aydin [1]

[1] Department of Radiology, Erzincan Binali Yidirim University, Erzincan 24100, Turkey; turkhuncetinmd@gmail.com (T.C.); sonay.aydin@erzincan.edu.tr (S.A.)
[2] Department of Radiology, Ankara Etlik City Hospital, Ankara 06170, Turkey; gokcecinar@gmail.com (G.C.); bernaucan@gmail.com (B.U.)
[3] Department of Internal Medicine, Erzincan Binali Yidirim University, Erzincan 24100, Turkey; fulyamemis@gmail.com
* Correspondence: barisirgul@gmail.com; Tel.: +90-554-482-71-25

Abstract: Background: Calcifications in the carotid and vertebral arteries may be present on cranial and temporal bone CT imaging of pediatric patients. Few studies have investigated the frequency, location, and patterns of carotid artery calcifications in this age group. However, these studies are outdated and do not include data on the vertebral artery. The aim of this study was to determine the frequency, location, and pattern of incidental carotid and vertebral artery calcifications on cranial CT and temporal bone CT images in children under 15 years of age. We also aimed to investigate possible associations between these calcifications and various diseases. **Methods:** A total of 300 CT images of the cranial and temporal bone of 300 pediatric patients were retrospectively evaluated for the presence of calcification in the carotid and vertebral arteries. The evaluation included determining the presence of calcification in the artery, the pattern of calcification, the degree of calcification, and its anatomical location. **Results:** In the current study, 300 CT images were analyzed, and calcifications were found in the vertebral artery in 17 patients (5.6%) and the carotid artery in 82 patients (27.3%). The supraclinoid segment and the carotid siphon regions are the most common locations of carotid artery calcifications, with 62 patients (20.7%). The V4 segment is also the most common location for vertebral artery calcifications, with 15 patients (5%). Focal punctate calcification is the most common pattern (65 patients, 21.7%). Incidental carotid and vertebral artery calcifications did not correlate with other diseases. **Conclusions:** Carotid and vertebral artery calcifications are common incidental findings in pediatric patients. In our study, no association was found between other diseases and incidental carotid and vertebral artery calcifications.

Keywords: carotid artery calcifications; vertebral artery calcifications; incidental cranial calcifications

1. Introduction

Incidental intracranial arterial calcifications detected on CT imaging of adult patients have attracted much attention due to their potential predictive value for atherosclerotic disease, hypercholesterolemia, diabetes mellitus, heart disease, carotid artery stenosis, and stroke [1–6].

Risk factors include diabetes mellitus, hypercholesterolemia, a history of cardiovascular disease in both sexes, excessive alcohol and smoking in males, and hypertension in women. The prevalence and volume of carotid artery calcification increases with age. Calcification is inversely related to mean flow velocity and associated with measures of vascular stiffness, such as pulse pressure, aortic pulse wave velocity, and pulsatility index [1,7–9]. Calcification has a significant negative predictive value for carotid bifurcation stenosis, but it is not a reliable indicator of stenosis in stroke suspects [10]. In stroke patients, there was a weak association between severe intracranial internal carotid artery stenosis and calcium burden [11]. After subarachnoid hemorrhage, severe calcification is associated with lower rates of vasospasm [10].

Age, pulse pressure, and a family history of vascular disease are all associated with carotid artery calcification, both intimal and medial. In addition, medial calcification is associated with diabetes mellitus and a history of vascular disease, while intimal calcification is associated with smoking and high blood pressure [12]. Intracerebral artery calcification can occur in any part of the brain and is commonly seen on CT imaging in the general population. In the large arteries, calcifications are a strong predictor of poor clinical outcomes and often become more common with age [1].

Just before entering the brain parenchyma, the ICA and its branches form a tortuous segment, often referred to as the carotid siphon, roughly corresponding to segments C4 and C5 (Figure 1). It is thought that this elastic and tortuous siphon compensates for the increased pulse pressure caused by the passage of the intracranial internal carotid artery through the skull [13]. In the general population, calcification of the carotid and vertebral arteries in the cervical and cranial regions is a common incidental finding on CT imaging [1]. The prevalence increases with age and is most common in the ICA [1].

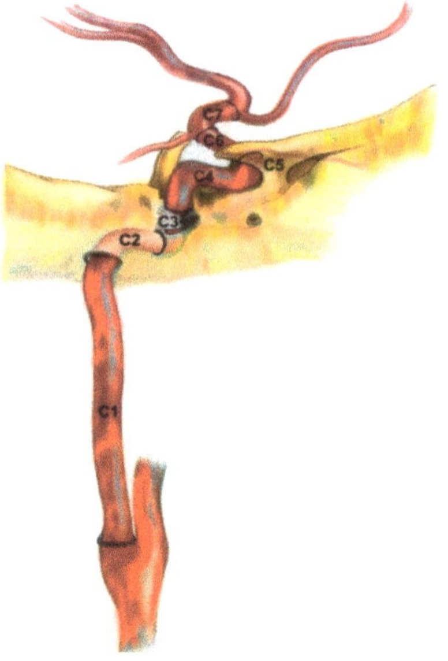

Figure 1. ICA segments.

In pediatric age groups, calcification in the ICA is more common in the supraclinoid segment and the carotid siphon regions [14,15]. And, calcification in the vertebral artery is more common in the V4 segment [14].

In population-based cohort studies, the prevalence of supraclinoid segment and siphon calcifications on CT has been reported to be 6% in pediatric age groups. For the vertebral artery, although no studies have been conducted in specific pediatric age groups, the prevalence of calcification in the adult age group has been evaluated together with the basilar artery, and it has been reported in a wide range from 2% to 13% in different study series [16].

In the Rotterdam Study, the most comprehensive study of the adult population, the prevalence and volume of cervical and intracranial arterial calcification increased with age in both sexes. In that study, age, smoking history, hypercholesterolemia, atherosclerotic vascular diseases, DM, and hypertension were the most important risk factors for calcification. Worldwide, Asian populations have the highest reported prevalence of intracranial arterial calcification [3,17,18].

ICA calcifications evolve with age from a few punctate calcifications or fine linear calcifications to large calcified plaques. It has been shown histologically that calcifications observed in the supraclinoid segment and ICA siphon in the pediatric age group are not associated with atherosclerosis and are located in the internal elastic lamina (IEL) [14–16]. Age-related increases in the volume and prevalence of ICA siphon calcification are substantial. Risk factors include excessive alcohol consumption and smoking in men, diabetes mellitus, hypercholesterolemia, history of cardiovascular disease, and early-onset hypertension in women [1–6].

Calcifications in intracranial arteries are usually localized in the intima and media of the arterial walls. Focal calcification in damaged or neoplastic brain tissue accounts for at least fifty per cent of all cases of intracranial calcification in all age groups [19]. Dystrophic calcification, particularly in the cerebral cortex, occurs after brain damage due to bacterial meningitis, encephalitis, hypoxic–ischemic injury and, occasionally, ischemic stroke. Vascular anomalies, including arteriovenous malformations and, less commonly, cavernomas, are often focally calcified. In pediatric age groups, cerebral infections caused by Mycobacterium tuberculosis, neurocysticercosis, Cryptococcus neoformans, and, more recently, the Zika virus can lead to many calcified lesions [19].

Calcification of the carotid and vertebral arteries can be seen on cranial and temporal bone CT scans in pediatric age groups. Studies investigating the incidence and pattern of carotid calcification in children are extremely rare in the medical literature. However, the studies that are currently available lack information on vertebral arteries and are out of date [14,19–23].

The aim of this study was to determine the frequency, location, and pattern of incidental carotid and vertebral artery calcifications on cranial CT and temporal bone CT images in children under 15 years of age. We also aimed to investigate the association of these findings with conditions that can cause intracranial calcification and additional risk factors for early atherosclerotic disease, such as hypercholesterolemia, diabetes, and chronic kidney disease.

2. Materials and Methods

CT images of the cranial and temporal bone obtained over a 15-month period were retrospectively analyzed to detect calcifications in the carotid and vertebral arteries in patients under 15 years of age. Evaluations included the extent of calcifications within the arteries, their anatomical location, and whether unilateral or bilateral calcifications were present.

After the ICA is separated from the common carotid artery, it is separated into 7 segments as C1–C7 (Figure 1). These are named cervical, petrous, lacerum, cavernous, clinoidal, ophthalmic, and communicating, respectively. C6 and C7 segments can also be classified as supraclinoid segments. Vertebral arteries, which mostly originate from the subclavian artery, are separated into 4 segments as V1–V4 (Figure 2). The first three segments (V1–V3) are extracranial, and the V4 segment is intradural. The V1 segment originates from the subclavian artery and extends to the entrance of the lowest transverse foramen, usually located at the 6th cervical vertebra. The V2 segment crosses the transverse foramen of the 6th cervical vertebra and terminates at the entrance of the transverse foramen of the 1st cervical vertebra. From here, the V3 segment continues until it reaches the dura. This is the beginning of the V4 segment, which continues to form the basilar artery at the pontomedullary junction.

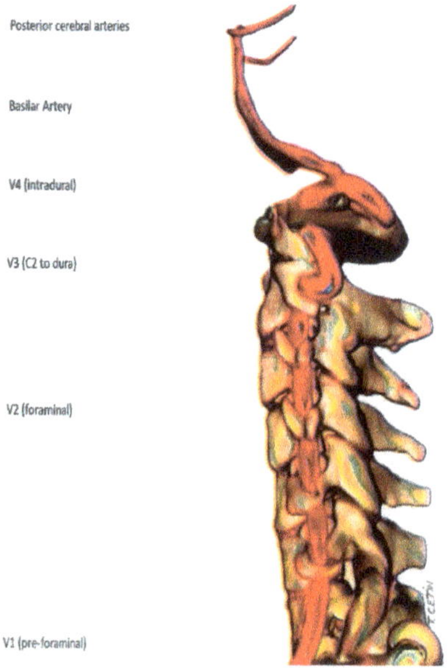

Figure 2. Vertebral artery segments.

In this study, cranial CT and temporal bone CT images of pediatric age groups in the computed tomography unit of our clinic in 2023 and 2024 were retrospectively reviewed. The anatomical segments of the carotid and vertebral arteries in the non-contrasted cranial CT and temporal bone CT images in consecutive axial–coronal–sagittal planes were evaluated for calcification findings. Twelve patients were excluded from the study due to inadequate evaluation of the bilateral supraclinoid segment and the cavernous and carotid siphon regions of the ICAs (X-ray hardening artefacts, motion artefacts, etc.) and inadequate anatomical or positional imaging of both the vertebral and ICA artery regions. As a result, CT examinations of a total of 300 pediatric patients (156 female, 144 male) were included in the final analysis. Finally, 300 cranial and temporal bone CT scans from 300 pediatric patients were retrospectively evaluated for the presence of carotid and vertebral artery calcification.

Computed tomography acquisition protocols were obtained using a 64-slice dual-source multi-detector CT scanner (Somatom Definition Flash, Siemens Healthcare, Forchheim, Germany) with a slice thickness of 0.1 or 0.2 mm. Image analysis was performed by two radiologists with 11 and 5 years of experience in pediatric imaging. Slices above and below the level of calcification were carefully reviewed to ensure that findings were not due to partial volume averaging of adjacent structures.

The presence of calcifications in the internal carotid and vertebral arteries was graded using a four-point grading scale developed specifically and uniquely for this study (Table 1). On this scale, hyperdense foci less than 1 mm in diameter were considered suspicious calcifications. Hyperdensities greater than or equal to 1 mm in diameter were considered prominent calcifications.

Table 1. Scale for grading the presence of ICA and vertebral artery calcifications (original EBYU Pediatric Classification Scale).

		Number and Percentage of Patients
Category 0	No evidence of calcification	201 (67%)
Category 1	Unilateral suspicious calcification focus	28 (9.3%)
Category 2	Prominent calcifications on one or more images, ranging from a single hyperdense focal point to peripheral areas of calcification	47 (15.6%)
Category 3	Prominent foci of calcification in bilateral ICA or vertebral arteries	24 (8.1%)

We evaluated the patient group according to this grading scale and included calcifications confirmed by both radiologists in the final analysis. We retrospectively reviewed the medical records of all patients who were found to have definite calcifications in the internal carotid artery and the vertebral artery segments by reviewing patient files. (In our study, we included only patient medical records that are currently available in the database system of our hospital. We did not have access to the medical records of some patients, and we also did not have access to examinations performed at an external center). To investigate possible associations between different pathological conditions associated with calcifications in pediatric patients and these arterial calcifications, we noted pathologies that may predispose to arterial calcifications, such as hypercholesterolemia, chronic kidney disease, and diabetes mellitus, from the patients' medical data. We also investigated possible associations between intracranial calcifications and various pathological conditions and diseases, listed in Table 2, in patients with ICA and vertebral artery calcifications [19,24]. This included previous cross-sectional radiological examinations of the patients.

Table 2. Summary of intracranial calcifications in childhood [19,24].

Intracranial Calcification	Etiologies	Anatomic Location/Calcification Pattern
Physiologic/Age-Related Intracranial Calcifications		Pineal gland, choroid plexus, falx cerebri, tentorium cerebelli, basal ganglia
Genetic Syndromes/Developmental Disorders	Sturge–Weber syndrome	Gyriform design with twin lines; similar to a tram track
	Tuberous sclerosis	Tubers that are subcortical and subependymal along the atrium and caudothalamic groove
	Neurofibromatosis	Choroid plexus calcifications in the latteral ventricles and cerebellar nodular calcifications
	Cockayne syndrome	Bilateral prominent or punctate calcifications at the level of the basal ganglia
	Krabbe disease	Corona radiata and internal capsule
	Pseudo-TORCH syndromes	Cortical bands, as well as in the thalamus, pons, and cerebellum
	Hyperphenylalaninemia	Basal ganglia
	Von Hippel–Lindau syndrome	Endolymphatic sac tumor
	Mitochondrial disorders	Dispersed or punctate in the thalamus and basal ganglia
	Fahr disease	Caudate, putamen, globus pallidus, thalamus, deep cortex, and dentate are all symmetrically involved

Table 2. *Cont.*

Intracranial Calcification	Etiologies	Anatomic Location/Calcification Pattern
Congenital Infection	Cytomegalovirus	The basal ganglia have mild punctate calcifications, and the periventricular region has thick, chunky calcifications
	Herpes	Dispersed
	Toxoplasmosis	Nodular calcification is seen in the periventricular and cortical regions Curvilinear calcification is seen in the thalamus and basal ganglia
	Rubella	The periventricular region and basal ganglia
	Zika	Subcortical punctate calcifications
	Human Immunodeficiency Virus	Subcortical tissue and basal ganglia
Acquired Infection	Neurocysticercosis	Calcific nodule within a calcified cyst
	Mycobacterium tuberculosis	Central calcific tuberculomas
	Cryptococcus neoformans	Parenchymal and leptomeningeal punctate calcifications
Vascular Malformations	Arteriovenous malformation	Punctate or curvilinear calcifications may be present
	Cavernous malformation	Amorphous/punctate calcifications
	Developmental venous anomaly	Dystrophic calcifications
Intra-Axial Neoplastic	Pilocytic Astrocytoma	Extensive calcification rarely occurs
	Oligodendroglioma	Nodular and grouped
	Ganglioglioma	Calcific mural nodules
	Medulloblastoma	Dispersed foci or grouped
Extra-Axial Neoplastic	Meningioma	Spherical and rim
	Craniopharyngioma	Thin and peripheral
	Germ cell tumors	Heterogeneous
	Lipoma	Eggshell calcifications
Intraventricular	Ependymoma	Point or mass-like
	Central neurocytoma	Variable, ranging from small punctate foci to large calcifications
Metabolic/Endocrine	Hypoparathyroidism	Basal ganglia
Inflammatory	Systemic lupus erythematosus	Most common in the cerebellum
	Sarcoidosis	Cerebellum, hypothalamus, and suprasellar regions

Statistical Analysis

Our study is descriptive. Therefore, descriptive statistics in the form of means, medians and percentiles were used. Advanced statistical methods were not used. Mean ± standard deviation was used as the descriptive statistic for numerical variables and the number and percentage (%) for categorical variables. SPSS 25.0 (IBM Corporation, Armonk, New York, NY, USA) was used for statistical analysis.

In this study, radiologist 1 and radiologist 2, experienced in cross-sectional imaging in pediatric age groups, independently evaluated CT images. Cohen's kappa coefficient was used to determine whether radiologists 1 and 2 agreed on the presence of pathology and quality assessment. The level of agreement was categorized as follows: $p < 0.05$ was considered statistically significant; a coefficient between 0 and 0.20 was considered low; a coefficient between 0.21 and 0.40 was considered moderate; a coefficient between 0.41 and 0.60 was considered moderate; a coefficient between 0.61 and 0.80 was considered substantial; and a coefficient between 0.81 and 1.00 was considered to be highly compatible.

The Ethics Committee approved our study. The following is the Ethics Committee approval number. Date: 12 December 2023. Number: 2023.12/003-128.6.

All methods used in studies involving human subjects complied with the Helsinki Declaration of 1964 and its subsequent amendments, the ethical standards of the institutional and/or national research committee, or similar ethical standards.

3. Results

In this study, cranial and temporal bone CT images of a total of 300 patients were analyzed in detail. The age of the patients ranged from 4 months to 15 years, with a mean age of 8.9 ± 0.2 years. The male to female ratio was approximately 1:1 (156 females, 144 males). Definite ICA and vertebral artery calcifications were seen in 23.6% (71/300) of the patients. Suspected calcifications were seen in 9.3% (28/300) of the analyzed CT sections. The proportion of patients with no evidence of arterial calcification was 67% (201/300). Definite calcifications were seen in 8.4% (6/71) of patients younger than 2 years, 26.7% (19/71) of patients aged 2–7 years, 39.4% (28/71) of patients aged 7–12 years, and 25.3% (18/71) of patients aged 12–15 years. Of the 71 patients with definite calcifications, 43% (31) were male and 56% (40) were female. Of the calcifications, 66% (47) were unilateral and 33% (24) were bilateral. In this study, a total of 300 CT images were analyzed, and definite and suspected foci of calcification were detected in the carotid artery in 82 patients (27.3%) and in the vertebral artery in 17 patients (5.6%). In our study, calcifications in the supraclinoid segment and the carotid siphon regions were observed in 62 patients (20.6%), and these were the most common anatomical locations of ICA calcifications (Table 3). V4 segment calcifications, which were observed in 15 cases (5%), were the most common anatomical location of vertebral artery calcifications (Table 4) (Figures 3–6). The most common vascular calcification pattern was focal–punctate calcification (65 patients, 21.6%).

Table 3. Sites of occurrence of ICA calcifications.

	Cervical	Petrous	Lacerum	Carotid Siphon	Supraclinoid
ICA Calcifications	7 (2.3%)	7 (2.3%)	6 (2%)	31 (10.3%)	31 (10.3%)

Table 4. Sites of occurrence of vertebral artery calcifications.

	V1	V2	V3	V4
Vertebral Artery Calcifications	1 (0.33%)	1 (0.33%)	0	15 (5%)

In our study, the agreement between the evaluations of radiologist 1 and radiologist 2 was measured between 0.81 and 1.00 in all cases and found to be highly compatible. For this reason, no image in our study was excluded from the study.

Medical records, clinical follow-up charts, and laboratory results of 71 patients with definite calcifications were available for review in the hospital database system. All medical data and results of these patients were carefully analyzed and recorded. Only two patients were found to have pre-existing and definitively diagnosed type 1 diabetes mellitus, which is known to contribute to early atherosclerosis. Two patients had a history of stage-I germinal matrix and intraventricular hemorrhage according to the Volpe classification in the neonatal period without any other known cause. However, there was no evidence of necrotic damage to the cerebral white matter or brain regions, such as the pons or hippocampus, or cerebral infarction in either patient. An analysis of the clinical findings and laboratory results of 71 patients with definite calcifications in the ICA and vertebral arteries found no evidence of diseases that may predispose to arterial calcifications, such as hypercholesterolemia, chronic kidney disease, and diabetes mellitus. Incident carotid and vertebral artery calcification did not correlate with other diseases.

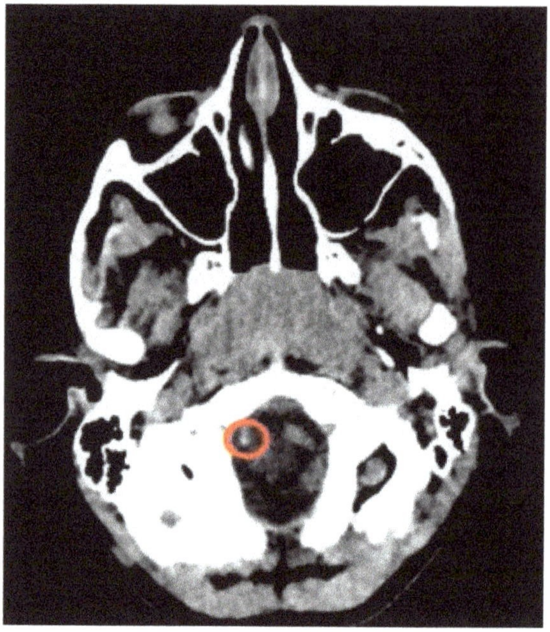

Figure 3. A 5-year-old girl with chronic otitis media; CT imaging of the temporal bone was performed. Hyperdense punctate calcification is shown in the V4 segment of the right vertebral artery (circle).

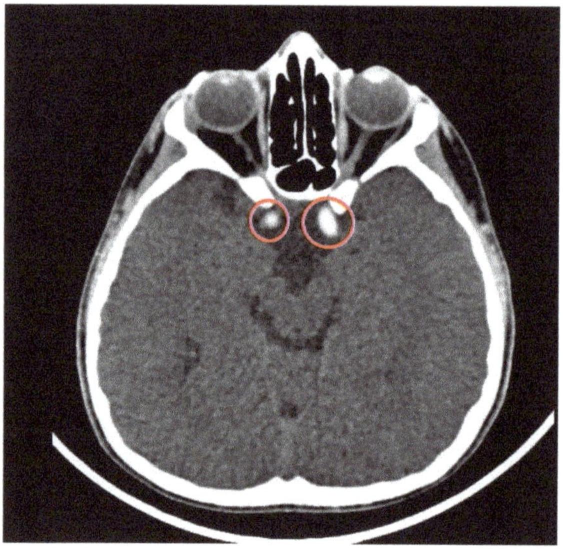

Figure 4. A 7-year-old boy patient had head trauma. Cranial CT shows hyperdense focal punctate calcifications in the supraclinoid segments of bilateral ICAs (circles).

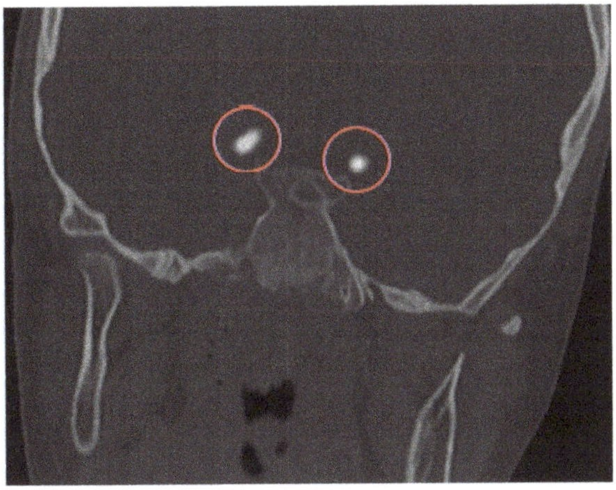

Figure 5. A 9-year-old male patient complained of severe headache and nausea and vomiting. Cranial CT imaging was performed. Hyperdense punctate calcification is shown in the V4 segment of the bilateral vertebral artery (circles).

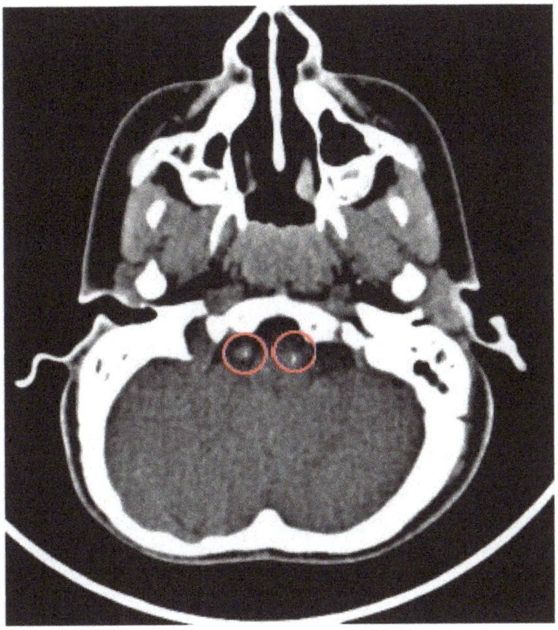

Figure 6. A 6-year-old male patient complained of headache and vomiting. Cranial CT imaging was performed. Hyperdense punctate calcifications are shown in the V4 segment of the bilateral vertebral artery (circles).

4. Discussion

In retrospective analyses performed to measure the frequency of identifiable calcifications in the carotid artery and vertebral artery walls of pediatric patients who underwent cranial CT and temporal bone CT imaging, it was noted that there was a significant increase of approximately 65% after the age of seven [14]. In a large series of adult patients, Ptak et al. concluded that there was a significant correlation between diabetes mellitus, hypercholesterolemia, and hypertension and the occurrence of carotid artery calcifications [25].

In a study of a patient population over 70 years of age, Katada et al. reported the incidence of incidental carotid and vertebral artery calcifications on cranial CT scans to be 15% [26]. This study also showed a significant association between vertebral artery calcification and aging. Vertebral artery calcification was not found in patients under 40 years of age. It has been reported that vertebral artery calcification started to be seen in patients over 50 years of age, and then the incidence increased with age [26].

B. Koch et al. hypothesized that well-defined foci of hyperdensity in the arterial wall in the ICA supraclinoid segment and the carotid siphon regions represent calcifications, and we accepted these imaging findings as suspicious foci of calcification in our pediatric age group series. And, we concluded that marked hyperdensities in the walls of the carotid arteries were likely to represent calcifications [14].

B. Koch et al. reported that definite calcifications were found in 25% and suspicious calcifications in 27.6% of the ICA structures of 663 patients in the pediatric age group [14]. It has been reported that the incidence of carotid calcifications increases with age in the pediatric age group. And, it has been reported that calcifications are more often localized, especially in the distal segment of the carotid siphon. This is because in the early stages of life, there is not much connective tissue around the carotid siphon, but, by the age of 5 years, this segment of the ICA becomes more rigid due to the increase in connective tissue surrounding the vascular structure, and the arterial vascular structure becomes more adherent to the bone cavity. For incidental vertebral artery calcifications, there is no study in the literature for specific pediatric age groups. Our research study is a first for vertebral arteries in this respect. The prevalence of vertebral artery calcifications in the adult period has been evaluated together with the basilar artery, and it has been reported in a wide range from 2% to 13% in various study series.

EM Peters et al. reported in a study that it is not always possible to exclude the presence of iron deposition in histopathological examinations of different intracranial arterial beds and calcification foci. They suggested the presence of calcifications in hemochromatosis and thalassemia as an example [27]. However, iron deposition usually exceeds 130 Hounsfield units density and can be clearly distinguished from calcifications on CT. We believe that the pathophysiology of calcifications in different vascular beds of the ICA and vertebral artery segments, where calcifications are common, should be the subject of a separate investigation.

John H. Livingston et al. report that intracranial calcifications are a common finding on neuroimaging in pediatric neurology practice and that calcifications occur in damaged, neoplastic, or malformed cerebral structures in approximately half of all cases. However, they do not propose a common physiopathological mechanism for pediatric vascular calcifications. They have not presented a systematic approach for the identification of characteristic vascular bed calcification patterns and their radiologic findings, especially in congenital infections and some genetic diseases. According to their research, congenital CMV infection accounts for a significant percentage of all cases. However, radiological and clinical aspects should be thoroughly assessed before concluding that cerebral calcifications are due to congenital infection, as several genetic diseases can mimic congenital infection, they noted. A methodical approach to identifying radiographic abnormalities allows for a diagnosis to be made in many cases, and characteristic patterns of calcification are observed in many cases. In the same study, John H. Livingston et al. said that some hereditary diseases, the origin of which has not yet been identified, are thought to be associated with cerebral calcification [19].

In our opinion, the main differences between physiological and pathological cases in pediatric ICA and vertebral artery calcifications should be investigated in large series in terms of physiopathological and radiological patterns. We also think that further investigations of the anatomical location and pattern correlations of histologically intracranial vascular bed calcification features in different neuroimaging modalities is an important issue. A comprehensive multidisciplinary approach is required to plan studies that emphasize the importance of whether there are interval changes in vascular calcifications with advancing age and in which cases they show progression.

The "Clinical Practice Guidelines on the Management of Atherosclerotic Carotid and Vertebral Artery Disease" established by the European Society for Vascular Surgery (ESVS) in 2023 aimed primarily to reduce the clinical impact of ICA and vertebral stenoses to prevent transient ischemic attack (TIA) or ischemic stroke [28]. However, there are no studies investigating the presence of plaque structures with calcifications that may lead to carotid and vertebral artery stenosis and their clinical effects in pediatric age groups. The most important factor in this regard is considered to be the infrequency of transient ischemic attacks in pediatric age groups.

Bergevin et al. stated that non-severe calcification may be due to vascular maturation and aging [20]. According to some studies, carotid artery calcification is a well-known sign of atherosclerosis and associated with significant morbidity and mortality. Intimal and medial calcification are the two categories of carotid calcification. It is now known that vascular calcification is an active, enzymatically controlled process involving endothelial dysfunction and early-stage dystrophic calcification. A pathogenic inflammatory response is triggered, leading to the deposition of calcium phosphate in the form of microcalcifications. This, in turn, leads to plaque formation and, ultimately, destabilization with the problems that follow. As the inflammation subsides, macrocalcifications and hydroxyapatite crystal formation take over, keeping the plaque stable. Early detection of carotid artery calcification through imaging has been found to be crucial [21–23]

In our study, the lack of association between incidental calcifications detected on CT imaging and risk factors for atherosclerotic disease in children under 15 years of age suggests that these incidental calcifications may be within physiological limits. We examined our study population for diseases associated with intracranial calcifications but found no association with these diseases. Therefore, it was suggested that the incidental calcifications in our study were not indicative of pathology and may develop under physiological conditions, such as arterial pressure differences or vascular maturation. We believe that the significance of incidental carotid artery wall calcifications in children can be analyzed in prospective studies of pediatric patients.

The main limitations of our study are that it was a single-center retrospective study and that the number of patients was limited. The number of patients under the age of 2 years in the database should be increased. In addition, because arterial vessel diameters show significant differences between age groups, we could not perform standardized measurements in this regard in our study, and we consider this to be one of the limitations of our study. In addition, the effect of epidemiological factors, such as ethnicity, on the occurrence of carotid and vertebral artery calcification was not evaluated in this study. Future studies in larger pediatric populations may provide additional information on epidemiological factors.

In addition, efforts are underway to integrate artificial intelligence into CT imaging and to achieve more advanced CT technologies over time. As a result of these studies, incidental carotid artery and vertebral artery calcifications will be easily detected in much larger patient groups with artificial intelligence. This will allow data to be collected in larger populations with lower error rates. We are excited about the new imaging techniques and trends that are constantly evolving in radiology [29].

5. Conclusions

Incidental calcifications in the ICA and the vertebral arteries are a common finding in cranial CT and temporal bone CT examinations in the pediatric age group, but they have not been associated with any disease or pathological manifestations. It is thought that these calcifications are not attributable to underlying conditions that may lead to early atherosclerotic calcification but are most likely a physiological response to turbulent flow in the natural anatomical curves of the arterial vascular structures.

As a result of this study, we suggest that calcifications in the supraclinoid segment and siphon of the ICA and calcification foci in the vertebral arteries may begin to develop at an early age, and the degree of ICA calcification may evolve with age from only a few focal punctate or fine linear patterns to large calcific plaques.

In conclusion, this study statistically analyzes the incidence, anatomical location, patterns, and possible etiological factors of incidental carotid and vertebral artery calcifications in pediatric age groups and provides concrete data to consider. These results may help to revive interest in incidental vascular calcifications in pediatric age groups.

Author Contributions: Conceptualization, T.C. and B.I.; methodology, S.A.; software, B.I.; validation, G.C., F.M., and B.U.; formal analysis, G.C.; investigation, B.U.; resources, B.I.; data curation, B.I.; writing—original draft preparation, T.C.; writing—review and editing, T.C.; visualization, S.A.; supervision, F.M.; project administration, T.C.; funding acquisition, B.I. All authors have read and agreed to the published version of the manuscript.

Funding: The APC was funded by the authors.

Institutional Review Board Statement: The study was conducted in accordance with the Declaration of Helsinki and approved by the Ethics Committee of Erzincan Binali Yildirim University. Date: 12 December 2023; number: 2023.12/003-128.6.

Informed Consent Statement: Informed consent was obtained from all subjects involved in the study.

Data Availability Statement: The data that support the findings of this study are available from the corresponding author (BI) upon reasonable request.

Conflicts of Interest: The authors declare no conflicts of interest.

References

1. Bartstra, J.W.; van den Beukel, T.C.; Van Hecke, W.; Mali, W.P.T.M.; Spiering, W.; Koek, H.L.; Hendrikse, J.; de Jong, P.A.; den Harder, A.M. Intracranial Arterial Calcification: Prevalence, Risk Factors, and Consequences: JACC Review Topic of the Week. *J. Am. Coll. Cardiol.* **2020**, *76*, 1595–1604. [CrossRef] [PubMed]
2. Olatunji, R.B.; Adekanmi, A.J.; Ogunseyinde, A.O. Intracranial Arterial Calcification in Black Africans with Acute Ischaemic Stroke. *Cerebrovasc. Dis. Extra* **2018**, *8*, 26–38. [CrossRef]
3. Bos, D.; Portegies, M.L.; van der Lugt, A.; Bos, M.J.; Koudstaal, P.J.; Hofman, A.; Krestin, G.P.; Franco, O.H.; Vernooij, M.W.; Ikram, M.A. Intracranial carotid artery atherosclerosis and the risk of stroke in whites: The Rotterdam Study. *JAMA Neurol.* **2014**, *71*, 405–411. [CrossRef]
4. Kamphuis, M.J.; van der Kamp, L.T.; Lette, E.; Rinkel, G.J.E.; Vergouwen, M.D.I.; van der Schaaf, I.C.; de Jong, P.A.; Ruigrok, Y.M. Intracranial arterial calcification in patients with unruptured and ruptured intracranial aneurysms. *Eur. Radiol.* **2024**, *34*, 7517–7525. [CrossRef] [PubMed]
5. Lee, J.G.; Lee, K.B.; Roh, H.; Ahn, M.Y.; Bae, H.J.; Lee, J.S.; Woo, H.Y.; Hwang, H.W. Intracranial arterial calcification can predict early vascular events after acute ischemic stroke. *J. Stroke Cerebrovasc. Dis. Off. J. Natl. Stroke Assoc.* **2014**, *23*, e331–e337. [CrossRef] [PubMed]
6. Cereda, A.; Franchina, A.G.; Tua, L.; Rocchetti, M.; Garattini, D.; D'Elia, E.; Lucreziotti, S. Coronary artery calcification as an incremental predictive risk: Research perspectives in primary prevention. *J. Cardiol.* 2025, *advance online publication.* [CrossRef]
7. Hussein, H.M.; Zacharatos, H.; Cordina, S.; Lakshminarayan, K.; Ezzeddine, M.A. Intracranial vascular calcification is protective from vasospasm after aneurysmal subarachnoid hemorrhage. *J. Stroke Cerebrovasc. Dis. Off. J. Natl. Stroke Assoc.* **2014**, *23*, 2687–2693. [CrossRef]

8. Park, K.Y.; Chung, P.W.; Kim, Y.B.; Moon, H.S.; Suh, B.C.; Yoon, W.T. Increased pulsatility index is associated with intracranial arterial calcification. *Eur. Neurol.* **2013**, *69*, 83–88. [CrossRef]
9. Del Brutto, O.H.; Mera, R.M.; Atahualpa Project Investigators. The Role of Brachial Pulse Pressure as an Indicator of Intracranial Atherosclerosis: The Atahualpa Project. *High Blood Press. Cardiovasc. Prev. Off. J. Ital. Soc. Hypertens.* **2017**, *24*, 419–424. [CrossRef]
10. Gotovac, N.; Išgum, I.; Viergever, M.A.; Biessels, G.J.; Fajdić, J.; Velthuis, B.K.; Prokop, M. Calcium at the carotid siphon as an indicator of internal carotid artery stenosis. *Eur. Radiol.* **2013**, *23*, 1478–1486. [CrossRef]
11. Baradaran, H.; Patel, P.; Gialdini, G.; Giambrone, A.; Lerario, M.P.; Navi, B.B.; Min, J.K.; Iadecola, C.; Kamel, H.; Gupta, A. Association between Intracranial Atherosclerotic Calcium Burden and Angiographic Luminal Stenosis Measurements. *AJNR. Am. J. Neuroradiol.* **2017**, *38*, 1723–1729. [CrossRef]
12. Vos, A.; Kockelkoren, R.; de Vis, J.B.; van der Schouw, Y.T.; van der Schaaf, I.C.; Velthuis, B.K.; Mali, W.P.T.M.; de Jong, P.A.; DUST study group. Risk factors for atherosclerotic and medial arterial calcification of the intracranial internal carotid artery. *Atherosclerosis* **2018**, *276*, 44–49. [CrossRef] [PubMed]
13. Sanders-Taylor, C.; Kurbanov, A.; Cebula, H.; Leach, J.L.; Zuccarello, M.; Keller, J.T. The carotid siphon: A historic radiographic sign, not an anatomic classification. *World Neurosurg.* **2014**, *82*, 423–427. [CrossRef] [PubMed]
14. Koch, B.; Blackham, A.; Jones, B. Incidental internal carotid artery calcifications on temporal bone CT in children. *Pediatr. Radiol.* **2007**, *37*, 141–144. [CrossRef]
15. Kobylinski, S. Häufigkeit und Lokalisation der Arterienverkalkungen im Kindesalter [Frequency and localisation of arterial calcifications during childhood (author's transl)]. *Zentralblatt Allg. Pathol. u. Pathol. Anat.* **1974**, *118*, 196–202.
16. Meyer, W.W.; Lind, J. Calcifications of the carotid siphon—A common finding in infancy and childhood. *Arch. Dis. Child.* **1972**, *47*, 355–363. [CrossRef]
17. Wu, X.H.; Chen, X.Y.; Wang, L.J.; Wong, K.S. Intracranial Artery Calcification and Its Clinical Significance. *J. Clin. Neurol.* **2016**, *12*, 253–261. [CrossRef]
18. Mak, H.K.; Wong, C.W.; Yau, K.K.; Wong, W.M.; Gu, J.; Khong, P.L.; Chan, B.P. Computed tomography evaluation of intracranial atherosclerosis in Chinese patients with transient ischemic attack or minor ischemic stroke—Its distribution and association with vascular risk factors. *J. Stroke Cerebrovasc. Dis. Off. J. Natl. Stroke Assoc.* **2009**, *18*, 158–163. [CrossRef]
19. Livingston, J.H.; Stivaros, S.; Warren, D.; Crow, Y.J. Intracranial calcification in childhood: A review of aetiologies and recognizable phenotypes. *Dev. Med. Child Neurol.* **2014**, *56*, 612–626. [CrossRef]
20. Bergevin, M.A.; Daugherty, C.C.; Bove, K.E.; McAdams, A.J. The internal carotid artery siphon in children and adolescents. *Hum. Pathol.* **1991**, *22*, 603–606. [CrossRef]
21. Ahmed, M.; McPherson, R.; Abruzzo, A.; Thomas, S.E.; Gorantla, V.R. Carotid Artery Calcification: What We Know So Far. *Cureus* **2021**, *13*, e18938. [CrossRef]
22. Agacayak, K.S.; Guler, R.; Sezgin Karatas, P. Relation Between the Incidence of Carotid Artery Calcification and Systemic Diseases. *Clin. Interv. Aging* **2020**, *15*, 821–826. [CrossRef] [PubMed]
23. Shi, X.; Gao, J.; Lv, Q.; Cai, H.; Wang, F.; Ye, R.; Liu, X. Calcification in Atherosclerotic Plaque Vulnerability: Friend or Foe? *Front. Physiol.* **2020**, *11*, 56. [CrossRef] [PubMed]
24. Gonçalves, F.G.; Caschera, L.; Teixeira, S.R.; Viaene, A.N.; Pinelli, L.; Mankad, K.; Alves, C.A.P.F.; Ortiz-Gonzalez, X.R.; Andronikou, S.; Vossough, A. Intracranial calcifications in childhood: Part 2. *Pediatr. Radiol.* **2020**, *50*, 1448–1475. [CrossRef]
25. Ptak, T.; Hunter, G.H.; Avakian, R.; Novelline, R.A. Clinical significance of cavernous carotid calcifications encountered on head computed tomography scans performed on patients seen in the emergency department. *J. Comput. Assist. Tomogr.* **2003**, *27*, 505–509. [CrossRef] [PubMed]
26. Katada, K.; Kanno, T.; Sano, H.; Shinomiya, Y.; Koga, S. Calcification of the vertebral artery. *Am. J. Neuroradiol.* **1983**, *4*, 450–453. [CrossRef]
27. Peters, M.E.M.; de Brouwer, E.J.M.; Bartstra, J.W.; Mali, W.P.T.M.; Koek, H.L.; Rozemuller, A.J.M.; Baas, A.F.; de Jong, P.A. Mechanisms of calcification in Fahr disease and exposure of potential therapeutic targets. *Neurol. Clin. Pract.* **2020**, *10*, 449–457. [CrossRef]
28. Naylor, R.; Rantner, B.; Ancetti, S.; de Borst, G.J.; De Carlo, M.; Halliday, A.; Kakkos, S.K.; Markus, H.S.; McCabe, D.J.H.; Sillesen, H.; et al. Editor's Choice—European Society for Vascular Surgery (ESVS) 2023 Clinical Practice Guidelines on the Management of Atherosclerotic Carotid and Vertebral Artery Disease. *Eur. J. Vasc. Endovasc. Surg. Off. J. Eur. Soc. Vasc. Surg.* **2023**, *65*, 7–111. [CrossRef]
29. Kantarcı, M.; Aydın, S.; Oğul, H.; Kızılgöz, V. New imaging techniques and trends in radiology. *Diagn. Interv. Radiol.* 2025, *advance online publication*. [CrossRef]

diagnostics

MDPI

Article

Procalcitonin, Presepsin, Endocan, and Interleukin-6 in the Early Diagnosis of Neonatal Sepsis—A Prospective Study

Maura-Adelina Hincu [1], Liliana Gheorghe [2,*], Cristina Dimitriu [3], Luminita Paduraru [1], Gabriela Zonda [4], Dan-Constantin Andronic [2], Ingrid-Andrada Vasilache [1], Luiza-Maria Baean [5] and Dragos Nemescu [1]

1 Department of Mother and Child Care, University of Medicine and Pharmacy "Grigore T. Popa", 700115 Iasi, Romania
2 Surgical Department, Faculty of Medicine, University of Medicine and Pharmacy "Grigore T. Popa", 700115 Iasi, Romania
3 Department of Morpho-Functional Sciences II, University of Medicine and Pharmacy "Grigore T. Popa", 700115 Iasi, Romania
4 Department of Neonatology, Centre Hospitalier Public du Cotentin, 50100 Cherbourg-en-Cotentin, France; ildikozonda@yahoo.com
5 Department of Fundamental Disciplines, Faculty of Midwifes and General Asistans, University of Medicine and Pharmacy "Carol Davila", 020021 Bucharest, Romania
* Correspondence: liliana.gheorghe@umfiasi.ro

Abstract: Background/Objectives: Neonatal early-onset sepsis (EOS) is a life-threatening condition, and numerous efforts have been invested in identifying the most promising biomarkers for its detection. In this prospective cohort study, we aimed to determine the diagnostic accuracy and optimal cut-off values of procalcitonin (PCT), presepsin, endocan, and interleukin (IL)-6 determined from the neonatal serum (0–12, 24–48, and 72–96 h), and umbilical blood cord for the diagnosis of EOS. **Methods**: A total of 122 patients were included in this study and were divided into two groups: group 1 (sepsis, n = 68 patients) and group 2 (without sepsis, n = 54 patients). Maternal and neonatal characteristics were assessed using descriptive statistics. Logistic regressions were used to evaluate the association between various biomarkers and the presence of EOS and to adjust for potential confounders. Using sensitivity analysis and Youden's index from the ROC curve, the biomarkers' diagnostic accuracy and optimal cut-off values were obtained. **Results**: PCT at 0–12 and 24–48 h of life exhibited the best diagnostic performance, with sensitivities (Ses) of 75% and 76.5% and specificities (Sps) above 74%. Presepsin demonstrated excellent performance at 24–48 h, with Ses of 68.42%, and Sps of 88.89%. IL-6 and endocan achieved modest results for the detection of EOS. **Conclusions**: PCT and presepsin measured at early neonatal timepoints demonstrated high diagnostic accuracy and favorable sensitivity–specificity balance for predicting EOS.

Keywords: early-onset sepsis; procalcitonin; presepsin; interleukin-6; endocan; diagnostic accuracy; cut-off values

1. Introduction

Neonatal early-onset sepsis (EOS) is characterized by the presence of a pathogenic bacterial species in a blood or cerebrospinal fluid culture collected within the first 72 h of life and continues to impact the neonatal morbidity and mortality rates worldwide [1]. However, various regions of the world have different mortality rates attributed to neonatal infections depending on specific factors related to demographic profile of the population, medical infrastructure, and financial resources [2]. Across the European continent, recent reports have highlighted persistent disparities in infant mortality rates, with significantly higher figures in Eastern Europe compared to Western Europe. For example, in 2023, infant mortality was reported at 3.3 deaths per 1000 live births in Western Europe, while rates in countries such as Romania and Slovakia reached 5.7 per 1000 live births [3]. These differences may reflect variations in access to timely and accurate diagnosis and management of neonatal sepsis.

A positive blood culture serves as the definitive diagnostic method, although the confirmation of its results occurs within a 36–48 h period. Despite the presence of particular signs and symptoms, fewer than 1% of newborns suspected of having sepsis yield a positive blood culture [4]. Although real-time polymerase chain reaction (PCR) assays could establish the diagnosis of neonatal sepsis faster than blood cultures, these are not routinely available [5]. The presence of sepsis biomarkers capable of notifying clinicians for the early detection of neonatal sepsis has the potential to improve both the immediate and future outcomes for actual sepsis patients, while simultaneously minimizing the unnecessary and detrimental use of preventative antibiotics [6].

Both C-reactive protein (CRP) and procalcitonin (PCT) are traditionally used serum markers for the diagnosis of neonatal sepsis. Other studied biomarkers include interleukin 6 (IL-6), presepsin, and endocan, all of which have exhibited significant variability in terms of diagnostic accuracy of the disease. For example, a recent systematic review and meta-analysis that evaluated the diagnostic accuracy of biomarkers determined maternal serum, umbilical cord blood, and neonatal serum for EOS and reported a pooled sensitivity (Se) of 79%, and a pooled specificity (Sp) of 91% for PCT, as well as a pooled Se of 83%, and a pooled Sp of 87% for IL-6, both determined from the umbilical cord blood [7]. Moreover, the authors reported a pooled Se of 82%, and an Sp of 86%, for presepsin determined from the neonatal serum. However, the diagnostic accuracy of combined biomarkers for the diagnosis of EOS is poorly studied, especially in various demographic regions where racial and ethnic disparities could influence their performance [8].

The primary aim of this prospective cohort study was to determine the diagnostic accuracy of PCT, presepsin, endocan, and IL-6 determined from the neonatal serum (0–12 h, 24–48 h, and 72–96 h) and umbilical blood cord for the diagnosis of EOS. The secondary aim of this study was to assess the diagnostic accuracy of the individual biomarkers for EOS using optimal cut-off values.

2. Materials and Methods

This prospective cohort study included patients diagnosed with or without a diagnosis of EOS who were born at "Cuza voda" Clinical Hospital of Obstetrics and Gynecology, Iasi, Romania, between 2019 and 2024. Inclusion criteria comprised the following: singleton neonates admitted to the neonatal intensive care unit (NICU) with or without suspected EOS diagnosis that was later confirmed according to the criteria proposed by the European Medicines Agency (EMA) [9], with a gestational age of 28 weeks or higher, for whom the serum samples could be collected at 0–12 h, 24–48 h, and 72–96 h post-birth, with available umbilical cord blood and/or maternal serum samples collected at birth and for whom informed consent was obtained from participants. For all participants in this study, the samples were processed if the EOS diagnosis was confirmed by positive hemocultures.

The exclusion criteria comprised severe congenital malformations or genetic syndromes, major perinatal complications unrelated to infection (i.e., hypoxic-ischemic encephalopathy-HIE, severe intraventricular hemorrhage-IVH), inadequate or missing serum sample volumes for biomarker analysis, mothers with known immunological, autoimmune diseases or chronic infections, and lack of informed consent.

Ethical approval for conducting this study was obtained from the Institutional Ethics Committees of the "Grigore T. Popa" University of Medicine and Pharmacy, Iasi (No. 175/17.04.2022) and "Cuza voda" Clinical Hospital of Obstetrics and Gynecology (No. 5750/09.05.2022 and No. 1405/02.02.2023).

The following data were recorded from the medical records: maternal and perinatal data (inadequate prenatal care, antepartum hemorrhage, antepartum antibiotics, corticosteroid therapy, maternal white blood cell count, CRP, fibrinogen, endocan levels, comorbidities such as gestational diabetes, pre-eclampsia, thrombophilia, etc.), delivery and perinatal factors (meconial amniotic fluid, duration of ruptured membranes, clinical or histological chorioamnionitis, amniotic fluid culture, vaginal secretion cultures, urine culture, lochia culture), birth and neonatal characteristics (sex, type of delivery, gestational age at birth, birth weight, intrauterine growth restriction, need for neonatal resuscitation, Apgar scores at 1 and 5 min, respiratory distress syndrome, and blood cultures), neonatal manifestations (fever, tachycardia, hypotension, inotropic support, renal impairment, metabolic acidosis, thrombocytopenia, hypoglycemia or hyperglycemia, persistent pulmonary hypertension), and neonatal complications (pneumothorax, pulmonary hemorrhage, feeding intolerance, intraventricular hemorrhage, retinopathy of prematurity).

Apart from these data, we determined a series of biochemical markers: white blood cell-WBC count (0–12 h, 24–48 h, and 72–96 h), fibrinogen (0–12 h, 24–48 h, and 72–96 h), CRP levels from cord blood, serum CRP values (0–12 h, 24–48 h, and 72–96 h), PCT levels from cord blood, serum PCT values (0–12 h, 24–48 h, and 72–96 h), IL-6 levels from cord blood and from serum of the neonates (0–12 h, 24–48 h, and 72–96 h), presepsin levels from the cord blood and from serum of the neonates (0–12 h, 24–48 h, and 72–96 h), as well as endocan levels from the cord blood and from the neonatal serum (0–12 h, 24–48 h, and 72–96 h).

The blood samples from mothers and newborns were stored in duplicates at −20 °C until processing. The PCT levels were determined using sandwich ELISA (Human PCT ELISA Kit, Elabscience, Houston, TX, USA) and reported as pg/mL. IL-6 determination from serum was performed according to the manufacturer's indications using sandwich ELISA (Human IL-6 ELISA Kit, Elabscience, USA) and the serum levels were expressed as pg/mL. The same method was used to determine the serum levels of endocan (MyBioSource Human Endocan ELISA kit, San Diego, CA, USA), which were expressed as pg/mL, as well as presepsin serum levels (MyBioSource Human Presepsin ELISA Kit, San Diego, CA, USA).

We performed a sample size calculation that would be able to detect a 20% difference in the mean values of the evaluated biomarkers between the septic and non-septic groups, considering a two-tailed alpha value of 0.05 and a power of 80%. The estimated sample size was 17 patients per group, totaling 34 participants. A total of 122 patients were included in this study and for statistical purposes were divided into two groups: group 1 (sepsis, n = 68 patients) and group 2 (without sepsis, n = 54 patients).

Descriptive statistics were used to assess both maternal and neonatal characteristics. Specifically, the Student's *t*-test was used to compare continuous variables with a normal distribution between groups, while the Wilcoxon rank-sum test was used to compare non-normally distributed continuous variables. On the other hand, categorical variables were compared between groups using chi-square test.

In the second stage of the analysis, we conducted multivariable logistic regression in order to evaluate the association between various biomarkers and the presence of EOS. We first performed univariable logistic regression analyses to estimate the crude association between each biomarker and EOS. Subsequently, multivariable logistic regression models were constructed to adjust for potential confounders, including gestational age at birth, duration of membrane rupture, and previous maternal antibiotic exposure. These covariates were selected based on their known or potential influence on neonatal sepsis risk and biomarker expression.

Adjusted odds ratios (aORs) and 95% confidence intervals (CIs) were reported to quantify the effect size of each biomarker on the odds of EOS. Confounding was assessed by comparing the crude and adjusted estimates; a change of $\geq$10% in the biomarker coefficient was considered indicative of confounding.

To evaluate the diagnostic accuracy of individual biomarkers in diagnosing EOS, we calculated standard performance metrics, including sensitivity (Se), specificity (Sp), positive predictive value (PPV), negative predictive value (NPV), accuracy, and the area under the receiver operating characteristic curve (AUC).

For each biomarker, optimal cut-off values were determined using Youden's index derived from the ROC curve. All analyses were conducted using Stata version 18.5 (StataCorp, College Station, TX, USA), and a two-tailed p-value < 0.05 was considered statistically significant.

3. Results

Mothers whose newborns developed sepsis presented with significantly higher rates of pre-eclampsia (8.82% versus 0%, p = 0.025) and thrombophilia (11.76% versus 0%, p = 0.009) than mothers whose newborns did not develop sepsis (Table 1). Also, these patients had significantly higher rates of positive vaginal cultures (20.59% versus 7.41%, p = 0.016). On the other hand, mothers whose newborns did not develop sepsis presented significantly higher rates of prolonged rupture of membranes (74.07% versus 38.24%, p < 0.001) in comparison with their counterparts. Also, this category of patients benefited significantly more frequently from antepartum antibiotic therapy (62.96% versus 35.29%, p = 0.002) and corticosteroid therapy (37.04% versus 14.71%, p = 0.004).

Table 1. Maternal clinical characteristics.

Variable	Sepsis (Group 1, 68 Patients)	No Sepsis (Group 2, 54 Patients)	p-Value
Inadequate prenatal care (%)	29.41	14.81	0.057
Antepartum hemorrhage (%)	2.94	3.70	0.814
Antepartum antibiotics (%)	35.29	62.96	0.002
Corticosteroid therapy (%)	14.71	37.04	0.004
Gestational diabetes (%)	5.88	3.70	0.580
Preeclampsia (%)	8.82	0.00	0.025
Thrombophilia (%)	11.76	0.00	0.009
Rupture of membranes > 18 h (%)	38.24	74.07	<0.001
Amniotic fluid culture (positive) (%)	44.12	25.93	0.235
Vaginal secretions culture (positive) (%)	20.59	7.41	0.016

Table 2 comprises a comparison of maternal biomarkers between the two groups, and our results indicated that only mean CRP values (15.94 $\pm$ 18.49 versus 8.22 $\pm$ 10.18 mg/L, p = 0.007) at admission and endocan levels (1279.15 $\pm$ 407.06 versus 970.01 $\pm$ 726.69 pg/mL, p = 0.007) were significantly higher for mothers whose newborns developed sepsis in comparison with the CRP values in the control group.

Neonates with a septic state experienced significantly higher rates of fever (8.82% versus 0%, p = 0.025), tachycardia (11.76% versus 0%, p = 0.009), hypotension (23.53% versus 3.70%, p = 0.002), and needed significantly more inotropic support (23.53% versus 3.70%, p = 0.020) in comparison with neonates without this condition (Table 3). Duration of parenteral feeding (8.59 $\pm$ 5.89 versus 6.00 $\pm$ 5.70 days,

$p = 0.0159$) and antibiotic treatment (7.44 ± 3.79 versus 4.81 ± 2.56, $p < 0.001$) were significantly higher for septic neonates in comparison with controls.

Table 2. Comparison of maternal biomarkers.

Variable	Sepsis (n = 68) Mean ± SD	No Sepsis (n = 54) Mean ± SD	Mean Difference (0–1)	*p*-Value
WBC ($\times 10^9$/L)	12.13 ± 4.65	12.35 ± 4.78	0.22	0.797
CRP (mg/L)	15.94 ± 18.49	8.22 ± 10.18	−7.72	0.007
Fibrinogen (mg/dL)	392.03 ± 147.41	380.81 ± 45.54	−11.21	0.591
Endocan (pg/mL)	1279.15 ± 407.06	970.01 ± 726.69	−309.14	0.04

Table legend: WBC—white blood cells; CRP—C-reactive protein; SD—standard deviation;

Table 3. Neonatal clinical characteristics and complications.

Variable	Sepsis (n = 68 Patients)	No Sepsis (n = 54 Patients)	*p*-Value
Sex (female) (%)	47.06	33.33	0.126
Type of delivery (cesarean) (%)	64.71	62.96	0.842
Gestational age at birth (weeks)	32.53 ± 4.60	32.04 ± 4.01	0.5358
Birthweight (g)	2001.47 ± 974.61	1907.04 ± 786.93	0.5645
Apgar score at 1 min	5.91 ± 2.37	5.81 ± 2.11	0.8144
Apgar score at 5 min	7.06 ± 1.66	6.81 ± 1.69	0.4252
SGA (%)	29.41	22.22	0.06
Fever (%)	8.82	0.00	0.025
Tachycardia (%)	11.76	0.00	0.009
Hypotension (%)	23.53	3.70	0.002
Inotropic support ≥ 1 day (%)	23.53	3.70	0.020
Renal impairment (%)	3.70	0.00	0.110
Metabolic acidosis (%)	26.47	3.70	0.001
Thrombocytopenia (%)	23.53	3.70	0.002
Hypoglycemia (%)	38.24	37.04	0.892
Hyperglycemia (%)	11.76	7.41	0.422
Persistent pulm. hypertension (%)	8.82	0.00	0.025
Blood culture positive (%)	17.65	0.00	0.032
Positive tracheal aspirate	61.76	0.00	0.001
Pneumothorax (%)	20.59	3.70	0.006
Pulmonary hemorrhage (%)	14.71	3.70	0.043
Feeding intolerance (%)	20.59	7.41	0.041
Intraventricular hemorrhage (%)	11.76	7.41	0.422
Retinopathy of prematurity (%)	11.76	11.11	0.124
Days of hospitalization	30.32 ± 26.59	36.93 ± 27.67	0.1834
Days of parenteral feeding	8.59 ± 5.89	6.00 ± 5.70	0.0159
Days of antibiotic therapy	7.44 ± 3.79	4.81 ± 2.56	<0.001
Death (%)	7.35	3.70	0.40

Legend: SGA—small for gestational age.

Also, as expected, this category of patients presented significantly higher rates of metabolic acidosis (26.47% versus 3.70%, $p = 0.001$), pneumothorax (23.53% versus 3.70%, $p = 0.002$), pulmonary hemorrhage (14.71% versus 3.70%, $p = 0.043$), and feeding intolerance (20.59% versus 7.41%, $p = 0.041$). No significant differences regarding death rates were encountered between the two groups ($p = 0.40$).

The paraclinical characteristics of the evaluated cohort indicated that neonates with sepsis presented significantly lower values of hemoglobin ($p = 0.003$), hematocrit ($p = 0.003$), and WBC in the first 12 h of life ($p = 0.0001$) compared with the values encountered in neonates without sepsis (Table 4).

Table 4. Neonatal paraclinical characteristics.

Variable	Sepsis (n = 68) Mean ± SD	No Sepsis (n = 54) Mean ± SD	*p*-Value
Hemoglobin (g/dL)	15.01 ± 2.72	16.47 ± 2.56	0.0031
Hematocrit (%)	46.00 ± 8.31	50.36 ± 7.76	0.0037
Platelets ($\times 10^3/\mu$L)	211.47 ± 92.11	260.74 ± 81.04	0.0025
WBC 0–12 h ($\times 10^3/\mu$L)	12.64 ± 7.27	18.69 ± 9.64	0.0001
WBC 24–48 h ($\times 10^3/\mu$L)	14.18 ± 8.10	16.91 ± 9.93	0.0964
WBC 72–96 h ($\times 10^3/\mu$L)	13.71 ± 8.66	13.23 ± 7.08	0.7400
Fibrinogen 24–48 h (mg/dL)	311.62 ± 128.20	198.48 ± 65.88	<0.0001
Fibrinogen 72–96 h (mg/dL)	325.56 ± 129.07	211.37 ± 66.06	<0.0001
I/T ratio 0–12 h	12.68 ± 71.43	0.20 ± 0.14	0.2022
I/T ratio 24–48 h	0.29 ± 0.16	0.19 ± 0.13	0.0001
I/T ratio 72–96 h	0.20 ± 0.10	0.12 ± 0.06	<0.0001
CRP from umbilical cord (mg/L)	10.04 ± 5.67	7.15 ± 4.40	0.0279
CRP 0–12 h (mg/L)	33.39 ± 36.03	9.91 ± 9.25	<0.0001
CRP 24–48 h (mg/L)	35.24 ± 24.28	7.79 ± 6.08	<0.0001
CRP 72–96 h (mg/L)	21.74 ± 27.64	6.56 ± 4.13	<0.0001

Legend: WBC—white blood cells; I/T—immature to totals ratio; CRP—C-reactive protein.

Also, this category of patients presented with significantly higher levels of fibrinogen at 24–48 h ($p < 0.001$), and at 72–96 h ($p < 0.001$), I/T ratios at 24–48 h ($p = 0.0001$) and 72–96 h ($p < 0.001$), and CRP serum levels determined from umbilical cord ($p = 0.02$), 0–12 h ($p < 0.001$), 24–48 h ($p < 0.001$), and 72–96 h ($p < 0.001$).

A comparison between the levels of biomarkers is presented in Table 5. Our data indicated that presepsin serum levels determined at 72–96 h of life ($p = 0.08$) and endocan levels determined from umbilical cord blood ($p = 0.255$) did not significantly differ between the evaluated groups. On the other hand, values of PCT, IL-6, presepsin, and endocan were significantly higher for neonates with sepsis.

Table 5. Comparisons of biomarkers' values between the evaluated groups.

Variable (Unit)	Sepsis (Mean ± SD)	No Sepsis (Mean ± SD)	*p*-Value
PCT (ng/mL)—umbilical cord	3.95 ± 10.24	0.47 ± 1.15	0.0151
PCT (ng/mL)—0–12 h	21.65 ± 23.77	3.63 ± 6.86	<0.001
PCT (ng/mL)—24–48 h	27.07 ± 23.93	7.69 ± 9.09	<0.001
PCT (ng/mL)—72–96 h	5.18 ± 8.45	1.72 ± 1.82	0.0037
IL-6 (pg/mL)—umbilical cord	529.01 ± 875.04	120.87 ± 135.08	0.0013
IL-6 (pg/mL)—0–12 h	939.83 ± 1570.05	138.81 ± 161.44	<0.001
IL-6 (pg/mL)—24–48 h	878.11 ± 2418.42	178.46 ± 281.67	0.0381
IL-6 (pg/mL)—72–96 h	907.60 ± 2455.13	118.59 ± 162.62	0.0200
Presepsin (ng/mL)—umbilical cord	12.39 ± 7.37	7.05 ± 5.90	0.0012
Presepsin (ng/mL)—0–12 h	24.65 ± 17.56	9.44 ± 7.36	<0.001
Presepsin (ng/mL)—24–48 h	41.50 ± 20.79	14.27 ± 13.46	<0.001
Presepsin (ng/mL)—72–96 h	19.52 ± 13.24	13.99 ± 11.19	0.087
Endocan (pg/mL)—umbilical cord	2406.79 ± 836.05	2714.40 ± 1137.98	0.255
Endocan (pg/mL)—0–12 h	3454.43 ± 1406.68	2606.93 ± 1149.44	0.0058
Endocan (pg/mL)—24–48 h	3619.92 ± 1055.10	2865.90 ± 1301.20	0.0108
Endocan (pg/mL)—72–96 h	3415.90 ± 914.09	2796.41 ± 1378.45	0.048

Legend: PCT—procalcitonin; IL-6—interleukin-6; SD—standard deviation.

In Table 6, we present the results from the univariate and multivariable logistic regression to evaluate the effect of predictors and covariates on the EOS occurrence. The results from univariate logistic regressions indicated that serum values of PCT at 0–12 h ($p < 0.001$), 24–48 h ($p < 0.001$), and 72–96 h ($p = 0.017$), IL-6 determined from umbilical cord ($p = 0.032$)

and serum at 0–12 h ($p = 0.001$), presepsin determined from umbilical cord ($p = 0.003$) and from serum at 0–12 h ($p < 0.001$) and 24–48 h ($p < 0.001$), as well as serum endocan levels at 0–12 h ($p = 0.007$) and at 24–48 h ($p = 0.011$) were significant predictors for EOS.

Table 6. Results from univariate and multivariable logistic regression to evaluate the effect of predictors and covariates on the EOS occurrence.

Variable	Covariate	Odds Ratio	Std. Error	*p*-Value	95% CI
PCT—umbilical cord	-	1.1497	0.1193	0.179	0.938–1.409
PCT—umbilical cord	Gestational age	1.109	0.0897	0.201	0.946–1.300
PCT—umbilical cord	ROM duration	1.1348	0.0975	0.141	0.959–1.343
PCT—umbilical cord	AB therapy duration	1.1514	0.1501	0.279	0.892–1.487
PCT—0–12 h	-	1.1373	0.0287	<0.001	1.082–1.195
PCT—0–12 h	Gestational age	1.1394	0.0291	<0.001	1.084–1.198
PCT—0–12 h	ROM duration	1.1447	0.0306	<0.001	1.086–1.206
PCT—0–12 h	AB therapy duration	1.13	0.0291	<0.001	1.074–1.188
PCT—24–48 h	-	1.112	0.0244	<0.001	1.065–1.161
PCT—24–48 h	Gestational age	1.1148	0.025	<0.001	1.067–1.165
PCT—24–48 h	ROM duration	1.1342	0.0285	<0.001	1.080–1.191
PCT—24–48 h	AB therapy duration	1.1355	0.0293	<0.001	1.079–1.195
PCT—72–96 h	-	1.171	0.0775	0.017	1.029–1.333
PCT—72–96 h	Gestational age	1.2178	0.0947	0.011	1.046–1.418
PCT—72–96 h	ROM duration	1.1911	0.0868	0.016	1.033–1.374
PCT—72–96 h	AB therapy duration	1.2218	0.0905	0.007	1.057–1.413
IL-6—umbilical cord	-	1.003	0.0014	0.032	1.000–1.006
IL-6—umbilical cord	Gestational age	1.0025	0.0013	0.06	0.999–1.005
IL-6—umbilical cord	ROM duration	1.0033	0.0015	0.023	1.000–1.006
IL-6—umbilical cord	AB therapy duration	1.0036	0.0017	0.031	1.000–1.007
IL-6—0–12 h	-	1.0044	0.0013	0.001	1.002–1.007
IL-6—0–12 h	Gestational age	1.0047	0.0015	0.001	1.002–1.008
IL-6—0–12 h	ROM duration	1.0047	0.0014	0.001	1.002–1.007
IL-6—0–12 h	AB therapy duration	1.0043	0.0021	0.044	1.000–1.008
IL-6—24–48 h	-	1.0004	0.0003	0.178	0.999–1.001
IL-6—24–48 h	Gestational age	1.0005	0.0004	0.158	0.999–1.001
IL-6—24–48 h	ROM duration	1.0021	0.0015	0.153	0.999–1.005
IL-6—24–48 h	AB therapy duration	1.0005	0.0003	0.156	0.999–1.001
IL-6—72–96 h	-	1.0005	0.0004	0.183	0.999–1.001
IL-6—72–96 h	Gestational age	1.0007	0.0004	0.133	0.999–1.002
IL-6—72–96 h	ROM duration	1.0032	0.0016	0.048	1.000–1.006
IL-6—72–96 h	AB therapy duration	1.0006	0.0004	0.162	0.999–1.001
Presepsin—umbilical cord	-	1.1202	0.0426	0.003	1.040–1.207
Presepsin—umbilical cord	Gestational age	1.1358	0.047	0.002	1.047–1.232

Table 6. *Cont.*

Variable	Covariate	Odds Ratio	Std. Error	*p*-Value	95% CI
Presepsin—umbilical cord	ROM duration	1.1399	0.0463	0.001	1.053–1.234
Presepsin—umbilical cord	AB therapy duration	1.137	0.0477	0.002	1.047–1.234
Presepsin—0–12 h	-	1.0967	0.0265	<0.001	1.046–1.150
Presepsin—0–12 h	Gestational age	1.1018	0.0266	<0.001	1.051–1.155
Presepsin—0–12 h	ROM duration	1.1037	0.0275	<0.001	1.051–1.159
Presepsin—0–12 h	AB therapy duration	1.103	0.0269	<0.001	1.051–1.157
Presepsin—24–48 h	-	1.0784	0.0161	<0.001	1.047–1.111
Presepsin—24–48 h	Gestational age	1.0898	0.0191	<0.001	1.053–1.128
Presepsin—24–48 h	ROM duration	1.086	0.0175	<0.001	1.052–1.121
Presepsin—24–48 h	AB therapy duration	1.0844	0.0177	<0.001	1.050–1.120
Presepsin—72–96 h	-	1.0383	0.0232	0.092	0.994–1.085
Presepsin—72–96 h	Gestational age	1.0316	0.024	0.181	0.986–1.080
Presepsin—72–96 h	ROM duration	1.0474	0.0249	0.052	1.000–1.097
Presepsin—72–96 h	AB therapy duration	1.0102	0.024	0.67	0.964–1.058
Endocan—umbilical cord	-	0.9997	0.0003	0.232	0.9991–1.0002
Endocan—umbilical cord	Gestational age	0.9997	0.0003	0.199	0.9991–1.0002
Endocan—umbilical cord	ROM duration	0.9997	0.0003	0.196	0.9991–1.0003
Endocan—umbilical cord	AB therapy duration	0.9996	0.0003	0.093	0.9991–1.0002
Endocan—0–12 h	-	1.0005	0.0002	0.007	1.0001–1.0009
Endocan—0–12 h	Gestational age	1.0005	0.0002	0.017	1.0001–1.0009
Endocan—0–12 h	ROM duration	1.0005	0.0002	0.011	1.0001–1.0009
Endocan—0–12 h	AB therapy duration	1.0005	0.0002	0.017	1.0001–1.0009
Endocan—24–48 h	-	1.0005	0.0002	0.011	1.0001–1.0009
Endocan—24–48 h	Gestational age	1.0005	0.0002	0.018	1.0001–1.0009
Endocan—24–48 h	ROM duration	1.0005	0.0002	0.032	1.0001–1.0008
Endocan—24–48 h	AB therapy duration	1.0005	0.0002	0.04	1.0001–1.0009
Endocan—72–96 h	-	1.0004	0.0002	0.052	1.0000–1.0008
Endocan—72–96 h	Gestational age	1.0004	0.0002	0.099	1.0000–1.0008
Endocan—72–96 h	ROM duration	1.0004	0.0002	0.101	1.0000–1.0008
Endocan—72–96 h	AB therapy duration	1.0005	0.0002	0.029	1.0000–1.0009

Legend: PCT—procalcitonin; IL-6—interleukin-6; ROM—rupture of membranes; AB—antibiotic therapy; CI—confidence intervals.

For PCT, across all time points, adjusted ORs remained close to unadjusted ORs, changing by less than approximately 7%, which indicates a minimal confounding effect of covariates. Across all the remaining biomarkers, adjustment for gestational age, ROM duration, and antibiotic therapy duration produced only an overall minimal confounding effect (between 0.05 and 6.5%).

In Table 7, we present the results from the testing for significant individual biomarkers for the prediction of EOS. PCT at 0–12 h (Se—75%, Sp—85.19%, and accuracy—79.51%) and 24–48 h (Se—76.47%, Sp—74.07%, and accuracy—75.41%) achieved the best performance metrics in terms of sensitivity, specificity, and accuracy for EOS detection.

Table 7. Performance of significant individual biomarkers for EOS diagnosis.

Biomarker	Timepoint	Sensitivity	Specificity	PPV	NPV	Accuracy
PCT	0–12 h	75.00%	85.19%	86.44%	73.02%	79.51%
PCT	24–48 h	76.47%	74.07%	78.79%	71.43%	75.41%
PCT	72–96 h	52.94%	55.56%	60.00%	48.39%	54.10%
IL-6	Cord	22.22%	100.00%	100.00%	79.41%	80.56%
IL-6	0–12 h	44.44%	96.30%	80.00%	83.87%	83.33%
Presepsin	Cord	30.43%	85.19%	46.67%	74.19%	68.83%
Presepsin	0–12 h	44.00%	92.59%	73.33%	78.12%	77.22%
Presepsin	24–48 h	68.42%	88.89%	81.25%	80.00%	80.43%
Endocan	0–12 h	24.00%	85.19%	42.86%	70.77%	65.82%
Endocan	24–48 h	22.22%	88.89%	50.00%	69.57%	66.67%

Legend: PCT—procalcitonin; IL-6—interleukin-6; PPV—positive predictive value; NPV—negative predictive value.

Even though IL-6 determined from the umbilical cord and from the neonatal serum at 0–12 h achieved better overall accuracy than PCT, it was characterized by low sensitivities (22.22% and 44.44%), and high specificity (100% and 96.3%).

Presepsin determined from the neonatal serum at 24–48 h achieved a moderate performance when used to diagnose EOS, with an Se of 68.42%, Sp of 88.89%, and accuracy of 80.43%. Also, endocan serum levels achieved the poorest performance for the detection of EOS (Se: 22.22–24%, Sp: 85.19–88.89%, and accuracy: 65.82–66.67%).

Finally, in Table 8, we present the calculated cut-offs for individual biomarkers that offer the best balance between sensitivity and specificity for EOS diagnosis. Our results indicated that PCT at 0–12 h (cutoff 7.81: Se—75%, Sp—85%, AUC value—0.80, J—0.60) and 24–48 h (cutoff 15.585: Se—74%, Sp—85%, AUC value—0.79, J—0.59) and presepsin at 24–48 h (cutoff 31.698: Se—68%, Sp—93%, AUC value—0.81, J—0.61) obtained the best values of Youden index.

Table 8. Performance of significant individual biomarkers for EOS occurrence.

Biomarker	Timepoint	Cutoff	Se	Sp	AUC	Youden Index (J)
PCT (ng/mL)	0–12 h	7.81	0.75	0.85	0.80	0.60
PCT (ng/mL)	24–48 h	15.585	0.74	0.85	0.79	0.59
PCT (ng/mL)	72–96 h	3.505	0.38	0.89	0.64	0.27
IL-6 (pg/mL)	Cord	309.928	0.44	0.93	0.69	0.37
IL-6 (pg/mL)	0–12 h	119.684	0.89	0.70	0.80	0.59
Presepsin (ng/mL)	Cord	8.789	0.65	0.77	0.76	0.42
Presepsin (ng/mL)	0–12 h	7.0825	1.00	0.56	0.78	0.56
Presepsin (ng/mL)	24–48 h	31.698	0.68	0.93	0.81	0.61
Endocan (pg/mL)	0–12 h	2795.009	0.76	0.67	0.71	0.43
Endocan (pg/mL)	24–48 h	2789.249	0.85	0.63	0.74	0.48

Legend: PCT—procalcitonin; IL-6—interleukin-6; Se—sensitivity; Sp—specificity; AUC—area under the curve.

4. Discussion

This prospective cohort study aimed to evaluate the diagnostic accuracy of PCT, presepsin, endocan, and IL-6 assessed at designated neonatal and maternal timepoints for the early detection of EOS in neonates. We also assessed the best cut-off values for achieving the highest diagnostic performance of individual biomarkers at specific timepoints. Our findings emphasize the clinical significance of PCT and presepsin as primary diagnostic tools of EOS while highlighting limitations in the predictive performance of endocan and IL-6, especially when used individually.

PCT is a prohormone of calcitonin, lacking hormonal activity, encoded by the CALC-I gene on chromosome 11, and secreted during sepsis and inflammation [10]. Its secretion commences within 2 h post-stimulation, reaches its peak at 12–24 h, and exhibits a half-life of around 24 h [11]. Our results indicated that among all the biomarkers assessed, PCT—particularly at 0–12 and 24–48 h of life—exhibited the best diagnostic performance, with sensitivities of 75% and 76.5%, specificities above 74%, and AUC values approaching 0.80. The estimated optimal cut-offs using the Liu approach validated the significant discriminative power of PCT, with Youden indices of 0.60 and 0.59 for the initial two timepoints, hence strengthening its utility in clinical triage and decision-making.

These findings align with the prior evidence suggesting that PCT rises rapidly in systemic infections and may serve as sensitive marker for EOS. A recent literature review performed by Eschborn et al., which evaluated the diagnosis performance of PCT and CRP for neonatal sepsis, indicated a mean sensitivity of 73.6% and a mean specificity of 82.8% of PCT for EOS sepsis, higher than the diagnostic performance of CRP (mean sensitivity: 65.6% and mean specificity: 82.7%) [12]. Moreover, a recent prospective cohort study by Rautela et al. that evaluated the diagnostic accuracy for EOS of IL-27 in comparison with CRP and PCT serum levels, indicated that PCT showed the highest sensitivity (82.93%) for EOS diagnosis, followed by IL-27 (sensitivity of 78.05%) and CRP (sensitivity of 73.17%) [13].

Presepsin, a marker of monocyte activation and innate immune response [14], demonstrated excellent performance at 24–48 h, with a Youden index of 0.61 and an AUC of 0.81. These values are comparable to PCT and suggest a strong role for presepsin in complementing clinical assessment, particularly in cases with ambiguous clinical presentation. Although its umbilical cord and 0–12 h values showed reduced sensitivity, its specificity remained high, offering potential utility in ruling-out sepsis as demonstrated by other studies [15–17].

IL-6 determined from umbilical cord blood or neonates' serum at 0–12 h of life, while biologically plausible as a sepsis marker as reported in several studies [18,19], showed limited sensitivity (22–44%), despite high specificity (93–100%). This reflects its brief half-life and highlights the critical importance of timing in biomarker sampling. These findings caution against relying on IL-6 alone as a screening tool, especially in settings where sepsis evolves sub-clinically.

Last, but not least, endocan demonstrated low sensitivity, moderate specificity, and modest overall diagnostic accuracies at 0–12 and 24–48 h after birth (65.82% and 66.67%). Its diagnostic performance (Youden indices ≤ 0.48) suggests limited clinical utility when used individually, despite its statistical associations in univariate analyses with EOS. Another prospective study conducted in Romania on a cohort of 59 patients indicated that for a calculated optimal threshold value of 1.62 ng/mL, serum endocan presented a sensitivity of 88% and a specificity of 50% for the diagnosis of EOS [20]. On the other hand, another study did not indicate endocan as a promising diagnostic marker for late-onset neonatal sepsis [21].

The literature data indicate tumor necrosis factor alpha (TNF-α), progranulin or neopterin as potential alternative diagnostic biomarkers. The cut-off value ranges of TNF-α for the diagnosis of EOS between 1.7 and 70 pg/mL have a sensitivity of 66–78% and a specificity of 41–76% according to recent reports [22–24]. A threshold of 18.94 pg/mL demonstrated a sensitivity of 79% and a specificity of 81% [23]. Given its moderate accuracy, this biomarker is considered a more reliable indicator for late-onset sepsis [23].

Another study pointed out that a cut-off value >37.89 ng/mL of progranulin achieved a diagnostic accuracy of 0.786 for EOS, with a sensitivity of 94.3%, specificity of 51.5%, positive predictive value of 61.7%, and negative predictive value of 91.7% [25]. Moreover, the combination of PRGN with PCT increased the diagnostic accuracy for EOS to 0.987 [25].

Last but not least, Shokry and colleagues evaluated the utility of neopterin in diagnosing EOS in full-term neonates. At a cut-off value of 499 nmol/L, this biomarker achieved an AUC value of 0.91 along with a sensitivity of 91%, specificity of 84.7%, positive predictive value of 91.9%, and negative predictive value of 88% [26]. A separate study conducted on both pre-term and full-term neonates reported excellent diagnostic accuracy for EOS, with an AUC of 0.992 at a threshold value of 100.3 nmol/L [27].

One strength of this study lies in the rigorous evaluation of confounding variables, including gestational age, duration of membrane rupture, and duration of maternal antibiotic therapy. Adjusting for these variables yielded minimal changes in effect estimates across all biomarkers (generally < 7%), indicating that these biomarkers retained independent predictive value. The stability of adjusted odds ratios further supports the robustness of the diagnostic signal, particularly for PCT and presepsin. Notably, these covariates may function more as effect modifiers, given their biological plausibility in influencing neonatal immune response and sepsis risk. Other strengths of this study include its prospective design, and a certain diagnosis of EOS based on blood culture confirmation.

On the other hand, the limitations of this study include small sample size, limited variability, inclusion of neonates admitted to the NICU, and lack of stratification based on specific gestational-age groups.

Further studies could use machine learning-based methods to explore the potential of individual biomarkers for EOS diagnosis along with specific maternal and neonatal risk factors. This could highlight the predictive performance of individual markers in specific clinical situations and at various time-points. Moreover, further validation of these algorithms would allow clinicians to establish the best approach for diagnosis EOS as soon as the first days of neonatal life, thus reducing the burden of unnecessary antibiotic administration.

5. Conclusions

PCT and presepsin measured at early neonatal timepoints—particularly at 0–12 h and 24–48 h—demonstrated high diagnostic accuracy and a favorable sensitivity–specificity balance for predicting EOS.

IL-6 and endocan may serve as adjunctive markers, though their performance is dependent on precise timing and clinical context.

Further multicenter validation and investigation of combined biomarker models are warranted to establish standardized, high-performance diagnostic algorithms for EOS.

Author Contributions: This paper is part of the doctoral research of M.-A.H. at "Grigore T. Popa" University of Medicine and Pharmacy, Iasi. Conceptualization, M.-A.H. and D.N.; methodology, L.P., G.Z. and M.-A.H.; software, I.-A.V., L.-M.B. and D.-C.A.; validation, L.G., C.D. and M.-A.H.; formal analysis, M.-A.H., L.G., C.D. and D.N.; investigation, L.P., G.Z., M.-A.H. and D.N.; resources, I.-A.V., L.-M.B., L.G. and D.-C.A.; data curation I.-A.V., L.-M.B., L.G. and D.-C.A.; writing—original draft preparation, M.-A.H. and D.N.; writing—review and editing, M.-A.H., L.G., C.D. and D.N.; supervision, D.N.; project administration, M.-A.H.; funding acquisition, M.-A.H. All authors have read and agreed to the published version of the manuscript.

Funding: This research was partially funded by the "Grigore T. Popa" University of Medicine and Pharmacy as a doctoral scholarship.

Institutional Review Board Statement: This study was conducted in accordance with the Declaration of Helsinki and approved by the Institutional Ethics Committee of "Grigore T. Popa" University of Medicine and Pharmacy, Iasi (No. 175/17.04.2022) and "Cuza voda" Clinical Hospital of Obstetrics and Gynecology (No. 5750/09.05.2022 and No. 1405/02.02.2023).

Informed Consent Statement: Informed consent was obtained from all subjects involved in this study.

Data Availability Statement: Dataset available on request from the authors.

Conflicts of Interest: The authors declare no conflicts of interest.

Abbreviations

The following abbreviations are used in this manuscript:

Abbreviation	Full Term
AB therapy	Antibiotic Therapy
aOR	Adjusted Odds Ratio
AUC	Area Under the Curve
CI	Confidence Interval
CRP	C-Reactive Protein
ELISA	Enzyme-Linked Immunosorbent Assay
EMA	European Medicines Agency
EOS	Early-Onset Sepsis
HIE	Hypoxic-Ischemic Encephalopathy
IL-6	Interleukin-6
IL-27	Interleukin-27
I/T ratio	Immature-to-Total Neutrophil Ratio
IVH	Intraventricular Hemorrhage
NICU	Neonatal Intensive Care Unit
NPV	Negative Predictive Value
OR	Odds Ratio
PCR	Polymerase Chain Reaction
PCT	Procalcitonin
PPV	Positive Predictive Value
ROM	Rupture of Membranes
SD	Standard Deviation
Se	Sensitivity
SGA	Small for Gestational Age
Sp	Specificity
WBC	White Blood Cells

References

1. Hayes, R.; Hartnett, J.; Semova, G.; Murray, C.; Murphy, K.; Carroll, L.; Plapp, H.; Hession, L.; O'Toole, J.; McCollum, D. Neonatal sepsis definitions from randomised clinical trials. *Pediatr. Res.* **2023**, *93*, 1141–1148. [CrossRef]
2. Vulcănescu, A.; Siminel, M.-A.; Dinescu, S.-N.; Dijmărescu, A.-L.; Manolea, M.-M.; Săndulescu, S.-M. Neonatal Mortality Due to Early-Onset Sepsis in Eastern Europe: A Review of Current Monitoring Protocols During Pregnancy and Maternal Demographics in Eastern Europe, with an Emphasis on Romania—Comparison with Data Extracted from a Secondary Center in Southern Romania. *Children* **2025**, *12*, 354. [PubMed]
3. Eurostat. Infant Mortality Rates. Available online: https://ec.europa.eu/eurostat/statistics-explained/index.php?title=Mortality_and_life_expectancy_statistics (accessed on 10 March 2025).
4. Helmbrecht, A.R.; Marfurt, S.; Chaaban, H. Systematic Review of the Effectiveness of the Neonatal Early-Onset Sepsis Calculator. *J. Perinat. Neonatal Nurs.* **2019**, *33*, 82–88. [CrossRef] [PubMed]
5. Kosmeri, C.; Giapros, V.; Serbis, A.; Baltogianni, M. Application of Advanced Molecular Methods to Study Early-Onset Neonatal Sepsis. *Int. J. Mol. Sci.* **2024**, *25*, 2258. [CrossRef] [PubMed]
6. De Rose, D.U.; Ronchetti, M.P.; Martini, L.; Rechichi, J.; Iannetta, M.; Dotta, A.; Auriti, C. Diagnosis and Management of Neonatal Bacterial Sepsis: Current Challenges and Future Perspectives. *Trop. Med. Infect. Dis.* **2024**, *9*, 199. [CrossRef]
7. van Leeuwen, L.M.; Fourie, E.; van den Brink, G.; Bekker, V.; van Houten, M.A. Diagnostic value of maternal, cord blood and neonatal biomarkers for early-onset sepsis: A systematic review and meta-analysis. *Clin. Microbiol. Infect.* **2024**, *30*, 850–857. [CrossRef]

8. Flannery, D.D.; Ramachandran, V.; Schrag, S.J. Neonatal Early-Onset Sepsis: Epidemiology, Microbiology, and Controversies in Practice. *Clin. Perinatol.* **2025**, *52*, 15–31. [CrossRef]
9. Tuzun, F.; Ozkan, H.; Cetinkaya, M.; Yucesoy, E.; Kurum, O.; Cebeci, B.; Cakmak, E.; Ozkutuk, A.; Keskinoglu, P.; Baysal, B. Is European Medicines Agency (EMA) sepsis criteria accurate for neonatal sepsis diagnosis or do we need new criteria? *PLoS ONE* **2019**, *14*, e0218002. [CrossRef]
10. Davies, J. Procalcitonin. *J. Clin. Pathol.* **2015**, *68*, 675–679. [CrossRef]
11. Reinhart, K.; Meisner, M.; Brunkhorst, F.M. Markers for sepsis diagnosis: What is useful? *Crit. Care Clin.* **2006**, *22*, 503–519. [CrossRef]
12. Eschborn, S.; Weitkamp, J.H. Procalcitonin versus C-reactive protein: Review of kinetics and performance for diagnosis of neonatal sepsis. *J. Perinatol.* **2019**, *39*, 893–903. [CrossRef] [PubMed]
13. Rautela, A.; Garg, J.; Agarwal, J.; Raj, N.; Das, A.; Sen, M. Evaluation of a novel serum marker, interleukin 27, in comparison to procalcitonin and C-reactive protein in the diagnosis of early-onset neonatal sepsis in a tertiary care center in north India. *Int. J. Crit. Illn. Inj. Sci.* **2024**, *14*, 181–187. [CrossRef] [PubMed]
14. Piccioni, M.G.; Del Negro, V.; Bruno Vecchio, R.C.; Faralli, I.; Savastano, G.; Galoppi, P.; Perrone, G. Is the Arabin Pessary really useful in preventing preterm birth? A review of literature. *J. Gynecol. Obstet. Hum. Reprod.* **2021**, *50*, 101824. [CrossRef]
15. Paraskevas, T.; Chourpiliadi, C.; Demiri, S.; Michailides, C.; Karanikolas, E.; Lagadinou, M.; Velissaris, D. Presepsin in the diagnosis of sepsis. *Clin. Chim. Acta* **2023**, *550*, 117588. [CrossRef] [PubMed]
16. Ruan, L.; Chen, G.Y.; Liu, Z.; Zhao, Y.; Xu, G.Y.; Li, S.F.; Li, C.N.; Chen, L.S.; Tao, Z. The combination of procalcitonin and C-reactive protein or presepsin alone improves the accuracy of diagnosis of neonatal sepsis: A meta-analysis and systematic review. *Crit. Care* **2018**, *22*, 316. [CrossRef]
17. Iskandar, A.; Arthamin, M.Z.; Indriana, K.; Anshory, M.; Hur, M.; Di Somma, S. Comparison between presepsin and procalcitonin in early diagnosis of neonatal sepsis. *J. Matern. Fetal Neonatal Med.* **2019**, *32*, 3903–3908. [CrossRef]
18. Qiu, X.; Zhang, L.; Tong, Y.; Qu, Y.; Wang, H.; Mu, D. Interleukin-6 for early diagnosis of neonatal sepsis with premature rupture of the membranes: A meta-analysis. *Medicine* **2018**, *97*, e13146. [CrossRef]
19. Eichberger, J.; Resch, B. Reliability of Interleukin-6 Alone and in Combination for Diagnosis of Early Onset Neonatal Sepsis: Systematic Review. *Front. Pediatr.* **2022**, *10*, 840778. [CrossRef]
20. Zonda, G.I.; Zonda, R.; Cernomaz, A.T.; Paduraru, L.; Avasiloaiei, A.L.; Grigoriu, B.D. Endocan—A potential diagnostic marker for early onset sepsis in neonates. *J. Infect. Dev. Ctries.* **2019**, *13*, 311–317. [CrossRef]
21. Gatseva, P.; Blazhev, A.; Yordanov, Z.; Atanasova, V. Early Diagnostic Markers of Late-Onset Neonatal Sepsis. *Pediatr. Rep.* **2023**, *15*, 548–559. [CrossRef]
22. Delanghe, J.R.; Speeckaert, M.M. Translational research and biomarkers in neonatal sepsis. *Clin. Chim. Acta* **2015**, *451*, 46–64. [CrossRef] [PubMed]
23. Celik, I.H.; Hanna, M.; Canpolat, F.E.; Mohan, P. Diagnosis of neonatal sepsis: The past, present and future. *Pediatr. Res.* **2022**, *91*, 337–350. [CrossRef] [PubMed]
24. Memar, M.Y.; Alizadeh, N.; Varshochi, M.; Kafil, H.S. Immunologic biomarkers for diagnostic of early-onset neonatal sepsis. *J. Matern. Fetal Neonatal Med.* **2019**, *32*, 143–153. [CrossRef] [PubMed]
25. Almonaem, A.; Rateb, E.; Ameen, S.G.; Elsharnoby, A. Progranulin Versus Procalcitonin as a Novel Biomarker in Diagnosis of Early-Onset Neonatal Sepsis. *Benha Med. J.* **2023**, *40*, 379–388.
26. Shokry, D.M.; Elbahiedy, R.M.; Abdelrahman, E.H. Serum Neopterin in Diagnosis of Early Onset Neonatal Sepsis. *Egypt. J. Hosp. Med.* **2023**, *91*, 5074–5080. [CrossRef]
27. Boseila, S.; Seoud, I.; Samy, G.; El-Gamal, H.; Ibrahim, T.S.; Ahmed, A.; El Kafoury, M.R.; Fathy, A. Serum neopterin level in early onset neonatal sepsis. *J. Am. Sci.* **2011**, *7*, 343–352.

diagnostics

MDPI

Article

Atypical Manifestations of Cowden Syndrome in Pediatric Patients

Ekaterina Zelenova [1,2,*], Tatiana Belysheva [1,3], Elena Sharapova [1], Irina Barinova [2], Alexandra Fedorova [1], Vera Semenova [1,2], Yana Vishnevskaya [1], Irina Kletskaya [4], Anna Mitrofanova [5], Denis Sofronov [1], Ivan Karasev [1], Denis Romanov [6,7], Timur Valiev [1] and Tatiana Nasedkina [2,5]

1 N.N. Blokhin National Medical Research Center of Oncology, Ministry of Health of the Russian Federation, 115478 Moscow, Russia; klinderma@bk.ru (T.B.); sharapovae.v@yandex.ru (E.S.); fedorova.ronc@gmail.com (A.F.); sulpiridum@yandex.ru (V.S.); yana_vishn@list.ru (Y.V.); mdsofronov@gmail.com (D.S.); i.karasev@ronc.ru (I.K.); timurvaliev@mail.ru (T.V.)
2 Engelhardt Institute of Molecular Biology, Russian Academy of Sciences, 119991 Moscow, Russia; irina.barinova.98@mail.ru (I.B.); tanased06@rambler.ru (T.N.)
3 Central State Medical Academy of the Administrative, Department of the President of Russia, 121359 Moscow, Russia
4 Russian Children's Clinical Hospital, Pirogov Russian National Research Medical University, 117997 Moscow, Russia; ikletskaya@gmail.com
5 Dmitry Rogachev National Medical Research Center of Pediatric Hematology, Oncology and Immunology, 117198 Moscow, Russia; ms.anna.mitrofanova@yandex.ru
6 Limited Liability Company, Center of Innovative Medical Technologies, 115191 Moscow, Russia; romanovronc@gmail.com
7 Federal Network of Expert Oncology Clinics "Euroonco", 115191 Moscow, Russia
* Correspondence: zelenovayeye@gmail.com

Abstract: Background/Objectives: Cowden syndrome (or *PTEN* hamartoma tumor syndrome) (CS/PHTS) belongs to a group of inherited disorders associated with the development of multiple hamartomas. The clinical presentation of patients may include dysmorphic facial features, macrocephaly, developmental delay, and multiple benign and malignant tumors of various localizations. At the same time, only thyroid cancer is thought to have an increased risk in childhood. Skin lesions in CS/PHTS occur in 90–100% of patients and include multiple tricholemmoma, papilloma, acral keratosis, pigmentation changes, as well as rarer forms like vascular malformations, fibromas, neuromas, melanoma, and basal cell carcinoma. **Methods:** Next-generation sequencing and Sanger sequencing were used to search for *PTEN* genetic variants. A histological and immunohistochemical examination of tumor biopsies and skin lesions was performed. **Results:** A total of 13 patients from six families with CS/PHTS, including 10 children, were described. Seven pediatric patients belonged to families with paternal transmission of the *PTEN* pathogenic variants, while three others were de novo cases. Atypical manifestations in CS/PHTS were diffuse large B-cell lymphoma in one adult, a renal cell carcinoma, three germ cell tumors, and a linear epidermal nevus in pediatric patients. A literature review of the identified pathogenic variants in the *PTEN* gene was performed, assessing their clinical significance and analyzing the traditional and modified diagnostic criteria as applied to the pediatric population. **Conclusions:** Taking into account the low incidence of CS/PHTS, the data presented significantly expand our current understanding of this disease and guide physicians to consider a wider range of possible malignant neoplasms in pediatric patients with CS/PHTS.

Keywords: Cowden syndrome; familial case; *PTEN*; epidermal nevus; diffuse B-cell lymphoma; germ cell tumors; renal cell carcinoma; thyroid cancer

1. Introduction

Cowden syndrome (CS) is a rare genodermatosis with autosomal dominant inheritance, rather high but incomplete penetrance, and marked variability in clinical presentation [1]. The incidence is thought to be about 1 case per 200,000 people, although this is most probably an underestimate because it is assumed that most patients are undiagnosed [2]. The majority of cases are due to germline pathogenic variants in the *PTEN* gene (CS type 1, OMIM #158350). Rarer types of the syndrome are associated with hypermethylation and abnormal expression of the *KLLN* gene (CS type 4), as well as germline variants in the *SDHB*, *SDHD*, *AKT1*, *PIK3CA*, and *SEC23B* genes [3]. In addition, cases due to somatic mosaicism have been described in the literature [4–6].

At the same time, pathogenic variants in the *PTEN* gene can be associated with the development of several inherited diseases of the *PTEN*-associated hamartoma tumor syndrome group. In addition to Cowden syndrome, they include Bannayan-Riley-Ruvalcaba syndrome (BRRS), Lhermitte–Duclos disease, macrocephaly/autism syndrome (OMIM #605309), Proteus-like syndrome, and juvenile polyposis of infancy caused by deletions of the *BMPR1* and *PTEN* genes [7,8]. Therefore, modern authors use the term CS/PHTS when describing patients with Cowden syndrome and a mutation in the *PTEN* gene. Currently, the NCCN diagnostic criteria (Table 1) are used to diagnose CS/PHTS in patients over 18 years of age [9].

Table 1. Diagnostic criteria for CS/PHTS.

<table>
<tr><th>Major Criteria</th><th>Minor Criteria</th></tr>
<tr><td>Macrocephaly (head circumference greater than 58 cm in women and greater than 60 cm in men)</td><td>Structural lesions of the thyroid gland (adenoma, adenomatous goiter, etc.)</td></tr>
<tr><td>Follicular carcinoma of the thyroid gland</td><td>Thyroid cancer (papillary carcinoma)</td></tr>
<tr><td>Breast cancer</td><td>Colorectal cancer</td></tr>
<tr><td>Endometrial cancer</td><td>Renal cell carcinoma</td></tr>
<tr><td>Gastrointestinal hamartomas (including ganglioneuromas but excluding hyperplastic polyps; ≥3)</td><td>Esophageal glycogen acanthosis (≥3)</td></tr>
<tr><td>Lhermitte–Duclos disease in adults (dysplastic gangliocytoma of the cerebellum)</td><td>Intellectual disability (IQ ≤ 75), autism spectrum disorder (ASD)</td></tr>
<tr><td>Macular pigmentation of the glans penis</td><td>Testicular lipomatosis</td></tr>
<tr><td rowspan="2">Multiple skin and mucous membrane lesions (≥3):
-tricholemmomas;
-acral keratosis;
-cutaneous mucosal neuromas;
-oral papillomas (especially on the gingiva and tongue).</td><td>Vascular anomalies</td></tr>
<tr><td>Lipoma (≥3)</td></tr>
</table>

The presence of a pathogenic variant in the *PTEN* gene and family history data are taken into account when calculating the criteria (Table 2) [4].

Adult patients with CS/PHTS have an increased risk of malignant neoplasms, primarily breast cancer, endometrial cancer, thyroid cancer, colorectal cancer, renal cell carcinoma, and rarely other carcinomas [10]. The median age of the first tumor detection is 36 years, and the risk of developing second tumors is 8 times higher than in the general population [11]. Sporadic cases of squamous cell carcinoma of the skin and mucosa, ovarian cancer, testicular cancer, prostate adenocarcinoma, hepatocellular carcinoma, and transitional cell carcinoma of the bladder have also been described in patients with CS/PHTS.

As the vast majority of symptoms of CS/PHTS manifest in adulthood, a number of authors have proposed their own criteria for the diagnosis in children. For example, Tan

MH et al. 2011 define macrocephaly as an obligatory sign, and the patients must also have at least one of four additional signs: ASD, gastrointestinal polyps, dermatological signs, arteriovenous malformations, and hemangiomas [8]. Bannayan–Riley–Ruvalcaba syndrome considered a phenotypic form of CS in children is characterized by a combination of macrosomia, macrocephaly with frontal bossing, autism spectrum disorders, intellectual disability, multiple hamartomas and skin lesions (pigmented spots and lentiginosis of the penis or vulva, lipomas, and vascular malformations) [12,13]. Among children, malignant tumors are diagnosed quite rarely. In pediatric patients, the risk of developing malignant neoplasia is significantly increased only for thyroid cancer and is 4–12% [14]. At the same time, a few authors highlight the association of germ cell tumors (testicular cancer and ovarian dysgerminoma) with CS/PHTS in the pediatric population [8]. Thus, to date, there is no clear data on the frequency and spectrum of malignant tumors in children with CS/PHTS.

Table 2. Application of diagnostic criteria in CS/PHTS.

Family History (at Least One Relative Fulfils the Diagnostic Criteria) and/or the Presence of a Pathogenic Variant in the *PTEN* Gene in the Patient	No Family History, Genetic Status of the Patient Is Unknown/*PTEN*-wt
(1) Any two major criteria with or without minor criteria; OR (2) One major criterion and two minor criteria; OR (3) Three minor criteria.	(1) Three major criteria (one of which is macrocephaly, Lhermitte–Duclos disease, or gastrointestinal malrotation); OR (2) Two major and three minor criteria.

This article analyzes six clinical cases of CS/PHTS, three of which are familial cases with paternal transmission of a pathogenic variant in the *PTEN* gene. The peculiarity of our patients is the presence of malignant tumors in childhood: ovarian germ cell tumors in three girls aged 4, 7, and 8 years; and a renal cell carcinoma in a boy aged 13 years. In one case, the patient's father developed diffuse large B-cell lymphoma, which is also uncommon in CS/PHTS. Another atypical feature was a linear epidermal nevus in a newborn as the first symptom of CS/PHTS. Based on the data, the applicability of modified criteria for the diagnosis and management of pediatric CS/PHTS patients is discussed.

2. Materials and Methods

2.1. Patients

A total of 13 patients (10 males and 3 females) aged between 1 month and 50 years at the time of examination and presenting with clinical manifestations characteristic of CS/PHTS were included in the study. All patients were seen by a dermatological oncologist and counseled by a geneticist. Some patients were additionally examined by other specialists (oncologist, neurologist, nephrologist, pulmonologist, cardiologist, and endocrinologist) due to concomitant pathology.

2.2. Histological Examination

A histological examination of paraffin-embedded tissues was performed for patients ID1 (linear epidermal nevus), ID12 (germ cell tumor), and ID13 (renal cell carcinoma and sclerosing pneumocytoma). Standard staining with hematoxylin and eosin was used. Immunohistochemistry (IHC) tests were applied for germ cell tumor (patient ID12) using four monoclonal antibodies: SALL4 (Cell Marque, Rocklin, CA, USA), oct3/4 (Cell Marque,

Rocklin, CA, USA), pan-cytokeratin C-11 (Abcam, Waltham, MA, USA), CD30 (Cell Marque, Rocklin, CA, USA).

2.3. Genetic Testing

Genomic DNA was isolated from blood leukocytes or nevus tissue and skin without lesions (patient ID1) using the QIAmp DNA Mini Kit (Qiagen, Hilden, Germany). NGS sequencing was performed for the probands in all families.

Libraries were prepared with KAPA HyperPrep Kit (Roche, Basel, Switzerland) as described earlier [15]. The libraries were hybridized with coding regions of 35 genes (Table S1), then pooled and sequenced on MiSeq (Illumina, San Diego, CA, USA) (paired-end sequencing, 300 cycles, and 250–300× coverage depth).

Sequencing data were processed and aligned to the reference genome sequence GRCh (hg38). The annotation of nucleotide sequence and variant discovery was performed using the GATK (Genome Analysis Toolkit) algorithm. Interpretation of the identified variants was carried out according to the ACMG guidelines (doi: 10.1038/gim.2015.30) using ClinVar (https://www.ncbi.nlm.nih.gov/clinvar, accessed on 18 September 2024), Varsome (https://varsome.com, accessed on 18 September 2024), or Franklin Genoox (https://franklin.genoox.com, accessed on 18 September 2024) databases. The identified pathogenic or likely pathogenic variants in all cases were verified by Sanger sequencing; primer pairs used are given in Table S2. For the relatives of the probands, only segregation analysis using Sanger sequencing was done.

3. Results

Atypical clinical manifestations were identified in six patients with CS/PHTS. Detailed clinical and anamnestic data were collected, and genetic testing of the patients and their available relatives was performed.

3.1. Case N°1

Patient ID1, a 2-year-old boy, was born to his mother's sixth pregnancy without peculiarities. At birth, there was marked macrosomia (4330 g/58 cm), and a soft epidermal nevus was apparent on the skin of the scalp and right temporal region. The nevus was a grayish-pink shade with irregular contours and a soft-elastic consistency (Figure 1A,B). The size of the nevus increased in proportion to the child's height. No other phenotypic manifestations were observed. At 2 months of age, the child was referred to a dermatologist-oncologist, and a nevus biopsy was performed. The morphological picture of the lesion corresponded to a soft epidermal nevus (Figure 1C–F).

A molecular genetic study of the nevus biopsy material was performed by NGS using a panel of skin cancer-associated genes. No pathogenic somatic variants in the *HRAS*, *KRAS*, *NRAS*, or *BRAF* genes were detected; however, in exon 5 of the *PTEN* gene, a variant c.309_312del (p.Phe104ValfsTer8) was found with an alternative allele frequency of 60%. The variant was likely pathogenic according to ACMG criteria (PM4 and PS2) and had not been described earlier. The same variant in the *PTEN* gene in the heterozygous state was detected in the patient's peripheral venous blood leukocytes, which indicated its germline origin, so the CS/PHTS was diagnosed.

In a family, the father (ID2) and two brothers (ID3 and ID4) were found to have macrocephaly. One of the brothers (ID3) had postnatal macrosomia (4350 g/53 cm), the other (ID4) had developmental delay and autism, and the father had lipomatosis. The same variant of the *PTEN* gene was found in the father and these two brothers by Sanger sequencing (Figure 2).

At the age of 2 years, the patient ID1 was found to have a colon polyp. Given the small size and single lesion, surgical treatment was not required; however, a colonoscopy was included in the further examination plan.

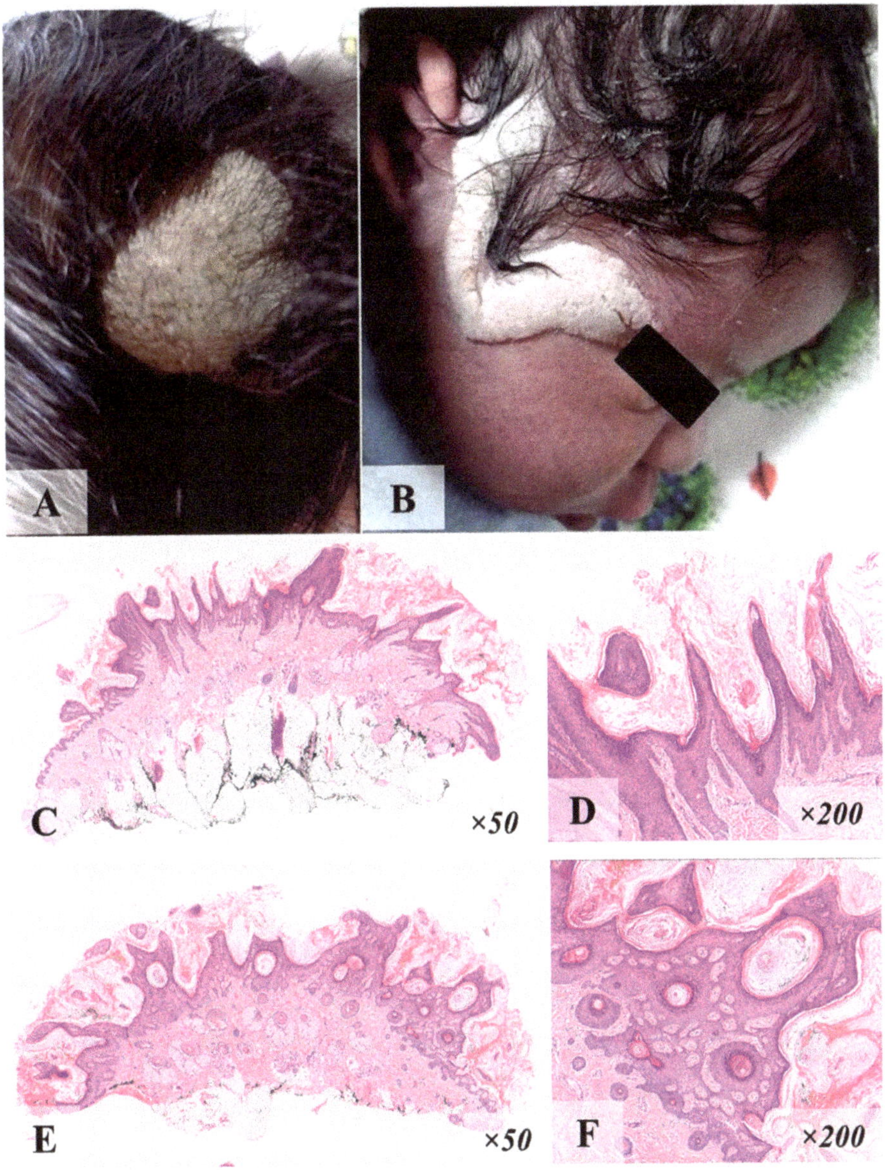

Figure 1. Epidermal nevus of a patient ID1 in the scalp (**A**), and right temporal region (**B**). Histological examination of biopsy (hematoxylin and eosin staining): (**C**,**D**)—papillomatous proliferation of multilayer squamous epithelium of the 'saw tooth' type; (**E**,**F**)—superficial layered keratotic masses, the formation of keratocysts of various sizes in the thickness of these outgrowths, and a loose connective tissue stroma at their base.

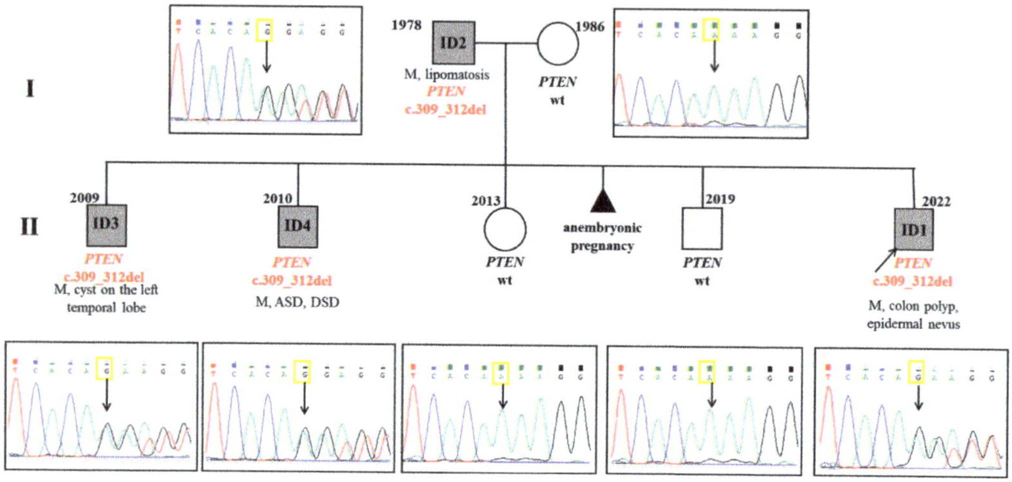

Figure 2. Pedigree of family from case N°1: ASD—autism spectrum disorder, DD—developmental delay, DSD—delayed speech development, M—macrocephaly, wt—wild type. The segregation analysis revealed a mutation in the *PTEN* gene in patients ID1–4, while the proband's mother, one brother, and a sister did not carry this pathogenic variant.

3.2. *Case N°2*

Patient ID5, a 14-year-old male, was born via cesarean section at 40 weeks due to macrosomia (4230 g/57 cm). In the first year of life, he experienced growth retardation, and a decrease in growth hormone levels in the blood; therefore, the patient received hormone replacement therapy until the age of 1 year. From the age of 11 months, the patient experienced recurrent loss of consciousness, cold sweats, marked weakness, and clonic tremors of the limbs; finally, hypoglycemia (less than 2 mmol/L) of unclear genesis was diagnosed.

The patient was under the dynamic observation of a neurologist for delayed psychomotor and speech development. At 1 year and 5 months of age, rhythm disturbances were noted, namely, continuous recurrent ventricular tachycardia and single- and paired-ventricular extrasystoles. First-degree circulatory insufficiency was diagnosed, and an additional chord of the left ventricle was detected. At the age of 5 years, the papilloma of the left palatine tonsil was surgically removed. During annual follow-up, lipomatosis and colon polyps were revealed at 11 years, and a thyroid nodule (TIRADS-3) was detected at 14 years.

A family history showed that the patient's younger brother (ID6) had normal height and weight characteristics at birth (3200 g/52 cm). However, there was a delay in speech and psychomotor development (he walked starting at 1 year and 9 months, but does not speak), and at the age of 2 years, this child was diagnosed with infantile cerebral palsy. Furthermore, he had macrocephaly, epicanthus, hypertelorism, cardiac (extra left ventricular chordae, incomplete right bundle-branch block, and resting bradycardia), and orthopedic problems (kyphoscoliosis and hallux valgus of the feet). At the age of 2 years and 10 months, a 4 cm lipoma was found on the skin in the right back region during an annual follow-up.

A comprehensive examination of the patients' father (ID7) revealed macrocephaly (head circumference 63 cm), multiple papillomas in the axillary and inguinal regions, polyposis of the colon, a lipoma of the jejunum, lymphofollicular hyperplasia of the colon, nodules in both lobes of the thyroid gland, and a vascular malformation in the left cerebellar hemisphere. At the age of 45 years, he was diagnosed with diffuse large

B-cell lymphoma, GCB (germinal center B-cell) type of stage IV-B (Ann Arbor classification) involving peripheral, intrathoracic, and intra-abdominal lymph nodes, and lesions of liver, spleen, lungs, and bone marrow. The father underwent polychemotherapy (PCT) according to the RB scheme (rituximab plus bendamustine), and further according to the R-CHOP scheme (rituximab plus cyclophosphamide, doxorubicin, vincristine, and prednisolone) with a positive effect.

Molecular genetic testing revealed a heterozygous pathogenic variant c.332G>A (p.Trp111Ter) in exon 5 of the *PTEN* gene in proband ID5, his brother ID6, and father ID7 (Figure 3).

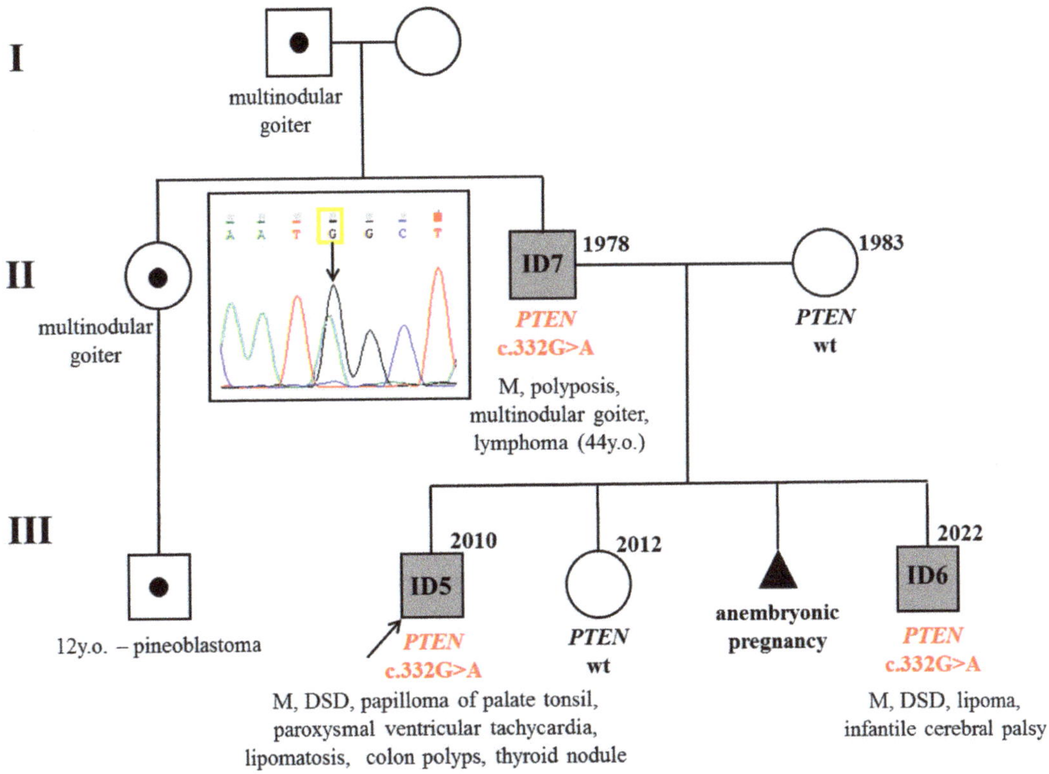

Figure 3. Pedigree from case N°2: M—macrocephaly, DSD—delayed speech development, wt—wild type. Segregation analysis revealed a mutation in patients ID5–7. Mother and sister of the proband are unaffected.

3.3. Case N°3

Patient ID8, a 15-year-old female (Figure 4A,B) was born with postnatal macrosomia (4350 g/54 cm), but early development was consistent with age. She was seen by a cardiologist until the age of 11 years due to an interventricular septal defect. At the age of 7, a voluminous mass was found in the right ovary and removed laparoscopically, which was defined as a mixed germ cell tumor consisting of mature teratoma (90%) and yolk sac tumor (10%). The patient received three courses of PCT according to the BEP scheme (bleomycin, etoposide, and cisplatin).

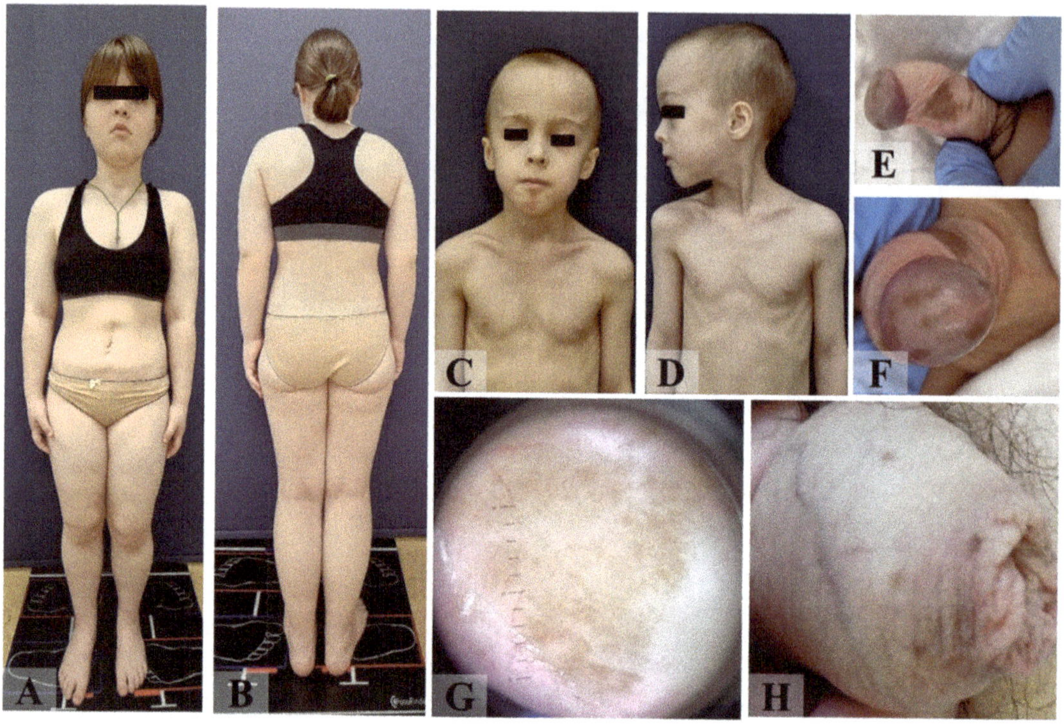

Figure 4. Phenotypic characteristics of the patients from clinical case N°3: proband (**A**,**B**); proband's brother—bird face, mandibular hypoplasia, microstomia, macrocephaly, high forehead (**C**,**D**), penile lentiginosis (**E**,**F**) with a homogeneous structure revealed by dermatoscopy (**G**); proband's father—penile lentiginosis (**H**).

At the age of 10 years, a hemithyroidectomy on the left lobe of the thyroid gland was performed due to a follicular adenoma. A year later, the patient underwent thyroidectomy for thyroid cancer in the right lobe, followed by radioactive iodine, and now there are no signs of progression. A more detailed description of the diagnosis and treatment of thyroid cancer in this patient is given by Bricheva E.B. et al., 2024 [16].

Genetic testing revealed a pathogenic variant c.380G>A (p.Gly127Glu) in exon 5 of the *PTEN* gene in the patient's blood, thus, the diagnosis of CS/PHTS was established. Further pedigree analysis revealed that the patient's younger brother (ID9) had macrosomia (4310 g/60 cm), macrocephaly, papillomatosis of the palatine tonsils, right-sided cryptorchidism, aplasia of the right testis, and macular pigmentation of the penis from birth (Figure 4C–G), while their father (ID10) has macrocephaly and penile lentiginosis (Figure 4H). The same pathogenic variant c.380G>A was detected in the father and brother, but not in other family members (Figure 5).

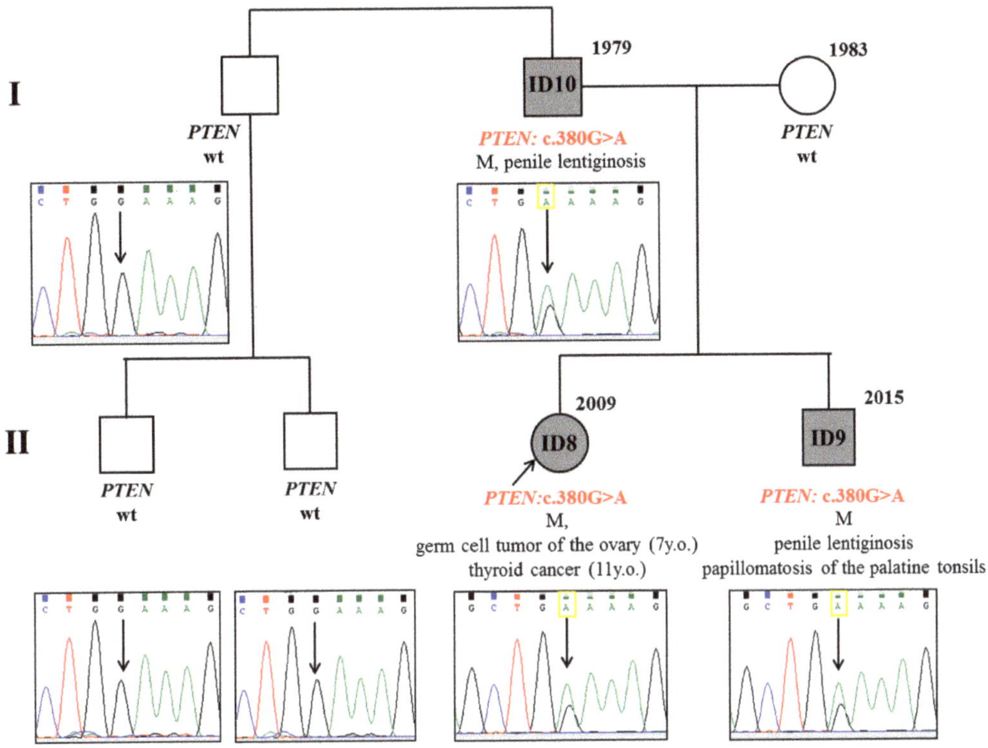

Figure 5. Pedigree of patients from case N°3: M—macrocephaly, wt—wild type. Also, there is the result of segregation analysis: ID8–10 have a mutation, while other family members are unaffected.

3.4. Case N°4

Patient ID11, a 14-year-old female, was delivered with vacuum extraction due to macrosomia (4060 g/54 cm). Her mother had a kidney doubling and at the age of 10 years underwent resection of the extra kidney.

The patient grew and developed according to her age; only intracranial hypertension was noted as a neurological symptom. At the age of 4, uterine extirpation with appendages, appendectomy, and resection of the greater omentum was performed because of a malignant germ cell tumor of the ovary, which consisted of embryonal tumor (85% of the tumor tissue), yolk sac tumor (10%), and immature teratoma (5%).

During the four courses of PCT, peritoneal carcinomatosis was noted, and the second surgical intervention aimed at removing metastatic foci was performed. No signs of recurrence were observed over the next 5 years. Since age 11, the patient had been receiving estrogen hormone replacement therapy. At the age of 10 years, multiple thyroid nodules up to 1 cm were detected and continued to grow, so a thyroidectomy was performed another 3 years later, and a multinodular goiter was diagnosed.

Considering multiple tumors, a molecular genetic study was recommended, and a pathogenic variant in the splice site of exon 8 of *PTEN* c.802-2A>T in the heterozygous state was detected. The variant was not found in both parents, so it was considered a *de novo* mutation in this family (Figure 6).

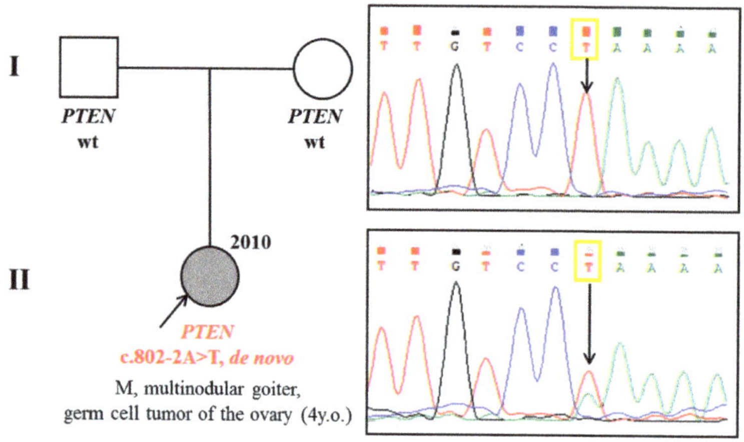

Figure 6. Pedigree and segregation analysis of a patient from clinical case N°4.

3.5. Case N°5

Patient ID12, a 10-year-old female, was born with macrosomia (4294 g/57 cm) and had intracranial hypertension since birth. A fibrolypoma of the supra scapular region appeared at 4 months and was surgically removed at 4 years of age.

At the age of 8, the proband had macrocephaly, scaphocephaly, and lymphatic malformation on her left thigh. Also, a left ovary tumor was detected on ultrasound. A histological and immunohistochemical examination of the biopsy identified this mass as a germ cell tumor (Figure 7).

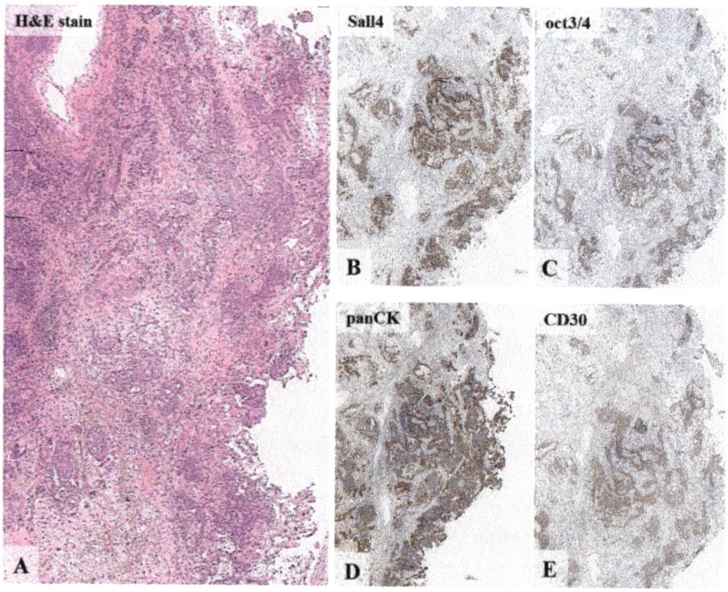

Figure 7. Histological ((**A**), eq. ×200) and immunohistochemical ((**B–E**), eq. ×100) examination of the patient's tumor from clinical case N°5: large cell adenomatoid tumor in fibrous stroma with hemorrhages (**A**); total expression of pangerminative cell marker (**B**); total expression of oct3/4 (**C**); panCK expression by all tumor cells (**D**); CD30 expression by all pathological elements (**E**).

The patient received PCT according to the MAKEI-96 scheme. After four courses, she underwent an MRI (Figure 8), followed by a salpingo-oophorectomy on the right side. No peritoneal dissemination was detected, the omentum was intact, and the germ cell tumor of mixed structure demonstrated complete therapeutic pathomorphosis.

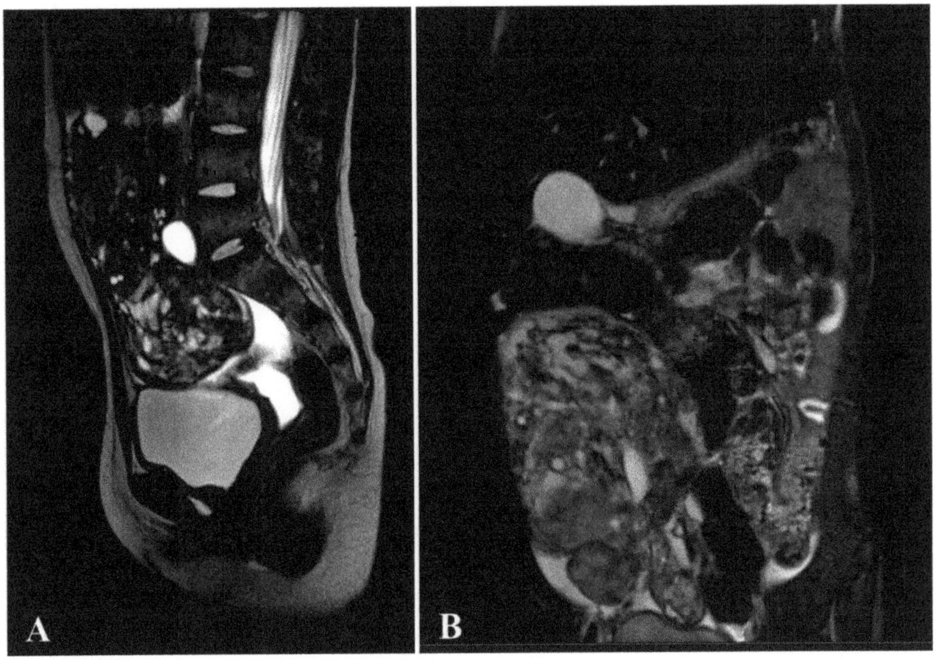

Figure 8. MRI of patient from case N° 5 ((**A**)—T2WI sag, (**B**)—T2 FS cor): massive pelvic tumor with intra-abdominal spread. The tumor has a cystic-solid structure with expansive growth. The upper pole of the tumor reaches the visceral surface of the liver, the lower pole pushes aside the bladder, right kidney, bowel loops, and inferior vena cava.

A molecular genetic study revealed a heterozygous pathogenic variant c.209T>C (p.Leu70Pro) in exon 3 of the *PTEN* gene, confirming the diagnosis of CS/PHTS. The parents refused to undergo segregation analysis.

3.6. *Case N°6*

Patient ID13, a 17-year-old male, had pronounced macrosomia (4800 g/58 cm) at birth. He was observed by a neurologist for delayed speech development (he started to speak at the age of 4.5) and intellectual disability. At the age of 2.5 years, he underwent an operation for lymphangioma of the right axillary region. At the age of 13, a renal cell carcinoma of the right kidney developed. The patient underwent nephrectomy (Figure 9), and one month later, a sclerosing pneumocytoma of the left lung was detected (Figure 10). The following phenotypic features were also presented: macrocephaly (head circumference 63 cm), genital lentiginosis, three "café-au-lait" spots on the trunk, gingival hypertrophy, enamel hypoplasia, chest deformity, and scoliosis. At the age of 14, the patient underwent thyroidectomy because of multiple follicular thyroid adenomas. Genetic testing revealed a pathogenic variant c.406T>C (p.Cys136Arg) in exon 5 of the *PTEN* gene in the heterozygous state, which indicated the presence of CS/PHTS.

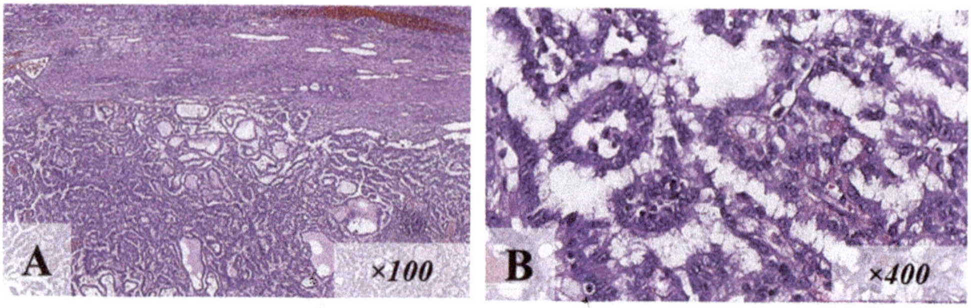

Figure 9. Renal cell carcinoma of patient ID13 (hematoxylin and eosin staining): tumor tissue of papillary structure (**A**); medium-sized cubic cells, nuclei are located basally (**B**).

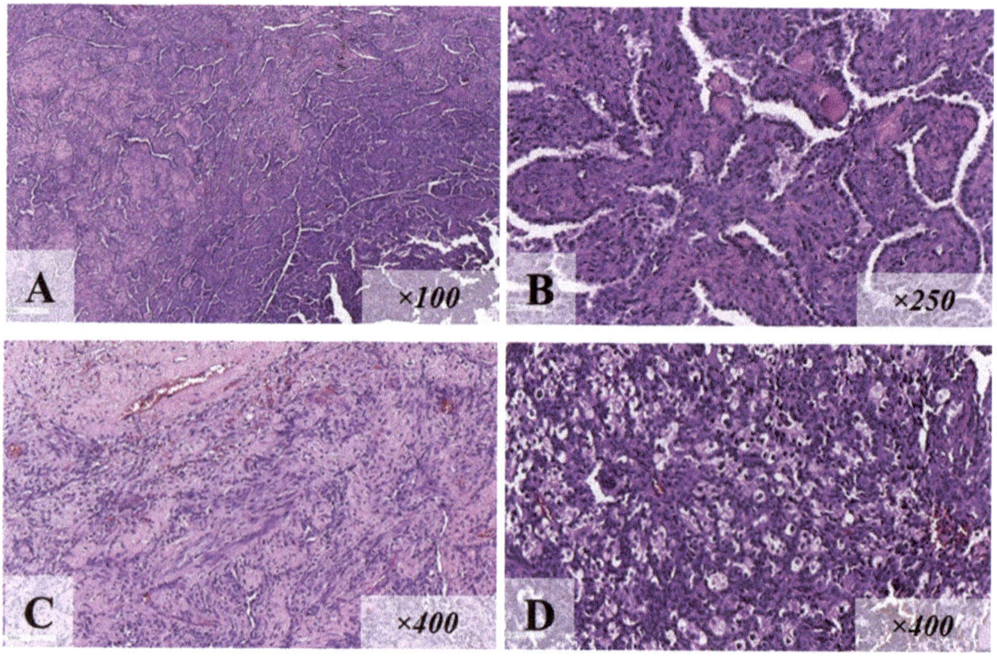

Figure 10. Histological examination (hematoxylin and eosin staining): Sclerosing pneumocytoma of the patient ID13 from clinical case N°6: tumor tissue of papillary and solid structure (**A**); the tumor is represented by superficial cubic cells lining the papillary structures, with rounded basophilic monomorphic nuclei with dispersed chromatin, and rounded cells with eosinophilic cytoplasm, and larger oval nuclei (**B**); there are areas of marked sclerotic changes (**C**) and extensive foci of xanthoma cell aggregations (**D**).

4. Discussion

Thus, the article presents 13 patients with CS/PHTS (Table 3): three familial cases with paternal transmission of the pathogenic variant, and three cases with *de novo* mutations in the *PTEN* gene. The results are summarized in Table 3.

When comparing the phenotype of pediatric patients in our sample with the generally accepted diagnostic criteria [9], we found that only one patient (ID9) could be diagnosed with CS/PHTS because he had a mutation in the *PTEN* gene and three major criteria (macrocephaly, penile lentiginosis, papillomatosis of the palatine tonsils).

Table 3. General characteristics of patients with CS/PHTS (major, minor, and additional criteria) [8,9]. Genomic coordinates are given according to the GRCh38 version.

Patient, Sex, Age	Major Criteria	Minor Criteria	Additional Pediatric Criteria	Atypical Features (Age of Diagnosis, Years)
Case N°1, g.87933068, c.309_312del (p.Phe104ValfsTer8)				
ID1 Male 2y.o.	Macrocephaly	-	Macrosomia (0)	Soft epidermal nevus (0), one hyperplastic polyp of the colon (2)
ID2 Male 47y.o.	Macrocephaly	Lipomatosis		
ID3 Male 16y.o.	Macrocephaly	-	Macrosomia (0), cyst on the skin in the left temporal region	
ID4 Male 15y.o.	Macrocephaly	ASD	DSD	
Case N°2, g.87933091, c.332G>A (p.Trp111Ter)				
ID5 Male 14y.o.	Macrocephaly, one papilloma of the palatine tonsil (5)	Lipomatosis (11) thyroid nodule (14)	DSD, epicanthus, hypertelorism, extra left ventricular chord, resting bradycardia, kyphoscoliosis, hallux valgus	Single hyperplastic polyps of the colon (11)
ID6 Male 3y.o.	Macrocephaly	Lipoma up to 4 cm in size (2y10m)	Macrosomia (0), DSD, paroxysmal ventricular tachycardia	
ID7 Male 47y.o.	Macrocephaly	Multinodular goiter, lipoma of the ileum, vascular malformation in the cerebellum	Lymphofollicular hyperplasia of the colon (18), papillomas in axillary and inguinal areas	Diffuse large B-cell lymphoma GCB type (44)
Case N°3, g.87933139, c.380G>A (p.Gly127Glu), rs398123322				
ID8 Female 15y.o.	Macrocephaly	Papillary thyroid cancer (11)	Macrosomia (0), ventricular septal defect, papillomas in the right axilla, and on the left hand	Germ cell tumor of the right ovary (7)
ID9 Male 10y.o.	Macrocephaly, penile lentiginosis, papillomatosis of the palatine tonsils (10)	-	Macrosomia (0), aplasia of the right testis	
ID10 Male 46y.o.	Macrocephaly, penile lentiginosis	-		
Case N°4, g.87960892, c.802-2A>T, rs587782455				
ID11 Female, 14y.o.	Macrocephaly	Multinodular goiter (10)	Macrosomia (0)	Germ cell tumor of the right ovary (4)

Table 3. *Cont.*

Patient, Sex, Age	Major Criteria	Minor Criteria	Additional Pediatric Criteria	Atypical Features (Age of Diagnosis, Years)
Case N°5, g.87925557, c.209T>C (p.Leu70Pro), rs121909226				
ID12 Female 10y.o.	Macrocephaly	Fibrolipoma of suprascapular region (4 months)	Macrosomia (0), scaphocephaly	Germ cell tumor of the left ovary (8)
Case N°6, g.87933165, c.406T>C (p.Cys136Arg), rs786201044				
ID13 Male 17y.o.	Macrocephaly	Lymphangioma of the right axillary region, follicular adenomas of the thyroid (14)	Macrosomia (0), MR, "café-au-lait" spots, gingival hypertrophy, chest deformation, scoliosis, pulmonary sclerosing pneumocytoma (13)	Papillary renal cell carcinoma (13)

Abbreviations: ASD—autism spectrum disorder; DSD—delayed speech development.

Meanwhile, all children in our sample fulfilled the modified pediatric criteria [8,17] and had macrocephaly and, at least, one of the following additional features:

- ASD/expressed developmental delay (ID4, ID5, ID6);
- dermatological features, namely, cyst (ID3), nevus of Jadassohn (ID1), lipoma (ID5, ID6), papillomas on the skin (ID8), fibrolipoma (ID12), and "café-au-lait" spots (ID13);
- anomalies of vascular development (ID13);
- gastrointestinal polyps (ID1, ID5);
- thyroid pathology including multinodular goiter (ID11), thyroid nodule (ID5) follicular adenoma (ID13), and papillary thyroid cancer (ID8);
- germ cell tumor (ID8, ID11, ID12).

Notably, the majority of pediatric patients in our sample had neonatal macrosomia. Thus, the present study emphasizes the need to use modified criteria when assessing the likely phenotypic features of patients with CS/PHTS in pediatric practice.

The spectrum of malignancies in CS/PHTS is quite extensive and includes solid tumors of various localizations in the older age group. Even though hematological malignancies are not typical for patients with CS/PHTS, there are single descriptions of lymphomas in the literature. For example, Galli E et al., 2020, describe Burkitt's lymphoma in a 57-year-old woman with CS/PHTS who presented with dysplastic cerebellar gangliocytoma at the age of 46 years, papillary thyroid cancer at 47 years, and breast cancer at 51 years [18]. Cavaillé M et al., 2018 described the parent of a patient with CS/PHTS with orbital lymphoma and MALT-lymphoma that developed between 40 and 50 years of age [19]. Another article presented a male patient with CS/PHTS, with B-cell lymphoblastic lymphoma at the age of 7 years and then breast cancer at the age of 31 years [20].

In our case, N°2, a pathogenic variant in the *PTEN* gene was identified in the patient ID7 with different phenotypic manifestations of CS/PHTS and diffuse large B-cell lymphoma diagnosed at the age of 44 years. Thus, the development of non-Hodgkin's lymphoma cannot be excluded in patients with CS/PHTS, which emphasizes the importance of publishing such cases.

In childhood, malignant tumors in patients with CS/PHTS are extremely rare and are mainly represented by thyroid cancer (TC). In carriers of pathogenic variants in the *PTEN* gene, the lifetime risk of TC is estimated to be 14–38%, with a debut usually in the third decade of life [21]. However, recent studies have demonstrated the possibility of developing TC as early as childhood [14]. The most frequent thyroid pathology in children with CS/PHTS includes nodular goiter and follicular adenomas [1]. Among the patients presented in this study, ID8 manifested TC at 11 years of age, while three other patients had benign thyroid neoplasms since childhood.

The prevalence of renal cell carcinoma (RCC) in carriers of pathogenic variants in the *PTEN* gene is relatively low (1.7 to 4%). Typically, these tumors are unilateral with a debut at the age of 40–50 years, and are predominantly papillary (I and II) or chromophobe histological types [18]. According to studies, the lifetime risk of RCC in patients with CS/PHTS is 34%, with a significant increase after 40 years of age [18,22,23]. At the same time, cases of earlier RCC manifestation have been described in the literature. For example, Kim RH et al., 2020, describe two cases of RCC at a young age in patients with CS/PHTS: a 22-year-old male with macrocephaly and benign thyroid lesions and a 21-year-old female with multiple hamartomas and developmental delay [24].

The development of RCC in childhood has only been presented in an article by Smpokou P, 2015 [25]. The patient described therein had multiple tumors: follicular TC at the age of 7 and then RCC at the age of 11. Our patient ID13 had RCC and a goiter, making these cases similar. Thus, our patient ID13 is the second published case of RCC in children with CS/PTHS. This work is particularly relevant in the context of current clinical guidelines, which recommend screening for RCC in patients with CS/PHTS after the age of 30 years. Consequently, there is no early diagnostics program for adolescents or young adults for RCC, significantly affecting the prognosis of this disease.

Germ cell tumors in CS/PHTS are represented by isolated observations in the literature without a clear correlation with the syndrome. Several cases of immature teratoma [26], ovarian dysgerminoma [27], malignant germ cell tumor of the ovary [28], and seminoma [29] have been described. Our clinical experience, including three cases of malignant germ cell tumors of the ovary in girls aged 4, 7, and 8 years, is the largest series reported in the literature. Such cases call for a revision of clinical guidelines to assess the risk of malignant tumors in patients with CS/PHTS in childhood and the development of a screening program.

Cutaneous manifestations in CS/PHTS are quite diverse [30], but the congenital nevus sebaceous of Jadassohn has been described in only one case with a mosaic variant in the *PTEN* gene [31]. The history of patient ID1 emphasizes the difficulty in the differential diagnosis of this syndrome. Congenital nevus along Blaschko lines is associated with epidermal nevus syndrome (Solomon's syndrome), which includes Schimmelpenning–Feuerstein–Mims syndrome, phakomatosis pigmentokeratotica, and others. In this regard, molecular genetic studies are an obligatory stage of diagnosis. In the case of our patient, the genetic diagnosis was established in time, which allowed us to take him under dynamic observation and detect colon polyps at the age of 2 years.

Gastrointestinal polyps are found in the majority of patients with CS/PHTS [32], and the lifetime risk of colorectal cancer is 9–16% [33]. This necessitates regular gastro- and colonoscopy; however, according to current standards, such investigations start at the age of 35 years. In this regard, the issue of dynamic follow-up for children with CS/PHTS, especially when polyposis is detected, remains open and requires multicenter studies to elaborate an individual approach to the treatment and management of patients.

Detailed recommendations for children and adolescents with CS/PHTS are presented in the article by Michaela Plamper et al., 2022 [17], but our data demonstrated the necessity of changing the age of beginning follow-up in some positions. For example, the authors suggested starting pelvic tumor screening (yearly testicular/uterine and ovarian ultrasound) at 10 years. Nevertheless, all three girls from our cases (ID8, 11, and ID12) were diagnosed with germ cell tumors at 4, 7, and 8 years. Lung and kidney examinations may also be added to the annual screening plan because of the possibility of pneumocytoma and renal cell carcinoma from puberty, as in the case of our patient ID13.

Establishing this diagnosis in adult patients can be difficult given the differential expression of clinical manifestations and incomplete penetrance, making it important to carefully analyze the pedigree and perform segregation analysis for the next of kin of patients with already verified CS/PHTS. Paternal transmission of pathogenic variants in the *PTEN* gene was noted in three of the six cases we describe. In all cases, the fathers were completely unaware of their diagnosis until the pathogenic variant of the *PTEN* gene was found in their children. At the same time, early diagnosis in these fathers would have decreased the birth of sick offspring using programs of prenatal diagnostics of the fetus or preimplantation diagnosis of embryos in cases of extracorporeal fertilization.

Genetic analysis is important not only for the further planning of pregnancy in patients but also for the prognosis of the disease. Clinical and genetic correlations in patients with CS/PHTS are now widely investigated. For example, in the article by Hendricks LA et al. 2022 [34], the largest number of mutations in patients with CS/PHTS was localized in exon 5 of the *PTEN* gene. Missense variants were associated with earlier disease manifestation, macrocephaly, and developmental delay, while variants leading to premature stop codon formation were more frequently observed in patients with later disease onset, as well as skin, thyroid, and cancer pathologies [34].

Among our patients, mutations in exon 5 were also predominant, and developmental delay was observed only in patients with nonsense mutations, coinciding with the data of the above study (Figure 11). However, all patients with malignancies in our sample had missense mutations or a splice site mutation (ID11), and only lymphoma was observed in a father at 44 years of age with a nonsense mutation from clinical case N°2 (ID7). The correlation with the cancer incidence, depending on the type of mutation, is probably not present in the pediatric population.

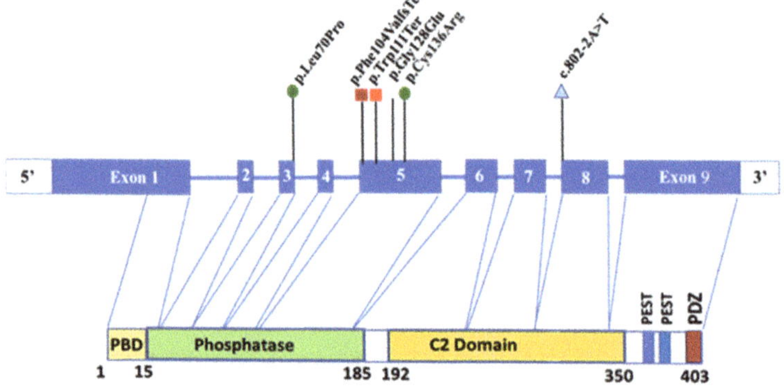

Figure 11. The distribution of pathogenic variants in the *PTEN* gene found in this study.

Additionally, we searched for articles mentioning mutations similar to those identified in our study to better compare phenotypic features. For the variants c.380G>A, c.332G>A, and c.802-2A>T, no clinical description of patients is provided.

The c.406T>C variant (p.Cys136Arg) has been mentioned more than 20 times (including in papers on molecular analyses of the altered function of the encoded protein and large statistical studies). Different clinical manifestations have been described: multiple spinal angiomas and follicular thyroid carcinoma on the background of multinodular goiter [35]; BRRS with arteriovenous malformation [36] and multinodular goiter in 18 years of age, multiple polyps, and ovarian cysts [37]. Our patient ID13 also had vascular pathology in the form of lymphangioma, follicular thyroid adenomas, and renal cell carcinoma. Multiple cancers in the form of thyroid cancer, endometrial cancer, and breast cancer were described in an adult female patient with this mutation [38], and a case of cancer metastasis to cancer in a 75-year-old patient is also known [39]. Cancer in childhood has been described in two patients: an endometrial cancer at 15 years of age and an ovarian tumor at 6 years of age [40]. However, other studies have not found an association with vascular pathology, thyroid pathology, and childhood malignancies in patients with this mutation [41].

The variant c.209T>C (p.Leu70Pro) is quite rare, and only one described case of follicular TC in a 31-year-old male was found in the literature. The patient's mother had breast cancer at 49 and 53 years of age and endometrial cancer at 63 years of age [42]. Our patient ID12 had no thyroid pathology but was treated for a malignant germ cell tumor of the left ovary at the age of 8 years. Considering the realization of most of the malignancies in CS/PHTS in adulthood, the clinical picture may be complementary; therefore, the patient is under dynamic follow-up with an oncologist.

Thus, even with the same *PTEN* mutation, an extremely wide range of clinical manifestations can be observed, both within the same family and between family cases.

This study has several limitations. Firstly, it is a small sample of CS/PHTS cases with atypical manifestations that were investigated in a single clinical center. Secondly, the NGS gene panel used in this study included only genes associated with cancer, while other genes that could have caused macrosomia were not investigated. Thirdly, only the probands were tested using targeted sequencing, whereas their relatives were examined using direct sequencing to identify a specific genetic defect. Fourth, in some cases, the parents or family members of patients with CS/PHTS were not available or refused to undergo genetic testing to determine the status of the *PTEN* gene.

5. Conclusions

The clinical cases described in this article raise the question of a possible expansion of the spectrum of cancers associated with Cowden syndrome by considering pediatric germ cell tumors. The clinical cases also highlight the importance of revising the current guidelines to include patients under 18 years of age in screening programs, not only for thyroid but also for renal cell carcinoma and polyposis. All patients should have their diagnosis verified by molecular genetic methods, as well as undergo a thorough examination for possible clinical manifestations and family history collection to identify all relatives with suspected Cowden syndrome.

Supplementary Materials: The following supporting information can be downloaded at https://www.mdpi.com/article/10.3390/diagnostics15121456/s1, Table S1. List of genes in the panel for DNA sequencing; Table S2. Pairs of primers for the mutations in the *PTEN* gene are described in the article.

Author Contributions: Conceptualization, T.B. and T.N., methodology, E.Z., V.S., I.K. (Irina Kletskaya) and D.S.; software, I.B. and V.S.; validation, E.Z., Y.V., I.K. (Irina Kletskaya) and A.M.; formal analysis, D.S., I.K. (Ivan Karasev) and T.V.; investigation, E.Z., I.B. and V.S.; resources, T.B., E.S., I.K. (Irina Kletskaya) and T.N.; data curation, D.R. and I.K. (Ivan Karasev); writing—original draft preparation, E.Z. and E.S.; writing—review and editing, A.F., I.K. (Ivan Karasev), T.V. and T.N.; visualization, T.B., I.B., A.F., V.S., Y.V., I.K. (Irina Kletskaya) and A.M.; supervision, T.B. and T.N.; project administration, T.B.; funding acquisition, T.B. and D.R. All authors have read and agreed to the published version of the manuscript.

Funding: This work was funded by the Ministry of Health of the Russian Federation (the project "Personalized approaches to the treatment of malignant neoplasms in children with genodermatoses", code NUYO-2023-0007).

Institutional Review Board Statement: The study was conducted according to the guidelines of the Declaration of Helsinki and approved by the Ethics Committee of N.N. Blokhin National Medical Research Center of Oncology (no. 2 from 29 February 2024).

Informed Consent Statement: Informed consent was obtained from all subjects involved in the study. The consent for publication has been obtained from their relatives or guardians.

Data Availability Statement: The original contributions presented in the study are included in the article. Further inquiries can be directed to the corresponding author.

Conflicts of Interest: Author Denis Romanov was employed by the company Limited Liability Company. The remaining authors declare that the research was conducted in the absence of any commercial or financial relationships that could be construed as a potential conflict of interest.

Abbreviations

CS/PHTS	Cowden syndrome (or *PTEN* hamartoma tumor syndrome)
CS	Cowden syndrome
ASD	Autism spectrum disorder
BRRS	Bannayan–Riley–Ruvalcaba syndrome
ACMG	American College of Medical Genetics and Genomics
PM	Pathogenic moderate
PS	Pathogenic strong
M	Macrocephaly
DD	Developmental delay
DSD	Delayed speech development
WT	Wild type
PCT	Polychemotherapy
R-CHOP	Rituximab, cyclophosphamide, doxorubicin hydrochloride, vincristine sulfate, prednisone
TIRADS	Thyroid Imaging Reporting and Data System
MRI	Magnetic resonance imaging
NGS	Next-generation sequencing
MALT	Mucosa-associated lymphoid tissue
RCC	Renal-cell carcinoma
TC	Thyroid cancer

References

1. Garofola, C.; Jamal, Z.; Gross, G.P. *Cowden Disease*; StatPearls Publishing: Treasure Island, FL, USA, 2023.
2. Nelen, M.R.; Kremer, H.; Konings, I.B.; Schoute, F.; van Essen, A.J.; Koch, R.; Woods, C.G.; Fryns, J.-P.; Hamel, B.; Hoefsloot, L.H.; et al. Novel PTEN mutations in patients with Cowden disease: Absence of clear genotype–phenotype correlations. *Eur. J. Hum. Genet.* **1999**, *7*, 267–273. [CrossRef] [PubMed]
3. Molvi, M.; Sharma, Y.K.; Dash, K. Cowden Syndrome: Case Report, Update and Proposed Diagnostic and Surveillance Routines. *Indian J. Dermatol.* **2015**, *60*, 255–259. [CrossRef] [PubMed]
4. Cavaillé, M.; Crampon, D.; Achim, V.; Bubien, V.; Uhrhammer, N.; Privat, M.; Ponelle-Chachuat, F.; Gay-Bellile, M.; Lepage, M.; Ouedraogo, Z.G.; et al. Diagnosis of PTEN mosaicism: The relevance of additional tumor DNA sequencing. A case report and review of the literature. *BMC Med. Genom.* **2023**, *16*, 166. [CrossRef] [PubMed]
5. Hendricks, L.A.; Schuurs-Hoeijmakers, J.; Spier, I.; Haadsma, M.L.; Eijkelenboom, A.; Cremer, K.; Mensenkamp, A.R.; Aretz, S.; Vos, J.R.; Hoogerbrugge, N. Catch them if you are aware: PTEN postzygotic mosaicism in clinically suspicious patients with PTEN Hamartoma Tumour Syndrome and literature review. *Eur. J. Med. Genet.* **2022**, *65*, 104533. [CrossRef]
6. Pritchard, C.C.; Smith, C.; Marushchak, T.; Koehler, K.; Holmes, H.; Raskind, W.; Walsh, T.; Bennett, R.L. A mosaic PTEN mutation causing Cowden syndrome identified by deep sequencing. *Anesthesia Analg.* **2013**, *15*, 1004–1007. [CrossRef]
7. Mester, J.; Charis, E. PTEN hamartoma tumor syndrome. *Handb. Clin. Neurol.* **2015**, *132*, 129–137.
8. Tan, M.-H.; Mester, J.; Peterson, C.; Yang, Y.; Chen, J.-L.; Rybicki, L.A.; Milas, K.; Pederson, H.; Remzi, B.; Orloff, M.S.; et al. A clinical scoring system for selection of patients for PTEN mutation testing is proposed on the basis of a prospective study of 3042 probands. *Am. J. Hum. Genet.* **2011**, *88*, 42–56. [CrossRef]

9. Takayama, T.; Muguruma, N.; Igarashi, M.; Ohsumi, S.; Oka, S.; Kakuta, F.; Kubo, Y.; Kumagai, H.; Sasaki, M.; Sugai, T.; et al. Clinical Guidelines for Diagnosis and Management of Cowden Syndrome/PTEN Hamartoma Tumor Syndrome in Children and Adults-Secondary Publication. *J. Anus Rectum Colon.* **2023**, *7*, 284–300. [CrossRef]
10. Tischkowitz, M.; Colas, C.; Pouwels, S.; Hoogerbrugge, N. PHTS Guideline Development Group; European Reference Network GENTURIS. Cancer Surveillance Guideline for individuals with PTEN hamartoma tumor syndrome. *Eur. J. Hum. Genet.* **2020**, *28*, 1387–1393. [CrossRef]
11. Hendricks, L.A.J.; Hoogerbrugge, N.; Schuurs-Hoeijmakers, J.H.M.; Vos, J.R. A review on age-related cancer risks in PTEN hamartoma tumor syndrome. *Clin. Genet.* **2021**, *99*, 219–225. [CrossRef]
12. Tuli, G.; Munarin, J.; Mussa, A.; Carli, D.; Gastaldi, R.; Borgia, P.; Vigone, M.C.; Abbate, M.; Ferrero, G.B.; De Sanctis, L. Thyroid nodular disease and PTEN mutation in a multicentre series of children with PTEN hamartoma tumor syndrome (PHTS). *Endocrine* **2021**, *74*, 632–637. [CrossRef] [PubMed]
13. Ciaccio, C.; Saletti, V.; D'Arrigo, S.; Esposito, S.; Alfei, E.; Moroni, I.; Tonduti, D.; Chiapparini, L.; Pantaleoni, C.; Milani, D. Clinical spectrum of PTEN mutation in pediatric patients. A bicenter experience. *Eur. J. Med. Genet.* **2019**, *62*, 103596. [CrossRef] [PubMed]
14. Jonker, L.; Lebbink, C.; Jongmans, M.; Nievelstein, R.; Merks, J.; van Dijkum, E.N.; Links, T.; Hoogerbrugge, N.; van Trotsenburg, A.; van Santen, H. Recommendations on surveillance for differentiated thyroid carcinoma in children with PTEN hamartoma tumor syndrome. *Eur. Thyroid. J.* **2020**, *9*, 234–242. [CrossRef]
15. Zelenova, E.; Belysheva, T.; Sofronov, D.; Semenova, V.; Radjabova, G.; Vishnevskaya, Y.; Kletskaya, I.; Sharapova, E.; Karasev, I.; Romanov, D.; et al. Cutaneous Metastasis of Rectal Cancer as a Diagnostic Challenge: A Clinical Case and Literature Review. *Diagnostics* **2024**, *14*, 2420. [CrossRef]
16. Bricheva, E.B.; Nagaeva, E.V.; Brovin, D.N.; Bondarenko, E.V.; Sheremeta, M.S.; Bezlepkina, O.B.; Olina, T.S.; Kovalenko, T.V. Thyroid cancer in a child with Cowden syndrome. *Probl. Endocrinol.* **2024**, *70*, 84–90. (In Russian) [CrossRef]
17. Plamper, M.; Gohlke, B.; Woelfle, J. PTEN hamartoma tumor syndrome in childhood and adolescence—A comprehensive review and presentation of the German pediatric guideline. *Mol. Cell. Pediatr.* **2022**, *9*, 3. [CrossRef] [PubMed] [PubMed Central]
18. Galli, E.; D'alò, F.; Cuccaro, A.; Alma, E.; Maiolo, E.; Brugnoletti, F.; Larocca, L.M.; Zollino, M.; Bacigalupo, A.P.; Hohaus, S. Burkitt Lymphoma as Fourth Neoplasia in a Patient Affected by Cowden Syndrome with a Novel PTEN Germline Pathogenic Variant. *Mediterr. J. Hematol. Infect. Dis.* **2020**, *12*, e2020034. [CrossRef]
19. Cavaillé, M.; Ponelle-Chachuat, F.; Uhrhammer, N.; Viala, S.; Gay-Bellile, M.; Privat, M.; Bidet, Y.; Bignon, Y.-J. Early Onset Multiple Primary Tumors in Atypical Presentation of Cowden Syndrome Identified by Whole-Exome-Sequencing. *Front. Genet.* **2018**, *9*, 353. [CrossRef]
20. Hagelstrom, R.T.; Ford, J.; Reiser, G.M.; Nelson, M.; Pickering, D.L.; Althof, P.A.; Sanger, W.G.; Coccia, P.F. Breast Cancer and Non-Hodgkin Lymphoma in a Young Male with Cowden Syndrome. *Pediatr. Blood Cancer* **2016**, *63*, 544–546. [CrossRef]
21. Bubien, V.; Bonnet, F.; Brouste, V.; Hoppe, S.; Barouk-Simonet, E.; David, A.; Edery, P.; Bottani, A.; Layet, V.; Caron, O.; et al. High cumulative risks of cancer in patients with PTEN hamartoma tumor syndrome. *J. Med. Genet.* **2013**, *50*, 255–263. [CrossRef]
22. Haibach, H.; Burns, T.W.; Carlson, H.E.; Burman, K.D.; Deftos, L.J. Multiple hamartoma syndrome (Cowden's disease) associated with renal cell carcinoma and primary neuroendocrine carcinoma of the skin (Merkel cell carcinoma). *Am. J. Clin. Pathol.* **1992**, *97*, 705–712. [CrossRef] [PubMed]
23. Mester, J.L.; Zhou, M.; Prescott, N.; Eng, C. Papillary renal cell carcinoma is associated with PTEN hamartoma tumor syndrome. *Urology* **2012**, *79*, 1187.e1–1187.e7. [CrossRef] [PubMed]
24. Kim, R.H.; Wang, X.; Evans, A.J.; Campbell, S.C.; Nguyen, J.K.; Farncombe, K.M.; Eng, C. Early-onset renal cell carcinoma in PTEN harmatoma tumor syndrome. *NPJ Genom. Med.* **2020**, *5*, 40. [CrossRef] [PubMed]
25. Smpokou, P.; Fox, V.L.; Tan, W.H. PTEN hamartoma tumor syndrome: Early tumor development in children. *Arch. Dis. Child.* **2015**, *100*, 34–37. [CrossRef]
26. Kouzuki, K.; Umeda, K.; Kawasaki, H.; Isobe, K.; Akazawa, R.; Tasaka, K.; Tanaka, K.; Kubota, H.; Saida, S.; Kato, I.; et al. Immature teratoma of the ovary associated with Cowden syndrome. *Pediatr. Blood Cancer* **2022**, *69*, e29555. [CrossRef]
27. Cho, M.Y.; Kim, H.S.; Eng, C.; Kim, D.S.; Kang, S.J.; Eom, M.; Yi, S.Y.; Bronner, M.P. First report of ovarian dysgerminoma in Cowden syndrome with germline PTEN mutation and PTEN-related 10q loss of tumor heterozygosity. *Am. J. Surg. Pathol.* **2008**, *32*, 1258–1264. [CrossRef]
28. Tullius, B.P.; Shankar, S.P.; Cole, S.; Triano, V.; Aradhya, S.; Huang, E.C.; Sanchez, T.; Pawar, A. Novel heterozygous mutation in the PTEN gene associated with ovarian germ cell tumor complicated by growing teratoma syndrome and overgrowth in a two-year-old female. *Pediatr. Blood Cancer* **2019**, *66*, e27788. [CrossRef]
29. Devi, M.; Leonard, N.; Silverman, S.; Al-Qahtani, M.; Girgis, R. Testicular mixed germ cell tumor in an adolescent with cowden disease. *Oncology* **2007**, *72*, 194–196. [CrossRef]
30. Hildenbrand, C.; Burgdorf, W.H.; Lautenschlager, S. Cowden syndrome-diagnostic skin signs. *Dermatology* **2001**, *202*, 362–366. [CrossRef]

31. Plana-Pla, A.; Condal, L.; Jaka, A.; Blanco, I.; Castellanos, E.; Bielsa, I. Verrucous epidermal nevus as a manifestation of a type 2 mosaic PTEN mutation in Cowden syndrome. *Pediatr. Dermatol.* **2023**, *40*, 179–181. [CrossRef]
32. Isa, H.M.; Mohamed, Z.S.; Isa, Z.H.; Busehail, M.Y.; Alaradi, Z.A. Cowden Syndrome: A Rare Cause of Intestinal Polyposis. *Cureus* **2024**, *16*, e64838. [CrossRef] [PubMed]
33. Tan, M.H.; Mester, J.L.; Ngeow, J.; Rybicki, L.A.; Orloff, M.S.; Eng, C. Lifetime cancer risks in individuals with germline PTEN mutations. *Clin. Cancer Res.* **2012**, *18*, 400–407. [CrossRef] [PubMed]
34. Hendricks, L.A.; Hoogerbrugge, N.; Venselaar, H.; Aretz, S.; Spier, I.; Legius, E.; Brems, H.; de Putter, R.; Claes, K.B.; Evans, D.G.; et al. Genotype-phenotype associations in a large PTEN Hamartoma Tumor Syndrome (PHTS) patient cohort. *Eur. J. Med. Genet.* **2022**, *65*, 104632. [CrossRef] [PubMed]
35. Jenny, B.; Radovanovic, I.; Haenggeli, C.A.; Delavelle, J.; Rüfenacht, D.; Kaelin, A.; Blouin, J.L.; Bottani, A.; Rilliet, B. Association of multiple vertebral hemangiomas and severe paraparesis in a patient with a PTEN hamartoma tumor syndrome: Case report. *J. Neurosurg.* **2007**, *107* (Suppl. S4), 307–313. [CrossRef]
36. Paparo, L.; Rossi, G.B.; Delrio, P.; Rega, D.; Duraturo, F.; Liccardo, R.; Debellis, M.; Izzo, P.; De Rosa, M. Differential expression of PTEN gene correlates with phenotypic heterogeneity in three cases of patients showing clinical manifestations of PTEN hamartoma tumour syndrome. *Hered. Cancer Clin. Pract.* **2013**, *11*, 8. [CrossRef]
37. Kubo, Y.; Urano, Y.; Hida, Y.; Ikeuchi, T.; Nomoto, M.; Kunitomo, K.; Arase, S. A novel PTEN mutation in a Japanese patient with Cowden disease. *Br. J. Dermatol.* **2000**, *142*, 1100–1105. [CrossRef]
38. Ngeow, J.; Stanuch, K.; Mester, J.L.; Barnholtz-Sloan, J.S.; Eng, C. Second malignant neoplasms in patients with cowden syndrome with underlying germline PTEN mutations. *J. Clin. Oncol.* **2014**, *32*, 1818–1824. [CrossRef]
39. Matsumoto, K.; Nosaka, K.; Shiomi, T.; Matsuoka, Y.; Umekita, Y. Tumor-to-tumor metastases in Cowden's disease: An autopsy case report and review of the literature. *Diagn. Pathol.* **2015**, *10*, 172. [CrossRef]
40. Pena-Couso, L.; Ercibengoa, M.; Mercadillo, F.; Gómez-Sánchez, D.; Inglada-Pérez, L.; Santos, M.; Lanillos, J.; Gutiérrez-Abad, D.; Hernández, A.; Carbonell, P.; et al. Considerations on diagnosis and surveillance measures of PTEN hamartoma tumor syndrome: Clinical and genetic study in a series of Spanish patients. *Orphanet J. Rare Dis.* **2022**, *17*, 85. [CrossRef]
41. Gervas, P.; Molokov, A.; Schegoleva, A.; Kiselev, A.; Babyshkina, N.; Pisareva, L.; Tyukalov, Y.; Choynzonov, E.; Cherdyntseva, N. New germline mutations in non-BRCA genes among breast cancer women of Mongoloid origin. *Mol. Biol. Rep.* **2020**, *47*, 5315–5321. [CrossRef]
42. Marsh, D.J.; Dahia, P.L.; Caron, S.; Kum, J.B.; Frayling, I.M.; Tomlinson, I.P.; Hughes, K.S.; Eeles, R.A.; Hodgson, S.V.; Murday, V.A.; et al. Germline PTEN mutations in Cowden syndrome-like families. *J. Med. Genet.* **1998**, *35*, 881–885. [CrossRef]

diagnostics

MDPI

Article

Growth Assessment and Nutritional Status in Children with Congenital Adrenal Hyperplasia—A Cross-Sectional Study from a Vietnamese Tertiary Pediatric Center

Thi Thuy Hong Nguyen [1], Khanh Minh Le [1], Thi Anh Thuong Tran [1,2], Khanh Ngoc Nguyen [1,2], Thi Bich Ngoc Can [1,2], Phuong Thao Bui [2], Dat Tien Tran [1] and Chi Dung Vu [1,2,*]

1 Department of Paediatrics, Hanoi Medical University, Hanoi 11521, Vietnam; bshong@hmu.edu.vn (T.T.H.N.); lekhanhminhmj111@gmail.com (K.M.L.); trananhthuong@hmu.edu.vn (T.A.T.T.); khanhnn@nch.gov.vn (K.N.N.); ngocctb@nch.gov.vn (T.B.N.C.); trantiendat1008@gmail.com (D.T.T.)

2 Center for Endocrinology, Metabolism, Genetic/Genomics and Molecular Therapy, Vietnam National Children's Hospital, Hanoi 11512, Vietnam; thaobp@nch.gov.vn

* Correspondence: dungvu@nch.gov.vn

Abstract: Background/Objectives: Children with congenital adrenal hyperplasia (CAH) face significant risks of impaired growth and metabolic disturbances despite standard glucocorticoid therapy. This cross-sectional study aimed to evaluate growth outcomes, nutritional status, and associated factors among children with CAH treated in a Vietnamese tertiary pediatric center. **Methods:** We assessed 201 children aged 1.1–16.5 years in a tertiary pediatric center in Vietnam for anthropometric parameters, biochemical markers (calcium, phosphate, 25-hydroxyvitamin D), and clinical features. Growth status was evaluated using WHO standards, and bone age was assessed radiographically. Statistical analyses explored associations between growth outcomes and clinical, biochemical, and treatment-related factors. **Results**: Stunting was present in 16.4% of children, while 53.3% were overweight or obese. Bone age advancement occurred in 51.7% of cases. Vitamin D insufficiency or deficiency was detected in 85.6% of patients, and hypocalcemia was present in 85.1%. Overweight/obesity, vitamin D deficiency, and bone age advancement were associated with older age, prolonged corticosteroid therapy, higher androgen levels, and clinical features of treatment imbalance (e.g., Cushingoid appearance, hyperpigmentation). Female sex was significantly associated with higher rates of stunting. **Conclusions**: Growth impairment, nutritional deficiencies, and skeletal maturation disturbances are prevalent among children with CAH in Vietnam. Early identification of risk factors and the implementation of tailored management strategies that address both endocrine and nutritional health are crucial for optimizing long-term outcomes.

Keywords: congenital adrenal hyperplasia; CAH; growth; bone age; obesity; vitamin D deficiency; calcium deficiency; Vietnamese children; glucocorticoid treatment

1. Introduction

Congenital adrenal hyperplasia (CAH) represents a group of autosomal recessive disorders characterized by enzymatic deficiencies in adrenal steroid biosynthesis [1]. Among these, 21-hydroxylase deficiency, caused by mutations in the *CYP21A2* gene, is the most prevalent, accounting for over 90% of cases globally [2]. This enzymatic defect disrupts cortisol and aldosterone production, leading to compensatory stimulation of adrenocorticotropic hormone (ACTH) and excessive adrenal androgen secretion. As a result, affected

 https://doi.org/10.3390/diagnostics15121534

children may exhibit clinical signs ranging from ambiguous genitalia at birth to early-onset puberty and metabolic disturbances [1].

The global incidence of CAH is estimated to range between 1 in 14,000 and 1 in 18,000 live births [1]. However, recent meta-analyses suggest that incidence rates may be increasing in certain populations, with reports as high as 1 in 9498 births [2,3]. Notably, incidence varies by geographic region and ethnic group, with higher rates observed in the Eastern Mediterranean and Southeast Asian populations [3].

The clinical presentation of CAH in infancy and childhood varies by the severity of the enzyme defect [4]. Classic CAH, particularly the salt-wasting form, often manifests during the neonatal period with vomiting, dehydration, hypotension, and hypoglycemia—hallmarks of adrenal insufficiency. Girls with classic 21-hydroxylase deficiency present with ambiguous genitalia, whereas affected boys exhibit subtle signs such as hyperpigmentation and penile enlargement. Without adequate treatment, prolonged androgen exposure leads to rapid growth, early pubic hair, and advanced bone age, and may trigger centrally mediated precocious puberty [5].

Beyond the endocrine abnormalities, CAH is increasingly recognized for its impact on somatic growth and nutritional health. A 2010 meta-analysis found that adult patients with CAH had a mean height approximately 10 cm below population norms, with a standard deviation score of −1.4 [6]. A 2018 study on children with congenital adrenal hyperplasia reported that 17.6% of patients were obese, and 25.7% exhibited short stature [7]. Obesity is another common finding in pediatric CAH. Approximately one-third of children are overweight or obese, with prevalence increasing markedly by age four [8–10].

Micronutrient deficiencies—especially vitamin D—have emerged as prevalent issues in CAH. A 2012 study of 244 patients revealed that 61% had suboptimal vitamin D levels, potentially due to the effects of prolonged corticosteroid therapy [8].

These outcomes are driven by both the disease pathology and its treatment. Excess adrenal androgens can prematurely advance skeletal maturation, compromising final height despite transient increases in growth velocity during early childhood. Studies have shown that affected children, especially those with the classic form, are prone to short stature, obesity, and altered body composition [11–13].

Simultaneously, managing the lifelong glucocorticoid therapy required for CAH presents a significant clinical challenge [14]. Clinicians must balance the consequences of undertreatment, such as androgen excess leading to virilization and premature bone age advancement, with the risks of overtreatment from the necessary supraphysiologic steroid doses. Excessive glucocorticoid exposure is well known to suppress linear growth and contributes to obesity, low bone mineral density, and other long-term cardiometabolic complications. These adverse effects tend to become more pronounced in children undergoing treatment for more than five years [10,15–18]. Furthermore, corticosteroids are known to impair vitamin D metabolism by increasing 24-hydroxylase activity, which accelerates the degradation of 25(OH)D [19].

While international studies have highlighted the long-term health risks in CAH, research in some regions remains limited. In Vietnam, for example, few studies have comprehensively evaluated physical development and nutritional status in children with CAH. A study by Nguyen et al. found that early diagnosis and adequate treatment adherence were critical to optimizing physical development in CAH children [20]. To our knowledge, this is the first study in Vietnam to simultaneously evaluate both growth development and nutritional status in children with CAH. Therefore, gaps remain regarding the long-term implications of glucocorticoid therapy on bone health, nutritional status, and growth outcomes, particularly in resource-limited settings. These challenges are often exacerbated by systemic barriers to care. For instance, a recent review by Eitel and

Fechner noted that access to universal newborn screening, widely recognized as the most effective strategy for early diagnosis, remains limited in many low- and middle-income countries [21]. In Vietnam, as of 2019, only an estimated 40% of newborns had access to comprehensive screening programs [22,23]. The potential for delayed diagnosis, combined with constrained access to multidisciplinary care, underscores the urgent need to assess real-world growth and nutritional outcomes in this specific population.

This study aimed to investigate the growth outcomes, nutritional indicators, and associated factors among 201 Vietnamese children with CAH at the Vietnam National Children's Hospital.

2. Materials and Methods

2.1. Subjects

This cross-sectional descriptive study was conducted on children diagnosed with congenital adrenal hyperplasia (CAH). Eligible participants were aged 1 to 17 years, in accordance with the World Health Organization's (WHO) child age classification (WHO, 2006) [24]. All patients included had a confirmed diagnosis of CAH in accordance with the Endocrine Society Clinical Practice Guidelines (2018) [2] (see Supplementary Materials S1) and had been undergoing treatment for at least 12 months.

Exclusion criteria included the presence of other chronic medical conditions or congenital malformations, such as congenital heart disease, epilepsy, or cancer.

The study was approved by the Institutional Review Board of Vietnam National Children's Hospital (protocol code 2685/BVNTW-HĐĐĐ, approved on 10 October 2024) in accordance with current legislation, the Declaration of Helsinki, and standards of good clinical practice. Informed consent was obtained from all parents or legal guardians of the children included in the study.

The study was conducted from July 2024 to April 2025 at the Center for Endocrinology, Metabolism, Genetics, and Molecular Therapy, Vietnam National Children's Hospital.

2.2. Clinical and Biochemical Assessments

Clinical data were collected through structured interviews, clinical examinations, and retrospective medical record reviews.

In alignment with the 2018 Endocrine Society Clinical Practice Guidelines for the management of congenital adrenal hyperplasia [2], we evaluated clinically relevant variables reflecting both undertreatment and overtreatment. These included signs of inadequate androgen suppression, such as hyperpigmentation, virilization (clitoromegaly in females, penile enlargement in males, hirsutism, acne, and other manifestations of androgen excess), as well as signs of glucocorticoid excess, like Cushingoid features (weight gain, truncal obesity, moon facies, facial plethora) [25] or acanthosis nigricans. Clinical history of adrenal crises was not formally quantified due to the retrospective nature of data collection and the potential for recall bias. Precocious puberty is defined as the appearance of secondary sexual characteristics before age 8 in girls and before age 9 in boys [26]. The diagnosis was based on clinical signs such as breast development in girls or testicular volume $\geq$ 4 mL in boys, rapid height growth, and bone age advanced by more than two standard deviations [26–31]. A baseline LH > 0.3 mIU/mL or stimulated peak LH > 5 mIU/mL confirms CPP, while suppressed LH/FSH with elevated sex steroid levels indicates PPP [32–37]. Imaging studies (pelvic/testicular ultrasound, brain MRI) and hormone testing (estradiol, testosterone, 17-OHP) were used to confirm the diagnosis and assess underlying etiologies [34,36,38–43].

Anthropometric assessments included weight, length/height, and body mass index (BMI), evaluated in accordance with the WHO Growth Standards (WHO 2006 for children under 5 years [24] and WHO 2007 for those aged 5 years and older [44]):

BMI: For children < 5 years—severe thinness (<−3 SD), thinness (−3 to <−2 SD), normal (−2 to +2 SD), overweight (>+2 to +3 SD), obesity (>+3 SD); for children ≥ 5 years—severe thinness (<−3 SD), thinness (−3 to <−2 SD), normal (−2 to +1 SD), overweight (>+1 to +2 SD), obesity (>+2 SD).

Height-for-age z-score (HAZ): normal (HAZ ≥ −2 SD), stunted (HAZ < −2 SD), and severely stunted (HAZ < −3 SD).

Weight was measured using a digital scale, and height or length was assessed using a stadiometer or recumbent length board, depending on the child's age and ability to stand.

Bone age was determined from standard radiographs of the left hand and wrist performed at the Department of Diagnostic Imaging using the Carestream DRX1-System (Carestream Health, Washington, DC, USA). All images were interpreted by trained radiologists employing the Greulich and Pyle atlas. BA-CA Classification: Categorization of skeletal maturation based on the comparison between bone age (BA) and chronological age (CA), where BA > CA indicates advanced bone age, BA = CA indicates bone age matches chronological age, and BA < CA indicates delayed bone age.

Biochemical analyses included measurements of total serum calcium, ionized calcium, and serum phosphate, performed using colorimetric absorption methods on a Beckman Coulter AU5800 analyzer (Beckman Coulter, Tokyo, Japan). Serum 25-hydroxyvitamin D [25(OH)D] levels were determined by electrochemiluminescence immunoassay on the same analyzer. Serum 17-hydroxyprogesterone was quantified using a semi-automated ELISA on a Biotek system (Biotek, Winooski, VT, USA), and testosterone levels were measured via electrochemiluminescence immunoassay on a Cobas E601 analyzer (Roche Diagnostics, Tokyo, Japan). All laboratory analyses were conducted at the Biochemistry Department. The reference ranges for each parameter were applied accordingly:

- 25-hydroxyvitamin D [25(OH)D]: deficiency: <50 nmol/L; insufficiency: 50–72.5 nmol/L [45].
- Total serum calcium, 2.2–2.7 mmol/L; ionized calcium, 1.12–1.23 mmol/L. Serum phosphate levels were interpreted using age-specific reference ranges as follows: 1.25–2.10 mmol/L for children aged 1–3 years, 1.20–1.80 mmol/L for ages 4–11 years, 0.95–1.75 mmol/L for ages 12–15 years, and 0.90–1.50 mmol/L for ages 16–19 years [46].
- 17-hydroxyprogesterone (17-OHP) and testosterone levels were interpreted according to age- and sex-specific reference standards.

The following treatment-related variables were collected: type of glucocorticoid, current daily dose, dosing frequency, and duration of therapy. All glucocorticoid doses were standardized by converting to hydrocortisone equivalents, using the following conversion ratios: 1 mg prednisolone = 5 mg hydrocortisone, and 1 mg dexamethasone = 80 mg hydrocortisone [19,47].

2.3. Data Analysis

All data were entered and processed using SPSS version 20.0 (IBM Corp., Armonk, NY, USA). The distribution of continuous variables was assessed using the Kolmogorov–Smirnov test, which is appropriate for sample sizes greater than 50. Continuous variables were presented as mean ± standard deviation (SD) if normally distributed or as median (minimum–maximum) if non-normally distributed. Categorical variables were expressed as frequencies and percentages.

Comparisons between groups were conducted using the following statistical tests: Independent *t*-test and ANOVA for normally distributed continuous variables; Mann–

Whitney U test and Kruskal–Wallis test for non-parametric variables; chi-squared test and Fisher's exact test for categorical variables depending on sample size. A p-value of <0.05 was considered statistically significant. In addition to p-values, effect sizes or measures of magnitude (e.g., mean differences, odds ratios, or relevant coefficients) were reported where applicable. Quality control measures included predefined inclusion/exclusion criteria, the use of standardized case report forms, and double data entry for validation. For variables with less than 20% missing data—including 17-hydroxyprogesterone (17OHP), ionized calcium, and the difference between bone age and chronological age (BA-CA)—missing values were imputed using the median of the respective variable. This approach was selected to preserve the distributional characteristics of non-normally distributed variables and to minimize potential bias. No variable exceeded the 20% missing data threshold that would require exclusion from analysis.

3. Results

3.1. Description of the Study Sample

A total of 201 children diagnosed with CAH were included in the study. The median age at valuation was 9.8 years, ranging from 1.1 to 16.5 years. Participants originated from 25 provinces across the northern and central regions of Vietnam (Figure 1). The geographic distribution analysis indicated regional variations in the number of reported CAH cases, with higher concentrations observed in certain provinces.

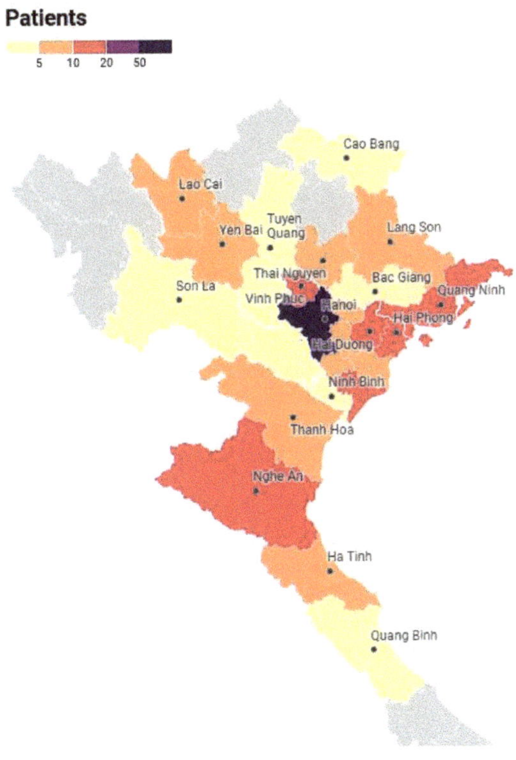

Figure 1. Geographic distribution of the CAH patient population (n = 201).

3.2. Growth Assessment and Nutritional Status

Anthropometric measurements revealed that the median height standard deviation score (SDS) was −0.7 (range: −4.0 to 4.3), and the median body mass index (BMI) SDS was 1.4 (range: −2.7 to 5.2). The median difference between bone age and chronological age (BA-CA) was 1.4 years (range: −8.3 to 8.6), indicating a general trend toward advanced skeletal maturation. Among the 201 patients, 51.7% had an advanced bone age (BA > CA), 38.3% had an age-appropriate bone age (BA = CA), and 10.0% had a delayed bone age (BA < CA). In terms of BMI, 1.5% were classified as thin, 45.3% had normal weight, 24.4% were overweight, and 28.9% were obese. Regarding height-for-age, 4.5% had severe stunting, 11.9% had moderate stunting, and 83.6% had normal stature. Vitamin D insufficiency or deficiency was observed in 85.6% of the sample, while 85.1% exhibited calcium deficiency. Among the 138 patients with available phosphate data, 6.5% were found to have phosphate deficiency (Figure 2). The baseline sociodemographic, clinical, biochemical, and anthropometric characteristics of the study population are presented in Table 1.

Table 1. Clinical characteristics of pediatric patients with CAH.

		Salt-Wasting	Simple Virilizing	Total
Sociodemographic	n	160	41	201
	Female, n (%)	50.6 (81)	56.1 (23)	104 (51.7)
	Age (year)	8.7 ± 4.3	9.8 ± 3.6	9.8 (1.1–16.5)
	Urban area, n (%)	92 (57.5)	20 (48.8)	112 (55.7)
Clinical characteristics	Height SDS	−0.9 (−4.0–2.9)	0.4 (−2.6–4.3)	−0.7 (−4.0–4.3)
	Normal, n (%)	130 (81.2)	38 (92.7)	168 (83.6)
	Moderate stunting, n (%)	21 (13.1)	3 (7.3)	24 (11.9)
	Severe stunting, n (%)	9 (5.6)	0 (0)	9 (4.5)
	BMI SDS	1.4 (−2.7–5.2)	1.2 (−1.0–3.4)	1.4 (−2.7–5.2)
	Thinness, n (%)	3 (1.9)	0 (0)	3 (1.5)
	Normal, n (%)	71 (44.4)	20 (48.8)	91 (45.3)
	Overweight, n (%)	41 (25.6)	8 (19.5)	49 (24.4)
	Obesity, n (%)	45 (28.1)	13 (31.7)	58 (28.9)
	Cushingoid appearance, n (%)	13 (8.1)	4 (9.8)	17 (8.5)
	Hyperpigmentation, n (%)	44 (27.5)	6 (14.6)	50 (24.9)
	Virilization, n (%)	23 (14.4)	8 (19.5)	31 (15.4)
	Central precocious puberty, n (%)	27 (16.9)	20 (48.8)	47 (23.4)
Biochemical and radiological markers	17OHP (nmol/L)	52.4 (0–1182)	57.1 (2.0–925)	52.4 (0–1182)
	Testosterone (nmol/L)	0.24 (0.1–26.3)	0.78 (0.1–29.8)	0.24 (0.1–29.8)
	Bone age (BA) − Chronological age (CA) (year) [1]	0.9 (−8.3–6.5)	2.5 (−1.4–8.6)	1.4 (−8.3–8.6)
	Advanced bone age (BA > CA), n (%)	70 (43.8)	34 (82.9)	104 (51.7)
	Age-appropriate bone age (BA = CA), n (%)	71 (44.4)	6 (14.6)	77 (38.3)
	Delayed bone age (BA < CA), n (%)	19 (11.9)	1 (2.4)	20 (10)
Treatment-related factors	Age at diagnosis and treatment (year) [2]	0 (0–3)	3 (0–9)	0 (0–9)
	Hydrocortisone ($mg/m^2/day$)	16.3 ± 4.4	18.7 ± 3.7	16.8 ± 4.4
	Duration of glucocorticoid therapy (year)	8.6 ± 4.3	6.7 ± 3.6	8.2 ± 4.2

[1] The difference between a patient's bone age and their chronological age; [2] Age at diagnosis and initiation of treatment occurred concurrently and is presented as a single variable.

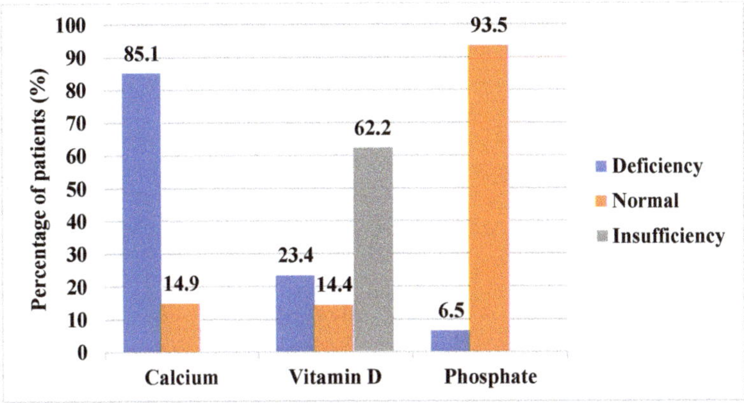

Figure 2. Distribution of calcium, vitamin D, and phosphate status.

3.3. Sociodemographic Factors

3.3.1. Age

Age was significantly associated with several key study outcomes. Children presenting with advanced bone age (BA > CA), higher BMI classifications (overweight/obesity), and vitamin D deficiency were significantly older than their respective comparison groups ($p < 0.001$ for each). A significant association was also observed with hypophosphatemia ($p = 0.039$). Conversely, no significant age differences were found for height-for-age classifications ($p = 0.183$) or the presence of hypocalcemia ($p = 0.24$). The distribution of age across nutritional and biochemical outcomes is summarized in Table 2.

Table 2. Median age and statistical comparisons across nutritional and biochemical outcomes in children with CAH.

Independent Factor	Variable Group	Subgroup	n	Median Age (Years)	*p*-Value
Age at evaluation	Hypocalcemia	Yes	171	0	0.24
		No	30	0	
	Hypophosphatemia	Yes	9	1.5	0.039 *
		No	129	0	
	Vitamin D Status	Deficiency	47	10.3	0.001 *
		Insufficiency	125	10.1	
		Sufficiency	29	5.6	
	BMI Classification	Thinness	3	2.5	<0.001 *
		Normal	91	7.5	
		Overweight	49	10.8	
		Obesity	58	10.5	
	Height-for-Age	Severe stunting	9	4.8	0.183
		Moderate stunting	24	12.7	
		Normal	168	9.7	
	BA-CA Classification	BA > CA	104	10.9	<0.001 *
		BA = CA	77	5.9	
		BA < CA	20	4.6	

* Variable with a significant effect.

3.3.2. Gender Differences

Gender-specific differences were observed in growth parameters among children with CAH. Both hypocalcemia and hypophosphatemia were highly prevalent in males and females, with no statistically significant differences between sexes ($p = 0.168$ and $p = 0.316$, respectively). Similarly, vitamin D status did not differ significantly by gender ($p = 0.875$).

Regarding nutritional status, obesity was more frequently observed in males than in females (35.1% vs. 23.1%), although this difference was not statistically significant ($p = 0.151$), indicating a trend toward significance ($p = 0.057$). In contrast, stunting was significantly more common among females, with 23.1% exhibiting moderate to severe stunting compared to 9.3% of males ($p = 0.003$).

In terms of bone age, delayed maturation was more frequent in females (13.5% vs. 6.2%), though the difference did not reach statistical significance ($p = 0.163$).

3.3.3. Residential Area

No significant differences were observed in the prevalence of hypocalcemia and hypophosphatemia between urban and rural children ($p = 0.073$ and $p = 0.186$, respectively). Vitamin D deficiency was more prevalent among urban children (28.6%) compared to their rural counterparts (16.9%), although the difference was not statistically significant ($p = 0.104$).

Similarly, the combined prevalence of overweight and obesity was higher in urban areas (59.8% combined) than in rural areas (49.4%), but the difference did not reach statistical significance ($p = 0.093$). No significant differences were found between urban and rural groups in height-for-age classification ($p = 0.218$) or patterns of bone age advancement ($p = 0.956$).

3.4. *Disease-Related Factors*

3.4.1. Clinical Phenotype

No significant differences were observed between salt-wasting and simple virilizing forms in the prevalence of hypocalcemia ($p = 0.298$), vitamin D status ($p = 0.337$), BMI classification ($p = 0.796$), or height-for-age classification ($p = 0.203$). In contrast, hypophosphatemia was significantly more prevalent in children with the simple virilizing form compared to those with the salt-wasting form (18.5% vs. 3.6%, $p = 0.014$). Moreover, bone age advancement was substantially more frequent in the simple virilizing group, with 82.9% of individuals showing advanced bone age, compared to 43.8% in the salt-wasting group ($p < 0.001$).

3.4.2. Clinical Disease Control Indicators

Obesity was significantly more prevalent among children with Cushingoid features (41.2% vs. 27.7%, $p = 0.001$, Cramer's V = 0.262) and among those with acanthosis nigricans (80.0% vs. 24.7%, $p < 0.001$, Cramer's V = 0.334) compared to their respective counterparts. Children with hyperpigmentation also demonstrated higher rates of obesity (40.0% vs. 25.2%, $p = 0.045$, Cramer's V = 0.201), as well as more frequent bone age advancement (70.0% vs. 45.7%, $p = 0.005$, Cramer's V = 0.227). Similarly, bone age advancement was more prevalent in children with virilization (77.4% vs. 47.1%, $p = 0.004$, Cramer's V = 0.231) and those with central precocious puberty (80.9% vs. 42.9%, $p < 0.001$, Cramer's V = 0.324).

The prevalence of hypocalcemia was significantly higher among children with hyperpigmentation compared to those without (96.0% vs. 81.5%, respectively; $p = 0.012$, OR = 5.46, 95% CI: 1.25–23.83). Similarly, children with central precocious puberty (CPP) had a significantly higher prevalence of hypocalcemia than those without CPP (95.7% vs. 81.8%; $p = 0.019$, OR = 5.00, 95% CI: 1.145–21.84). Hypophosphatemia was also significantly more common in the CPP group compared to the non-CPP group (14.7% vs. 3.8%; $p = 0.041$, OR = 4.31, 95% CI: 1.086–17.103). No other significant associations were found between the clinical features and the assessed nutritional or growth outcomes (Table 3).

Table 3. Associations between clinical features and nutritional or growth outcomes in children with CAH.

	Cushingoid Appearance		Acanthosis Nigricans		Hyperpigmentation		Virilization		Central Precocious Puberty	
	p-Value	OR (95% CI)	*p*-Value	OR (95% CI)	*p*-Value	OR (95% CI)	*p*-Value	OR (95% CI)	*p*-Value	OR (95% CI)
Hypocalcemia	1 (FET)	0.803 (0.22–2.98)	0.704 (FET)	2.59 (0.33–20.43)	0.012 (X^2) *	5.46 (1.25–23.83)	0.054 (FET)	6.17 (0.81–47.07)	0.019 (X^2) *	5 (1.145–21.84)
Hypophosphatemia	1 (FET)	NA	1 (FET)	NA	0.121 (FET)	3.357 (0.85–13.22)	0.626 (FET)	1.65 (0.319–8.572)	0.041 (FET) *	4.31 (1.086–17.103)
	p-value	Cramer's V	*p*-value	Cramer's V	*p*-value	Cramer's V	*p*-value	Cramer's V	*p*-value	Cramer's V
Vitamin D Status	0.933 (FET)	0.053	0.741 (FET)	0.073	0.131 (X^2)	0.142	0.128 (FET)	0.139	0.142 (X^2)	0.139
BMI Classification	0.001 (FET) *	0.262	< 0.001 (FET) *	0.334	0.045 (FET) *	0.201	0.779 (FET)	0.083	0.392 (FET)	0.132
Height-for-age	0.64 (FET)	0.059	0.852 (FET)	0.08	0.74 (FET)	0.069	0.206 (FET)	0.129	0.168 (FET)	0.138
BA-CA Classification	0.43 (FET)	0.088	0.205 (FET)	0.135	0.005 (FET) *	0.227	0.004 (FET) *	0.231	<0.001 (FET) *	0.324

* Variable with a significant effect. Values in the table represent *p*-values. Statistical tests used include the chi-squared test (χ^2) and Fisher's exact test (FET), depending on expected cell counts. NA indicates comparisons where odds ratios could not be calculated due to zero counts in one or more cells.

3.4.3. Biochemical Markers

Median 17-hydroxyprogesterone (17-OHP) levels were higher in children with hypocalcemia (52.4 nmol/L) than in those without hypocalcemia (39.7 nmol/L), although this difference approached but did not reach statistical significance ($p = 0.137$). In contrast, median testosterone concentrations were significantly elevated in the hypocalcemia group (0.24 nmol/L) compared to the non-hypocalcemia group (0.09 nmol/L, $p = < 0.001$).

Regarding hypophosphatemia, children with the condition had slightly lower median 17-OHP levels compared to those without (47.8 vs. 55.1 nmol/L); however, this difference was not statistically significant ($p = 0.103$). Likewise, testosterone levels did not differ significantly between the groups ($p = 0.543$). Testosterone levels also varied significantly by vitamin D status ($p = 0.027$), with lower median concentrations observed in children with normal vitamin D levels (0.09 nmol/L) compared to those with deficiency or insufficiency (both 0.24 nmol/L). In contrast, median 17-OHP levels did not differ significantly across vitamin D categories: 55.8 nmol/L in the deficient group, 52.35 nmol/L in the insufficiency group, and 31.3 nmol/L in the normal group ($p = 0.317$).

Regarding growth parameters, 17-OHP levels differed significantly across BMI categories ($p = 0.014$), with the highest median concentration observed in children with obesity (107.5 nmol/L). In contrast, testosterone levels did not significantly vary by BMI classification ($p = 0.083$).

In relation to height-for-age, children with severe stunting showed a trend toward lower testosterone levels (median 0.09 nmol/L) compared to those with moderate stunting or normal status (both 0.24 nmol/L), although the difference did not reach statistical significance ($p = 0.053$). No significant differences were observed in 17-OHP levels across height-for-age groups ($p = 0.131$).

Bone age advancement was significantly associated with hormonal levels. Children with an advanced bone age (BA > CA) had the highest median testosterone levels

(0.78 nmol/L, $p < 0.001$) and 17-OHP levels (69.6 nmol/L, $p = 0.005$) compared to those whose BA was equal to or less than their chronological age.

3.5. Treatment-Related Factors

Children with hypocalcemia had a significantly longer treatment duration compared to those without (median, 8.9 vs. 2.8 years; $p < 0.001$; r = 0.447), indicating a moderate to large effect size. In contrast, there was no significant difference in treatment duration for children with or without hypophosphatemia ($p = 0.942$; r = 0.006). Treatment duration also varied by vitamin D status ($p = 0.007$; $\eta^2 = 0.04$). Children with vitamin D deficiency had the longest treatment (median 9.7 years), followed by those with insufficiency (8.5 years) and normal levels (5.3 years). This suggests a small but relevant effect.

Regarding BMI, treatment was longer in obese (10.1 years) and overweight (9.1 years) children compared to those with a normal BMI (5.8 years) or thinness (2.5 years; $p < 0.001$; $\eta^2 = 0.08$), reflecting a moderate effect. No significant difference was found by height-for-age classification ($p = 0.108$; $\eta^2 = 0.01$). For bone age, children with advanced bone age (BA > CA) had a longer treatment duration (median, 10.2 years) compared to those with bone age equal to chronological age (5.8 years) or delayed bone age (4.6 years; $p < 0.001$; $\eta^2 = 0.10$). This indicates a moderate effect. These associations between glucocorticoid treatment duration and growth or nutritional parameters are summarized in Table 4.

Table 4. Associations between glucocorticoid treatment duration and nutritional or growth outcomes in children with congenital adrenal hyperplasia (CAH).

	Outcome Variable	p-Value	Effect Size
Glucocorticoid treatment duration	Hypocalcemia	<0.001 *	r = 0.447
	Hypophosphatemia	0.942	r = 0.006
	Vitamin D status	0.007 *	$\eta^2 = 0.04$
	BMI classification	<0.001 *	$\eta^2 = 0.08$
	Height-for-age classification	0.108	$\eta^2 = 0.01$
	BA-CA classification	<0.001 *	$\eta^2 = 0.10$

* Variable with a significant effect.

3.6. Associations Between Subclinical Nutritional and Growth Outcomes

In the BA-CA classification groups, hypocalcemia was significantly more prevalent among children with advanced bone age (BA > CA) at 96.2%, compared to those with age-appropriate (72.7%) or delayed bone age (75.0%) ($p < 0.001$). Vitamin D deficiency was also more frequent in the advanced bone age group (26.9%) than in those with bone age equal to (19.5%) or delayed relative to chronological age (20.0%). This trend was statistically significant, as confirmed by linear-by-linear association ($p = 0.036$). In contrast, no significant association was found between bone age classification and the prevalence of hypophosphatemia ($p = 0.457$).

When stratified by height-for-age categories, no significant differences were observed in the prevalence of hypocalcemia, hypophosphatemia, or vitamin D status. However, analysis by BMI classification revealed a significantly higher prevalence of hypocalcemia among overweight (93.9%) and obese (91.4%) children compared to those with normal BMI (76.9%) or thinness (66.7%) ($p = 0.016$). The distribution of vitamin D status across BMI categories showed a trend toward significance ($p = 0.063$) and a significant linear association ($p = 0.012$); vitamin D deficiency was more common in overweight (29.3%) and obese children (30.6%) than in those with normal weight (16.5%). No significant association was found between BMI classification and hypophosphatemia ($p = 0.76$). Children with hypocalcemia had a significantly different distribution of vitamin D status compared to those without hypocalcemia ($p = 0.016$), characterized by a higher prevalence of vitamin D deficiency (25.7% vs. 10%) and a lower proportion of normal vitamin D status (11.7% vs. 30%).

4. Discussion

This study provides a detailed clinical and biochemical profile of 201 Vietnamese children with congenital adrenal hyperplasia (CAH), highlighting growth impairment, skeletal maturation disturbances, nutritional deficits, and treatment-related effects. Our findings are generally consistent with international literature while offering novel insights from a Southeast Asian context.

4.1. Growth and Nutritional Outcome

In our study, the median height standard deviation score (SDS) was −0.7 (range: −4.0 to 4.3), and 16.4% of participants were classified as stunted (11.9% moderate, 4.5% severe). This finding aligns with previous studies, where Muthusamy et al. reported a pooled mean height standard deviation (SDS) of −1.03 in a meta-analysis [6] and Gidlöf et al. found a final height SDS of −0.78 in an extensive European registry [48]. Moreover, studies have indicated that during adrenarche and early puberty, children with CAH may initially appear taller than their peers due to accelerated skeletal maturation, but ultimately achieve a lower final adult height if skeletal advancement persists [49]. In our study, although early bone age advancement was common (51.7%), this did not necessarily translate into preserved final height, emphasizing the need for careful longitudinal growth monitoring. A key finding in our study was the significantly higher rate of stunting among females (23.1%) compared to males (9.3%). This gender dichotomy is strongly supported by previous longitudinal research. A study by Patel et al. specifically evaluating growth trajectories in children with 21-hydroxylase deficiency found that growth curves for height, weight, and BMI differed significantly by gender [50]. They reported that females, in contrast to males, showed a pattern of disproportionately greater adiposity and increasing BMI but had shorter stature during adolescence. In their cohort, females with salt-wasting CAH initially experienced less growth retardation than males but ultimately developed a greater discrepancy between their weight and height scores. Meanwhile, females with non-salt-wasting CAH showed only a slight gain in height SDS, while their weight and BMI SDS progressively increased throughout childhood.

In an attempt to explain this, Patel et al. noted that both sexes in their study received comparable doses of corticosteroids, indicating that the difference in height outcome was not simply related to steroid treatment. The authors speculated that other factors, such as prenatal programming due to androgen excess in utero, may contribute to these different postnatal growth patterns, with a more pronounced adverse effect on height in females.

Overweight and obesity were highly prevalent in our cohort, with 24.4% classified as overweight and 28.9% as obese, totaling 53.3%, similar to rates reported by Abdel Meguid et al., who observed a 60% prevalence among Egyptian CAH children [17]. This is notably higher than the 16.5% prevalence found by Völkl et al. in a German cohort [51], possibly reflecting differences in genetic background, treatment regimens, or lifestyle factors. Importantly, we found that obesity was more frequent in males (35.1%) than in females (23.1%) and increased significantly with age (median age of obese children: 10.5 years, $p < 0.001$), which supports the findings of Gidlöf et al. [48]. The pathophysiological mechanisms underlying obesity in CAH are multifactorial, including supraphysiological glucocorticoid exposure leading to central adiposity [52], altered insulin sensitivity [53], and the anabolic effects of chronic hyperandrogenism [54].

However, those findings should be interpreted within the context of the current nutritional landscape in Vietnam. According to the 2019–2020 General Nutrition Survey, the nationwide prevalence of stunting in children aged 5 to 19 years was 14.8%, a figure comparable to the rate in our cohort [55]. This suggests that stunting may be a persistent public health challenge in the region, potentially exacerbated by the effects of CAH and its treatment. More strikingly, the 53.3% prevalence of overweight and obesity in our study is substantially higher than the national average of 19.0% reported for school-aged children in the same survey. While rising obesity rates are a general concern in Vietnam, particularly in urban areas, the markedly higher prevalence in our patients strongly suggests that disease-specific factors, such as supraphysiologic glucocorticoid dosing and metabolic alterations inherent to CAH, are major contributors to this adverse outcome.

Skeletal maturation disturbances were also prominent. In our study, 51.7% of patients had an advanced bone age, which was more common in the simple virilizing form (82.9%) compared to the salt-wasting form (43.8%, $p < 0.001$), consistent with the findings by Bomberg et al. [56]. Furthermore, we found that children with advanced bone age exhibited higher median testosterone and 17-OHP levels. This observation is supported by Finkielstain et al., who reported a significant correlation between bone age advancement and elevated concentrations of androstenedione and testosterone [9]. Such findings reflect the pathophysiological mechanism of chronic ACTH stimulation, leading to excess adrenal androgen production and promoting premature epiphyseal fusion, thereby compromising linear growth potential.

Vitamin D insufficiency or deficiency, as well as hypocalcemia, were prevalent, affecting 85.6% and 85.1% of our patients, respectively. This finding mirrors the high prevalence of vitamin D insufficiency (74.9%) reported by Demirel et al. in children with CAH [57] and aligns with the findings by Finkielstain et al., who noted that 19% of classic CAH patients were vitamin D deficient and 42% were insufficient [8]. However, to provide a direct comparative context for our findings, a key study by Laillou et al. on healthy Vietnamese children reported that 58% had 25(OH)D levels below 50 nmol/L [58]. This figure comprised 21% of children classified as deficient (<30 nmol/L) and 37% classified as insufficient (30–49.9 nmol/L). When more liberal diagnostic thresholds were applied (25(OH)D <75 nmol/L), approximately 90% of healthy Vietnamese children were classified as having hypovitaminosis D. Furthermore, the same study found that 97% of children had mild hypocalcemia. These deficiencies in the general pediatric population were linked to extremely low dietary intake, with children consuming only about 1% of the recommended nutrient intake for vitamin D and less than 43% for calcium. Given this high baseline prevalence of vitamin D and calcium deficiencies in the general Vietnamese pediatric population, it is likely that the rates observed in our CAH cohort are compounded by these widespread environmental and dietary factors rather than being solely a consequence of CAH or its treatment.

Additionally, vitamin D deficiency increased with age and BMI, being more prevalent in older children (10.3 vs. 5.6 years, $p = 0.001$) and those with obesity (29.3% vs. 16.5%, $p = 0.012$), consistent with patterns in steroid-treated pediatric populations [38].

4.2. Related Factors

Prolonged corticosteroid therapy was found to have a significant impact on growth and metabolic outcomes in children with CAH. In our study, children with obesity had a longer median treatment duration (10.1 years) compared to those with a normal BMI (5.8 years, $p < 0.001$). Additionally, children with hypocalcemia received corticosteroids for a median of 8.9 years, compared to 2.8 years for those without ($p < 0.001$). Additionally, corticosteroid duration varied significantly with vitamin D status ($p = 0.007$), being longest in children with deficiency (9.7 years) and shortest in those with normal levels (5.3 years). These findings are consistent with previous studies. Abdel Meguid et al. reported that children who had been treated with corticosteroids for more than five years exhibited a markedly higher prevalence of overweight and obesity, reaching 60% [17]. Similarly, Finkielstain et al. observed that 35% of children with CAH were obese, with a higher proportion receiving long-acting glucocorticoid formulations compared to non-obese peers [8]. In addition to its impact on body composition, corticosteroid therapy adversely affected linear growth. Stikkelbroeck et al. demonstrated that higher cumulative glucocorticoid doses were significantly associated with reduced height-for-age z-scores (HAZ) during critical periods of growth, specifically between 6 and 12 months and between 8 and 14 years of age [16]. These findings support the well-established notion that supraphysiological glucocorticoid exposure suppresses chondrocyte proliferation and disrupts the growth plate, ultimately impairing linear growth potential. Moreover, corticosteroid use was associated with disturbances in vitamin D metabolism. Demirel et al. reported that children receiving supraphysiological steroid doses (>15 mg/m^2/day) exhibited lower serum 25-hydroxyvitamin D levels compared to those on physiological doses, although the difference did not reach statistical significance [57]. These findings suggest that glucocorticoid therapy may contribute to impaired vitamin D status through indirect mechanisms, thereby exacerbating the risk of bone mineral disturbances and hypocalcemia observed in patients with CAH.

Higher BMI categories were significantly associated with a greater prevalence of vitamin D deficiency in this study. Among obese children, the deficiency rate was 29.3%, compared to 16.5% in those with normal BMI, with a significant linear trend across BMI classifications (p = 0.012). The proportion of vitamin D sufficiency was also lower in obese participants (10.3%) than in their normal-weight peers (22%), reinforcing the link between adiposity and impaired vitamin D status. These findings are consistent with those of Demirel et al., who reported that children with higher BMI tended to have lower 25-hydroxyvitamin D concentrations. However, the association did not reach statistical significance [57]. This relationship is biologically plausible, given that vitamin D, as a fat-soluble vitamin, may be sequestered in adipose tissue, thereby reducing its circulating bioavailability [59]. Consequently, children with higher BMI may be at greater risk for hypovitaminosis D, compounding the nutritional and skeletal challenges already faced by CAH patients.

Among our patients, elevated 17-hydroxyprogesterone (17-OHP) and testosterone levels were significantly associated with adverse growth and skeletal outcomes. Median 17-OHP was higher in children with hypocalcemia (52 vs. 39.7 nmol/L, p = 0.317) and obesity (107.5 nmol/L in obese children, p = 0.014). Testosterone levels were significantly higher in individuals with hypocalcemia (p < 0.001), vitamin D deficiency (p = 0.027), and advanced bone age (p < 0.001). These findings reflect the impact of poor biochemical control on mineral metabolism, body composition, and skeletal maturation. Children with advanced bone age exhibited the highest median 17-OHP and testosterone levels, reinforcing the contribution of androgen excess to accelerated skeletal development. This is consistent with prior studies, where elevated 17-OHP concentrations (>30 nmol/L) during adrenarche were associated with lower estimated final height [49], and testosterone elevations were significantly linked to bone age advancement [8]. Although children with central precocious puberty (CPP) demonstrated higher testosterone concentrations, this was not associated with significant height impairment at the time of evaluation in our cohort.

In our cohort, several clinical features demonstrated significant associations with adverse growth and nutritional outcomes. Cushingoid appearance and acanthosis nigricans were strongly associated with higher BMI classifications, reflecting the impact of chronic glucocorticoid excess and consequent insulin resistance. Indicators of poor biochemical control, particularly hyperpigmentation, were also linked to multiple systemic disturbances. Hyperpigmentation was associated with a higher prevalence of obesity, more frequent bone age advancement, and a significantly increased prevalence of hypocalcemia, suggesting that chronic ACTH elevation may exacerbate these conditions. Among undertreatment indicators, virilization correlated substantially with advanced bone age classification, consistent with the effect of androgen excess on premature skeletal maturation. The presence of CPP was significantly associated not only with profound bone age advancement but also with a higher prevalence of both hypocalcemia and hypophosphatemia. These results underscore that inadequate androgen suppression, particularly to the point of inducing CPP, has profound effects on both skeletal and mineral metabolism in children with CAH.

Our findings complement earlier Vietnamese studies. Nguyen et al. [20] conducted a study of 124 pediatric CAH patients and found that early diagnosis, sufficient steroid dosing, and treatment adherence were key to achieving good treatment outcomes. However, their study did not include biochemical or nutritional indicators [18].

The limitations of this study include its cross-sectional design, which precludes causal inference, and the absence of bone mineral density assessments, genotypic data, and lipid or insulin profiling. In our study, we did not observe statistically significant differences in calcium, phosphorus, or vitamin D levels between the salt-wasting and simple virilizing forms of CAH. However, genotypic data were not available for this cohort, and thus, we could not evaluate whether biochemical differences exist across specific 21-hydroxylase mutation types. Given the established correlation between genotype and phenotype severity, future studies should incorporate molecular characterization to determine whether certain mutations are associated with distinct patterns of micronutrient abnormalities or bone mineral status. Additionally, pubertal development was not assessed using Tanner staging, limiting the ability to precisely interpret hormone levels and skeletal maturation in relation to pubertal status. Although we evaluated biochemical markers of nutritional status, dietary intake data, such as food frequency questionnaires or detailed nutrient intake records, were not collected, which limited our ability to directly correlate micronutrient deficiencies with dietary patterns. Phosphate measurements were available in a subset of patients, which limited the statistical power for analyses involving phosphate deficiency. While this did not affect the primary study objectives, the results related to phosphate status should be interpreted with caution. Another significant limitation of this study is the lack of established local pediatric biochemical reference intervals for the Vietnamese population. To maintain consistency, we adopted age-stratified reference ranges from a major pediatric textbook (Nelson Textbook of Pediatrics) for our definitions of deficiency [46]. We fully acknowledge that these international ranges, likely based on Western populations, may not perfectly reflect the biochemical norms for Vietnamese children. This limitation introduces the potential for misclassification, either overestimating or underestimating the true prevalence of nutritional deficiencies in our cohort. Future research should aim to fill this gap by conducting population-based studies to define national biochemical reference values. Additionally, standardized pubertal staging, comprehensive dietary assessments, and behavioral evaluations should be integrated into future studies to elucidate better the complex nutritional and metabolic risk profiles of children with CAH. Nonetheless, the study's large sample size, integrated clinical and hormonal data, and inclusion of both urban and rural populations provide valuable insights into CAH management in resource-constrained settings.

5. Conclusions

In a Vietnamese pediatric cohort with congenital adrenal hyperplasia, we identified a high prevalence of overweight/obesity, vitamin D deficiency, hypocalcemia, and advanced bone age, despite standard treatment. Significant associations were found between adverse outcomes and clinical indicators of treatment imbalance, androgen excess, prolonged corticosteroid exposure, and residential area. These findings reflect not only disease-specific challenges but also broader nutritional and healthcare disparities within the Vietnamese context. Our results underscore the urgent need for individualized, comprehensive management strategies that address both endocrine control and nutritional status to improve long-term health outcomes in this population.

Supplementary Materials: The following supporting information can be downloaded at: https://www.mdpi.com/article/10.3390/diagnostics15121534/s1.

Author Contributions: Conceptualization, T.T.H.N. and C.D.V.; methodology, T.T.H.N., K.M.L., T.A.T.T. and C.D.V.; software, T.T.H.N., K.M.L. and D.T.T.; validation, T.T.H.N., K.N.N. and P.T.B.; formal analysis, T.T.H.N., K.M.L. and D.T.T.; investigation, T.T.H.N., K.M.L. and T.B.N.C.; data curation, T.T.H.N., P.T.B., T.B.N.C. and K.N.N.; writing—original draft preparation, T.T.H.N., K.M.L. and T.A.T.T.; writing—review and editing, T.T.H.N., K.M.L., T.A.T.T., K.N.N., T.B.N.C., P.T.B. and C.D.V.; visualization, T.T.H.N. and K.M.L.; supervision, C.D.V. All authors have read and agreed to the published version of the manuscript.

Funding: This research received no external funding.

Institutional Review Board Statement: The study was conducted in accordance with the Declaration of Helsinki and approved by the Institutional Review Board National Children's Hospital (protocol code 2685/BVNTW-HĐĐĐ, on 10 October 2024).

Informed Consent Statement: Informed consent was obtained from all legal guardians of the children included in the study.

Data Availability Statement: The original contributions presented in this study are included in the article. Further inquiries can be directed to the corresponding authors.

Acknowledgments: The authors would like to thank the staff of the Center for Endocrinology, Metabolism, Genetics, and Molecular Therapy at Vietnam National Children's Hospital for their support in data collection. The authors also acknowledge the families who participated in this study.

Conflicts of Interest: The authors declare no conflicts of interest.

Abbreviations

The following abbreviations are used in this manuscript:

ACTH	Adrenocorticotropic hormone
BA	Bone age
BMI	Body mass index
CA	Chronological age
CAH	Congenital adrenal hyperplasia
CPP	Central precocious puberty
ELISA	Enzyme-linked immunosorbent assay
HAZ	Height-for-age
SD	Standard deviation
SDS	Standard deviation score
SV	Simple virilizing
SW	Salt-wasting
WHO	World Health Organization
17OHP	17-hydroxyprogesterone
25(OH)D	25-hydroxyvitamin D

References

1. Gruñeiro-Papendieek, L.; Chiesa, A.; Mendez, V.; Prieto, L. Neonatal Screening for Congenital Adrenal Hyperplasia: Experience and Results in Argentina. *J. Pediatr. Endocrinol. Metab.* **2008**, *21*, 73–78. [CrossRef] [PubMed]
2. Speiser, P.W.; Arlt, W.; Auchus, R.J.; Baskin, L.S.; Conway, G.S.; Merke, D.P.; Meyer-Bahlburg, H.F.L.; Miller, W.L.; Murad, M.H.; Oberfield, S.E.; et al. Congenital Adrenal Hyperplasia Due to Steroid 21-Hydroxylase Deficiency: An Endocrine Society* Clinical Practice Guideline. *J. Clin. Endocrinol. Metab.* **2018**, *103*, 4043–4088. [CrossRef] [PubMed]
3. Navarro-Zambrana, A.N.; Sheets, L.R. Ethnic and National Differences in Congenital Adrenal Hyperplasia Incidence: A Systematic Review and Meta-Analysis. *Horm. Res. Paediatr.* **2023**, *96*, 249–258. [CrossRef] [PubMed]
4. Sharma, L.; Momodu, I.I.; Singh, G. Congenital Adrenal Hyperplasia. In *StatPearls*; StatPearls Publishing: Treasure Island, FL, USA, 2025.
5. Speiser, P.W.; White, P.C. Congenital Adrenal Hyperplasia. *N. Engl. J. Med.* **2003**, *349*, 776–788. [CrossRef]
6. Muthusamy, K.; Elamin, M.B.; Smushkin, G.; Murad, M.H.; Lampropulos, J.F.; Elamin, K.B.; Abu Elnour, N.O.; Gallegos-Orozco, J.F.; Fatourechi, M.M.; Agrwal, N.; et al. Adult Height in Patients with Congenital Adrenal Hyperplasia: A Systematic Review and Metaanalysis. *J. Clin. Endocrinol. Metab.* **2010**, *95*, 4161–4172. [CrossRef]
7. Alzanbagi, M.A.; Milyani, A.A.; Al-Agha, A.E. Growth Characteristics in Children with Congenital Adrenal Hyperplasia. *Saudi Med. J.* **2018**, *39*, 674–678. [CrossRef]
8. Finkielstain, G.P.; Kim, M.S.; Sinaii, N.; Nishitani, M.; Van Ryzin, C.; Hill, S.C.; Reynolds, J.C.; Hanna, R.M.; Merke, D.P. Clinical Characteristics of a Cohort of 244 Patients with Congenital Adrenal Hyperplasia. *J. Clin. Endocrinol. Metab.* **2012**, *97*, 4429–4438. [CrossRef]
9. Huang, M.; Ma, H.; Du, M.; Chen, H.; Li, Y.; Chen, Q.; Zhang, J.; Guo, S. Metabolic Status in Children with Classic Congenital Adrenal Hyperplasia Due to 21-Hydroxylase Deficiency. In *Proceedings of the ESPE Abstracts*; Bioscientifica: Bristol, UK, 2023; Volume 97.
10. Bonfig, W.; Dalla Pozza, S.B.; Schmidt, H.; Pagel, P.; Knorr, D.; Schwarz, H.P. Hydrocortisone Dosing during Puberty in Patients with Classical Congenital Adrenal Hyperplasia: An Evidence-Based Recommendation. *J. Clin. Endocrinol. Metab.* **2009**, *94*, 3882–3888. [CrossRef]
11. Merke, D.P.; Auchus, R.J. Congenital Adrenal Hyperplasia Due to 21-Hydroxylase Deficiency. *N. Engl. J. Med.* **2020**, *383*, 1248–1261. [CrossRef]
12. Halper, A.; Sanchez, B.; Hodges, J.S.; Kelly, A.S.; Dengel, D.; Nathan, B.M.; Petryk, A.; Sarafoglou, K. Bone Mineral Density and Body Composition in Children with Congenital Adrenal Hyperplasia. *Clin. Endocrinol.* **2018**, *88*, 813–819. [CrossRef]
13. Nicolaides, N.C.; Charmandari, E. Chrousos Syndrome: From Molecular Pathogenesis to Therapeutic Management. *Eur. J. Clin. Investig.* **2015**, *45*, 504–514. [CrossRef] [PubMed]
14. Anisowicz, S.K.; Vogt, K.S. Congenital Adrenal Hyperplasia. *Pediatr. Ann.* **2025**, *54*, e74–e77. [CrossRef] [PubMed]
15. Balsamo, A.; Cicognani, A.; Baldazzi, L.; Barbaro, M.; Baronio, F.; Gennari, M.; Bal, M.; Cassio, A.; Kontaxaki, K.; Cacciari, E. CYP21 Genotype, Adult Height, and Pubertal Development in 55 Patients Treated for 21-Hydroxylase Deficiency. *J. Clin. Endocrinol. Metab.* **2003**, *88*, 5680–5688. [CrossRef] [PubMed]
16. Stikkelbroeck, N.M.M.L.; Van'T Hof-Grootenboer, B.A.E.; Hermus, A.R.M.M.; Otten, B.J.; Van'T Hof, M.A. Growth Inhibition by Glucocorticoid Treatment in Salt Wasting 21-Hydroxylase Deficiency: In Early Infancy and (Pre)Puberty. *J. Clin. Endocrinol. Metab.* **2003**, *88*, 3525–3530. [CrossRef]

17. Abdel Meguid, S.E.; Soliman, A.T.; De Sanctis, V.; Abougabal, A.M.S.; Ramadan, M.A.E.F.; Hassan, M.; Hamed, N.; Ahmed, S. Growth and Metabolic Syndrome (MetS) Criteria in Young Children with Classic Congenital Adrenal Hyperplasia (CAH) Treated with Corticosteroids (CS). *Acta Bio-Medica Atenei Parm.* **2022**, *93*, e2022304. [CrossRef]
18. Nimkarn, S.; Lin-Su, K.; New, M.I. Steroid 21 Hydroxylase Deficiency Congenital Adrenal Hyperplasia. *Pediatr. Clin. N. Am.* **2011**, *58*, 1281–1300. [CrossRef]
19. Kurahashi, I.; Matsunuma, A.; Kawane, T.; Abe, M.; Horiuchi, N. Dexamethasone Enhances Vitamin D-24-Hydroxylase Expression in Osteoblastic (UMR-106) and Renal (LLC-PK1) Cells Treated with 1α,25-Dihydroxyvitamin D_3. *Endocrine* **2002**, *17*, 109–118. [CrossRef]
20. Nguyen, T.G.; Nguyen, P.D. Treatment Outcome and Some Affecting Factors of Congenital Adrenal Hyperplasia. *J. Med. Res.* **2011**, *74*, 102–106.
21. Eitel, K.B.; Fechner, P.Y. Barriers to the Management of Classic Congenital Adrenal Hyperplasia Due to 21-Hydroxylase Deficiency. *J. Clin. Endocrinol. Metab.* **2025**, *110*, S67–S73. [CrossRef]
22. Therrell, B.L.; Padilla, C.D.; Borrajo, G.J.C.; Khneisser, I.; Schielen, P.C.J.I.; Knight-Madden, J.; Malherbe, H.L.; Kase, M. Current Status of Newborn Bloodspot Screening Worldwide 2024: A Comprehensive Review of Recent Activities (2020–2023). *Int. J. Neonatal Screen.* **2024**, *10*, 38. [CrossRef]
23. Vietnam+ (VietnamPlus) Prenatal, Newborn Screening Programme Helps Improve Population Quality. Available online: https://en.vietnamplus.vn/prenatal-newborn-screening-programme-helps-improve-population-quality-post250241.vnp (accessed on 12 June 2025).
24. WHO. *Length/Height-for-Age, Weight-for-Age, Weight-for-Length, Weight-for-Height and Body Mass Index-for-Age: Methods and Development*; de Onis, M., Ed.; WHO child growth standards; WHO Press: Geneva, Switzerland, 2006; ISBN 978-92-4-154693-5.
25. Nieman, L.K.; Biller, B.M.K.; Findling, J.W.; Newell-Price, J.; Savage, M.O.; Stewart, P.M.; Montori, V.M. The Diagnosis of Cushing's Syndrome: An Endocrine Society Clinical Practice Guideline. *J. Clin. Endocrinol. Metab.* **2008**, *93*, 1526–1540. [CrossRef] [PubMed]
26. Brito, V.N.; Spinola-Castro, A.M.; Kochi, C.; Kopacek, C.; Silva, P.C.A.d.; Guerra-Júnior, G. Central Precocious Puberty: Revisiting the Diagnosis and Therapeutic Management. *Arch. Endocrinol. Metab.* **2016**, *60*, 163–172. [CrossRef] [PubMed]
27. Jørgensen, A.; Rajpert-De Meyts, E. Regulation of Meiotic Entry and Gonadal Sex Differentiation in the Human: Normal and Disrupted Signaling. *Biomol. Concepts* **2014**, *5*, 331–341. [CrossRef] [PubMed]
28. Perluigi, M.; Di Domenico, F.; Buttterfield, D.A. Unraveling the Complexity of Neurodegeneration in Brains of Subjects with Down Syndrome: Insights from Proteomics. *Proteom. Clin. Appl.* **2014**, *8*, 73–85. [CrossRef]
29. Avramis, V.I.; Sencer, S.; Periclou, A.P.; Sather, H.; Bostrom, B.C.; Cohen, L.J.; Ettinger, A.G.; Ettinger, L.J.; Franklin, J.; Gaynon, P.S.; et al. A Randomized Comparison of nativeEscherichia Coli Asparaginase and Polyethylene Glycol Conjugated Asparaginase for Treatment of Children with Newly Diagnosed Standard-Risk Acute Lymphoblastic Leukemia: A Children's Cancer Group Study. *Blood* **2002**, *99*, 1986–1994. [CrossRef]
30. Korkmaz, O.; Sari, G.; Mecidov, I.; Ozen, S.; Goksen, D.; Darcan, S. The Gonadotropin-Releasing Hormone Analogue Therapy May Not Impact Final Height in Precocious Puberty of Girls with Onset of Puberty Aged 6–8 Years. *J. Clin. Med. Res.* **2019**, *11*, 133–136. [CrossRef]
31. Macedo, D.B.; Cukier, P.; Mendonca, B.B.; Latronico, A.C.; Brito, V.N. Advances in the etiology, diagnosis and treatment of central precocious puberty. *Arq. Bras. Endocrinol. Metabol.* **2014**, *58*, 108–117. [CrossRef]
32. Chaudhary, S.; Walia, R.; Bhansali, A.; Dayal, D.; Sachdeva, N.; Singh, T.; Bhadada, S.K. FSH-Stimulated Inhibin B (FSH-iB): A Novel Marker for the Accurate Prediction of Pubertal Outcome in Delayed Puberty. *J. Clin. Endocrinol. Metab.* **2021**, *106*, e3495–e3505. [CrossRef]
33. Soriano-Guillén, L.; Argente, J. Central precocious puberty: Epidemiology, etiology, diagnosis and treatment. *An. Pediatr. Barc. Spain 2003* **2011**, *74*, e1–e336. [CrossRef]
34. Tomlinson, C.; Macintyre, H.; Dorrian, C.; Ahmed, S.; Wallace, A. Testosterone Measurements in Early Infancy. *Arch. Dis. Child. Fetal Neonatal Ed.* **2004**, *89*, F558–F559. [CrossRef]
35. Johannsen, T.H.; Main, K.M.; Ljubicic, M.L.; Jensen, T.K.; Andersen, H.R.; Andersen, M.S.; Petersen, J.H.; Andersson, A.-M.; Juul, A. Sex Differences in Reproductive Hormones During Mini-Puberty in Infants with Normal and Disordered Sex Development. *J. Clin. Endocrinol. Metab.* **2018**, *103*, 3028–3037. [CrossRef] [PubMed]
36. Alotaibi, M.F. Physiology of Puberty in Boys and Girls and Pathological Disorders Affecting Its Onset. *J. Adolesc.* **2019**, *71*, 63–71. [CrossRef] [PubMed]
37. Koskenniemi, J.J.; Virtanen, H.E.; Toppari, J. Testicular Growth and Development in Puberty. *Curr. Opin. Endocrinol. Diabetes Obes.* **2017**, *24*, 215–224. [CrossRef] [PubMed]
38. Sultan, C.; Gaspari, L.; Maimoun, L.; Kalfa, N.; Paris, F. Disorders of Puberty. *Best Pract. Res. Clin. Obstet. Gynaecol.* **2018**, *48*, 62–89. [CrossRef]

39. Muerköster, A.-P.; Frederiksen, H.; Juul, A.; Andersson, A.-M.; Jensen, R.C.; Glintborg, D.; Kyhl, H.B.; Andersen, M.S.; Timmermann, C.A.G.; Jensen, T.K. Maternal Phthalate Exposure Associated with Decreased Testosterone/LH Ratio in Male Offspring during Mini-Puberty. Odense Child Cohort. *Environ. Int.* **2020**, *144*, 106025. [CrossRef]
40. Latronico, A.C.; Brito, V.N.; Carel, J.-C. Causes, Diagnosis, and Treatment of Central Precocious Puberty. *Lancet Diabetes Endocrinol.* **2016**, *4*, 265–274. [CrossRef]
41. Willemsen, R.H.; Elleri, D.; Williams, R.M.; Ong, K.K.; Dunger, D.B. Pros and Cons of GnRHa Treatment for Early Puberty in Girls. *Nat. Rev. Endocrinol.* **2014**, *10*, 352–363. [CrossRef]
42. Spaziani, M.; Lecis, C.; Tarantino, C.; Sbardella, E.; Pozza, C.; Gianfrilli, D. The Role of Scrotal Ultrasonography from Infancy to Puberty. *Andrology* **2021**, *9*, 1306–1321. [CrossRef]
43. Lloyd, C.; McHugh, K. The Role of Radiology in Head and Neck Tumours in Children. *Cancer Imaging Off. Publ. Int. Cancer Imaging Soc.* **2010**, *10*, 49–61. [CrossRef]
44. World Health Organization. *WHO Child Growth Standards: Head Circumference-for-Age, Arm Circumfer-ence-for-Age, Triceps Skinfold-for-Age and Subscapular Skinfold-for-Age: Methods and Development*; World Health Organization Child Growth Standard: Geneva, Switzerland, 2007.
45. Holick, M.F.; Binkley, N.C.; Bischoff-Ferrari, H.A.; Gordon, C.M.; Hanley, D.A.; Heaney, R.P.; Murad, M.H.; Weaver, C.M. Evaluation, Treatment, and Prevention of Vitamin D Deficiency: An Endocrine Society Clinical Practice Guideline. *J. Clin. Endocrinol. Metab.* **2011**, *96*, 1911–1930. [CrossRef]
46. Kliegman, R.M.; Blum, N.J.; Tasker, R.C.; Wilson, K.M.; St. Geme, J.W.; Schuh, A.M.; Mack, C.L.; Deardorff, M.A.; Nelson, W.E. (Eds.) *Nelson Textbook of Pediatrics*, 22nd ed.; Elsevier: Philadelphia, PA, USA, 2025; ISBN 978-0-323-88305-4.
47. Hindmarsh, P.C. Management of the Child with Congenital Adrenal Hyperplasia. *Best Pract. Res. Clin. Endocrinol. Metab.* **2009**, *23*, 193–208. [CrossRef] [PubMed]
48. Gidlöf, S.; Hogling, D.E.; Lönnberg, H.; Ritzén, M.; Lajic, S.; Nordenström, A. Growth and Treatment in Congenital Adrenal Hyperplasia: An Observational Study from Diagnosis to Final Height. *Horm. Res. Paediatr.* **2024**, *97*, 445–455. [CrossRef] [PubMed]
49. Troger, T.; Sommer, G.; Lang-Muritano, M.; Konrad, D.; Kuhlmann, B.; Zumsteg, U.; Flück, C.E. Characteristics of Growth in Children with Classic Congenital Adrenal Hyperplasia Due to 21-Hydroxylase Deficiency During Adrenarche and Beyond. *J. Clin. Endocrinol. Metab.* **2022**, *107*, e487–e499. [CrossRef] [PubMed]
50. Patel, L.; Chandrashekhar, S.R.; Gemmell, I.; O'Shea, E.; Jones, J.; Banerjee, I.; Amin, R.; Clayton, P. Gender Dichotomy in Long Term Growth Trajectories of Children with 21-Hydroxylase Deficiency Congenital Adrenal Hyperplasia. *Horm. Res. Paediatr.* **2011**, *75*, 206–212. [CrossRef]
51. Völkl, T.M.K.; Simm, D.; Beier, C.; Dörr, H.G. Obesity Among Children and Adolescents with Classic Congenital Adrenal Hyperplasia Due to 21-Hydroxylase Deficiency. *Pediatrics* **2006**, *117*, e98–e105. [CrossRef]
52. Geer, E.B.; Islam, J.; Buettner, C. Mechanisms of Glucocorticoid-Induced Insulin Resistance. *Endocrinol. Metab. Clin. N. Am.* **2014**, *43*, 75–102. [CrossRef]
53. Kim, M.S.; Fraga, N.R.; Minaeian, N.; Geffner, M.E. Components of Metabolic Syndrome in Youth with Classical Congenital Adrenal Hyperplasia. *Front. Endocrinol.* **2022**, *13*, 848274. [CrossRef]
54. Ben Simon, A.; Brener, A.; Segev-Becker, A.; Yackobovitch-Gavan, M.; Uretzky, A.; Schachter Davidov, A.; Alaev, A.; Oren, A.; Eyal, O.; Weintrob, N.; et al. Body Composition in Children and Adolescents with Non-Classic Congenital Adrenal Hyperplasia and the Risk for Components of Metabolic Syndrome: An Observational Study. *Front. Endocrinol.* **2022**, *13*, 1022752. [CrossRef]
55. Ministry of Health Vietnam. *General Nutrition Survey 2019–2020*; Medical Publishing House: Hanoi, Vietnam, 2021.
56. Bomberg, E.M.; Addo, O.Y.; Kyllo, J.; Gonzalez-Bolanos, M.T.; Ltief, A.M.; Pittock, S.; Himes, J.H.; Miller, B.S.; Sarafoglou, K. The Relation of Peripubertal and Pubertal Growth to Final Adult Height in Children with Classic Congenital Adrenal Hyperplasia. *J. Pediatr.* **2015**, *166*, 743–750. [CrossRef]
57. Demirel, F.; Kara, O.; Tepe, D.; Esen, I. Bone Mineral Density and Vitamin D Status in Children and Adolescents with Congenital Adrenal Hyperplasia. *Turk. J. Med. Sci.* **2014**, *44*, 109–114. [CrossRef]
58. Laillou, A.; Wieringa, F.; Tran, T.N.; Van, P.T.; Le, B.M.; Fortin, S.; Le, T.H.; Pfanner, R.M.; Berger, J. Hypovitaminosis D and Mild Hypocalcaemia Are Highly Prevalent among Young Vietnamese Children and Women and Related to Low Dietary Intake. *PLoS ONE* **2013**, *8*, e63979. [CrossRef] [PubMed]
59. Vranić, L.; Mikolašević, I.; Milić, S. Vitamin D Deficiency: Consequence or Cause of Obesity? *Medicina* **2019**, *55*, 541. [CrossRef] [PubMed]

diagnostics MDPI

Article

Evaluation of Nailfold Capillaroscopic Findings in Pediatric Patients with Celiac Disease: A Cross-Sectional and Comparative Study

Gül Çirkin [1,†] and Raziye Burcu Taskin [2,*,†]

1 Department of Pediatric Gastroenterology, Hepatology and Nutrition, Health Sciences University, Tepecik Training and Research Hospital, Izmir 35020, Turkey; gul_cirkin@hotmail.com
2 Department of Pediatric Rheumatology, Health Sciences University, Tepecik Training and Research Hospital, Yenişehir Neighborhood, Gaziler Street Number: 468, Izmir 35020, Turkey
* Correspondence: raziyeburcu.taskin@saglik.gov.tr; Tel.: +90-5334907182
† These authors contributed equally to this work.

Abstract

Background/Objectives: Celiac disease (CD) is a chronic autoimmune enteropathy with increasing recognition of systemic involvement, including potential microvascular alterations. While nailfold videocapillaroscopy (NVC) is an established tool in rheumatology for assessing microcirculation, its application in pediatric CD remains unexplored. Our aim was to investigate capillaroscopic abnormalities in children with CD and assess their associations with clinical and laboratory parameters, including dietary adherence. **Methods:** This cross-sectional study included 76 pediatric CD patients and 76 age- and sex-matched healthy controls. All participants underwent standardized NVC evaluation, assessing capillary density, dilatation, morphology, and microhemorrhages. Clinical data, laboratory values, and dietary adherence (based on clinical symptoms and tissue transglutaminase-IgA levels) were recorded. **Results:** Compared to controls, CD patients exhibited significantly lower capillary density and increased frequencies of dilated capillaries, microhemorrhages, and abnormal morphologies ($p < 0.001$). A nonspecific NVC pattern predominated among CD patients. Capillary abnormalities were more pronounced in patients without tTG-IgA normalization (>10 U/mL) and with symptoms suggestive of gluten exposure. Additionally, the number of dilated capillaries positively correlated with age and disease duration. No significant differences were found based on ANA status. **Conclusions:** This is the first study to demonstrate NVC-detectable microvascular alterations in pediatric CD. Findings suggest subclinical microvascular involvement, which may be potentially modifiable through dietary adherence. NVC may serve as a non-invasive tool to detect early vascular changes and monitor systemic manifestations in pediatric CD. Longitudinal studies are warranted to clarify the reversibility and prognostic implications of these abnormalities.

Keywords: celiac disease; pediatrics; nailfold videocapillaroscopy; gluten; dietary

1. Introduction

Celiac disease (CD) is an autoimmune condition, which can be triggered by gluten intake in genetically predisposed individuals, and results in chronic damage to the small intestinal mucosal barrier [1]. Beyond involvement in the gastrointestinal tract, it is now recognized that celiac disease has a broader impact on multiple organ systems, including an increased risk of cardiovascular manifestations [2]. Furthermore, it is frequently accompanied by other autoimmune diseases, such as connective tissue disorders, which themselves confer an elevated risk of vascular involvement [1,3]. However, the risk of vascular involvement in children with CD remains controversial.

Recent experimental data from a humanized mouse model suggest that CD induces systemic vascular alterations through activation of intestinal immunity [4]. Although direct human evidence is limited, these findings imply that CD may contribute to microvascular dysfunction and endothelial injury. Supporting this view, several studies have demonstrated that there is an increased risk of the development of microvascular complications in children with concomitant type 1 diabetes mellitus (T1DM) and CD, regardless of their glycemic control status [5]. In addition, recent pediatric evidence has indicated vascular alterations, such as increases in carotid intima-media thickness and arterial stiffness, which can occur in individuals with CD, even in the absence of elevated blood pressure [6]. Nonetheless, the current body of evidence on CD-associated vasculopathy remains limited, restricting the development of specific vascular screening protocols.

Nailfold videocapillaroscopy (NVC) is a rapid, non-invasive, cost-effective technique that allows direct visualization of the microcirculation. It has recently gained prominence as a valuable diagnostic and prognostic tool in the field of rheumatology, especially for monitoring patients with Raynaud's phenomenon who are at risk of developing autoimmune disorders [7,8]. This technique is commonly applied in both the initial evaluation and longitudinal follow-up of juvenile systemic sclerosis (jSSc) and juvenile dermatomyositis (JDM). Beyond rheumatological diseases, its application has been extended to various non-rheumatological conditions associated with inflammation-mediated microvascular dysfunction, such as hypertension, diabetes mellitus, and Crohn's disease [9–11]. Nonetheless, there is a notable gap in the literature concerning pediatric populations with celiac disease, with existing knowledge primarily derived from a single adult study [12].

In light of the possible microvascular alterations associated with celiac disease, we aimed to test the hypothesis that microvascular changes detected by NVC in children with celiac disease are more prevalent than in healthy controls and are associated with non-compliance with a gluten-free diet.

2. Materials and Methods

2.1. Study Design and Participants

From January 2024 to June 2025, a cross-sectional comparative study was conducted in the Pediatric Gastroenterology and Rheumatology Departments of Tepecik Training and Research Hospital to investigate whether microvascular involvement is present in CD and to assess its association with clinical features, particularly adherence to a gluten-free diet. Pediatric patients aged <18 years who were diagnosed with CD in the Pediatric Gastroenterology Department of Tepecik Training and Research Hospital and had no accompanying systemic illnesses were included. The diagnoses of the patients were made according to the guidelines of the European Society for Pediatric Gastroenterology, Hepatology and Nutrition (ESPGHAN). Accordingly, patients with serum tissue transglutaminase (tTG) immunoglobulin A (IgA) (tTG-IgA) levels exceeding 10 U/mL underwent upper gastrointestinal endoscopy. Duodenal biopsy samples were obtained and evaluated using the Marsh classification, and only those with Type 3 lesions were included in the study [13,14].

Inclusion criteria also required that the diagnosis be established at our center, disease onset occur before 18 years of age, tTG-IgA values be available at both diagnosis and at the most recent follow-up visit (when the capillaroscopy assessment was performed), and that patients had provided consent to participate in the study. To avoid potential confounding factors, patients with systemic autoimmune connective tissue diseases such as systemic lupus erythematosus (SLE), juvenile Sjögren's syndrome (jSS), and jSSc that could influence nailfold capillaroscopic findings were excluded after a detailed rheumatological history and examination. Patients with coexisting T1DM, selective IgA deficiency, or incomplete records were also excluded from the study.

To compare the NVC findings, a healthy control group was formed with the same number of children who had no history of systemic disease or gastrointestinal symptoms and showed no evidence of growth retardation, selected from those attending the same hospital outpatient clinic for routine health examinations. However, for ethical reasons, invasive procedures or serological testing for celiac disease were not performed in these asymptomatic children.

2.2. Data Collection

Data on demographics, clinical features, baseline laboratory results, and histopathology from diagnosis to the last visit were systematically recorded using standardized forms, with all assessments performed by a pediatric gastroenterologist. Demographic variables included sex, current age, age at CD diagnosis, duration of follow-up, and family history. Clinical data encompassed gastrointestinal symptoms (diarrhea, constipation, abdominal pain, distension, bloating, vomiting, and weight loss) and extraintestinal symptoms (irritability, fatigue/lethargy, rash, and joint pain/inflammation). Anthropometric parameters included weight (kg), height (cm), and body mass index (BMI) standard deviation score (SDS). Among the baseline laboratory investigations assessed at diagnosis, erythrocyte sedimentation rate (ESR), C-reactive protein (CRP), prothrombin time (PT), international normalized ratio (INR), and antinuclear antibody (ANA) levels were recorded. All laboratory tests were performed in the hospital's central laboratory, and tTG-IgA levels were measured using the enzyme-linked immunosorbent assay (ELISA) method.

The rheumatologist who performed the NVC was blinded to the participants' group allocation. NVC was conducted without knowledge of whether the subject was a patient or control. Subsequently, the same rheumatologist, still blinded, obtained a rheumatologic history and performed a physical examination for connective tissue diseases in all participants.

At the last visit, when capillaroscopy was performed, all patients underwent clinical evaluation, physical examination (including anthropometric measurements), and tTG-IgA testing. Based on tTG-IgA levels and clinical findings from this assessment, patients were categorized into two groups: Group 1 included those without tTG-IgA normalization (>10 U/mL) and with symptoms suggestive of gluten exposure, while Group 2 included those with normalized tTG-IgA ($\leq$10 U/mL) and no symptoms [15].

2.3. Nailfold Capillaroscopy Assessment

NVC was performed using a standardized protocol as previously described in the literature [16,17]. All evaluations were conducted under standardized environmental conditions. Before image acquisition, the study participants rested for at least 20 min in a quiet room with an ambient temperature of 20–24 °C. A single experienced rheumatologist, blinded to the clinical status of the subjects, performed all the examinations using a Dino-Lite Capillary Scope (MEDL4N Pro, AnMo Electronics Corporation, Hsinchu, Taiwan) with ×200 magnification and fiberoptic illumination. It was ensured that none of the children in either the patient group or the control group had undergone any dermatological or cosmetic procedures involving the nailfold area within 15 days before the nailfold capillaroscopy assessment.

NVC was applied to eight fingers of each participant, excluding the thumbs. Two adjacent images were obtained from each finger, yielding a total of sixteen images per subject. Image acquisition and analysis were conducted using DinoXcope software (version 2.6).

The capillaroscopic parameters listed below were evaluated according to internationally accepted definitions [16,17].

- Capillary density: The number of capillaries per linear millimeter; a density of <7/mm was considered abnormal.
- Capillary morphology:
    - Normal: Hairpin-shaped, crossing once or twice, or tortuous capillaries with a convex tip.
    - Abnormal: Branching or bushy morphology, features suggestive of neoangiogenesis, non-convex tips, or capillaries exhibiting three or more crossings.
- Capillary dilations: Capillaries with an apical loop diameter of 20–50 μm (normal: <20 μm).
- Giant capillaries: Homogeneously dilated capillaries with an apical diameter of ≥50 μm.
- Microhemorrhages: Presence or absence of punctate or flame-shaped hemorrhagic spots in the pericapillary area.

For quantitative analysis, the mean values of capillary density, number of dilated capillaries, tortuous forms, and capillary morphology, including abnormal shapes and normal features such as capillaries with crossings or tortuosity, were calculated by averaging values across all 16 images per participant. Giant capillaries and microhemorrhages were noted as either present or absent.

For qualitative analysis, each image was categorized as one of the following.

- Scleroderma pattern: The presence of giant capillaries and/or multiple architectural irregularities, typically accompanied by a significant decrease in capillary density. (≤3/mm).
- Non-scleroderma patterns:
    - Normal pattern: Homogeneous capillary size (<20 μm), normal morphology, and capillary density ≥7/mm.
    - Nonspecific pattern: Features including abnormal morphology, presence of dilations, or a density <7/mm without fulfilling criteria for the scleroderma pattern.

Classification was determined based on the image findings. If at least one image demonstrated a scleroderma pattern, the subject was assigned to that category. In the absence of scleroderma findings, the predominant non-scleroderma pattern (normal or nonspecific) was recorded. In cases where both non-scleroderma patterns were equally represented, the nonspecific pattern was prioritized.

2.4. Ethical Approval and Informed Consent

Approval for this study was granted by the Ethics Committee of İzmir Tepecik Training and Research Hospital (Decision No: 2025/01-16, Date: 5 February 2025). The parents or legal guardians of all the children provided written informed consent for participation in the study.

2.5. Statistical Analysis

Data obtained in the study were analyzed statistically using IBM SPSS Statistics for Windows, version 25.0 (IBM Corp., Armonk, NY, USA, 2017) Descriptive statistics were stated as the mean ± standard deviation (SD) or median and interquartile range (IQR: 25th–75th percentiles) values, depending on their distributional characteristics for continuous variables and as number (n) and percentage (%) for categorical variables. The conformity of continuous variables to a normal distribution was examined using the Kolmogorov–Smirnov test. In the comparisons of two independent groups of data, the

Mann–Whitney U test was used when the data did not show a normal distribution or when sample sizes were small (n < 30). The Kruskal–Wallis H test was applied in the comparisons of three or more independent groups. When this test indicated significant differences, the Dunn test with Bonferroni correction was used as post hoc analysis to control for multiple comparisons. Relationships between categorical variables were examined using the Pearson Chi-Square test, Fisher's exact test, or Yates' correction, depending on data characteristics and expected frequencies. The relationships between capillaroscopic parameters and clinical variables in the celiac disease group were examined with Spearman's rank correlation coefficient (Spearman's rho), as these data did not exhibit a normal distribution. A value of $p < 0.05$ was accepted as the level of statistical significance.

3. Results

3.1. Demographic and Clinical Features of the Participants

The study enrolled 76 children diagnosed with CD [median age: 13 years (range: 4–18); 57.9% female] and 76 age- and gender-matched healthy control subjects [median age: 11 years (range: 5–17); 48.7% female]. There were no significant differences between the groups in terms of age or sex ($p > 0.05$). The BMI SDS values were significantly lower in the CD group compared to the control group ($p = 0.005$).

Group 1 patients, those without tTG-IgA normalization (>10 U/mL) and with symptoms suggestive of gluten exposure, accounted for 57.9% of the CD cohort, and ANA positivity was observed in 13.2% of patients (Table 1).

Table 1. Characteristics of study participants.

Variables	Celiac Disease (*n*:76)	HCs (*n*:76)	*p* Value
Age years, median (min–max)	13 (4–18)	11 (5–17)	0.08 $^{\mu}$
Gender (male/female)	32/44	39/37	0.25 *
BMI-SDS median (min–max)	0.2 (−3.2–2.1)	0.45 (−2.1–2.2)	0.005 $^{\mu}$
Disease duration months, median (min–max)	23.5 (0–156)	-	-
tTG-IgA value U/mL, median (min–max)	52 (10–200)	-	-
Patients without tTG-IgA normalization, *n* (%)	44 (57.9)	-	-
ANA: Negative *n* (%)	66 (86.8)	-	-

BMI: body mass index; SDS: Standard Deviation Score; HCs: healthy controls; tTG-IgA: tissue transglutaminase IgA; ANA: antinuclear antibody. $^{\mu}$ Mann Whitney U test. * Pearson Chi-Square test with Yates' correction.

3.2. Nailfold Videocapillaroscopy Findings

3.2.1. Capillaroscopic Differences Between CD Patients and Healthy Controls

Quantitative analysis of NVC demonstrated a significantly lower median capillary density in the CD group compared to the control group ($p < 0.001$). A markedly higher prevalence of dilated capillaries ($p < 0.001$) and microhemorrhages ($p = 0.006$), and an increase in capillary length ($p = 0.026$) were determined in the CD group.

In terms of capillary morphology, a significantly higher rate of both abnormal shapes ($p < 0.001$) and normal morphological variants, such as crossing ($p < 0.001$) and tortuous capillaries ($p < 0.001$), was observed in the CD group than in the control group.

Qualitative evaluation showed a significantly higher rate of nonspecific NVC patterns in the CD group ($p < 0.001$). The detailed capillaroscopic findings are presented in Table 2, with capillaroscopy image examples shown in Figure 1.

Table 2. Comparison of capillaroscopic findings between patients and controls.

Variables	Celiac Disease (*n*:76)	HCs (*n*:76)	*p* Value
Capillaroscopic Findings (per mm)			
Capillary density, median (IQR)	7(6.813–7.063)	7.063 (7–7.125)	<0.001 $^{\mu}$
Dilated capillaries, median (IQR)	0 (0–0.094)	0 (0–0)	<0.001 $^{\mu}$
Abnormal shapes, median (IQR)	0.13 (0–0.19)	0 (0–0)	<0.001 $^{\mu}$
Crossing capillaries, median (min–max)	0.184 (0–0.938)	0 (0–0.375)	<0.001 $^{\mu}$
Tortuous capillaries, median (min–max)	0.125 (0–0.93)	0 (0–0.313)	<0.001 $^{\mu}$
Capillary length (μm), median (IQR)	275 (246.5–306.5)	255 (230–290)	0.026 $^{\mu}$
Reduced capillary density (<7), *n* (%)	33 (43.4)	5 (6.6)	<0.001 *
Presence of dilated capillaries, *n* (%)	25 (32.9)	3 (3.9)	<0.001 *
Presence of giant capillaries, *n* (%)	0	0	>0.05
Presence of abnormal shapes, *n* (%)	45 (59.2)	0 (0)	<0.001 *
Presence of microhemorrhages, *n* (%)	8 (10.5)	0 (0)	0.006 *
Presence of crossing capillaries, *n* (%)	62 (81.6)	15 (19.7)	<0.001 *
Presence of tortuous capillaries, *n* (%)	45 (59.2)	19 (25)	<0.001 *
Overall NVC pattern			
Normal pattern, *n* (%)	22 (28.9)	68 (89.5)	<0.001 *
Nonspecific pattern, *n* (%)	54 (71.1)	8 (10.5)	

NVC: Nailfold videocapillaroscopy, HCs: healthy controls, IQR: interquartile range. $^{\mu}$ Mann–Whitney U test.
* Pearson Chi-Square test, Yates' correction, Fisher's exact test.

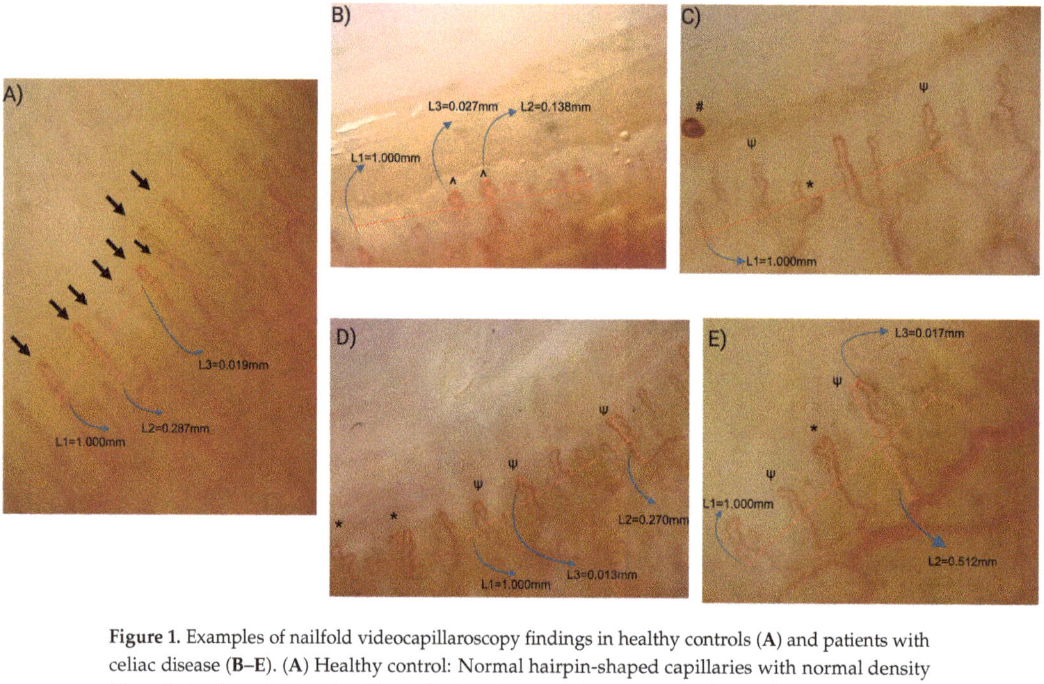

Figure 1. Examples of nailfold videocapillaroscopy findings in healthy controls (**A**) and patients with celiac disease (**B–E**). (**A**) Healthy control: Normal hairpin-shaped capillaries with normal density (8 capillaries/mm; ≥7/mm), without dilation, abnormal shapes, or microhemorrhages, representing a normal pattern. (**B**) Celiac disease: Two crossing capillaries (^) and one dilated capillary (>20 μm, <50 μm) as shown in L3 (27 μm), with reduced density (6/mm), representing a nonspecific pattern. (**C**) Celiac disease: Abnormal shaped capillary (*), tortuous capillaries (ψ) and microhemorrhage (#) with normal density (7/mm), representing a nonspecific pattern. (**D**) Celiac disease: Abnormal shaped capillaries (*) and tortuous capillaries (ψ) with normal density (7/mm), representing a nonspecific pattern. (**E**) Celiac disease: Abnormal-shaped capillary (*) and tortuous capillary (ψ) with reduced density (6/mm), representing a nonspecific pattern. Measurement references: L1—grid representing 1 mm nailfold in real life; L2—capillary length; L3—apical loop diameter.

3.2.2. Correlations and Subgroup Analyses

When the CD patients were analyzed according to disease duration (newly diagnosed ≤3 months vs. established diagnosis >3 months) or ANA positivity, there were observed to be no significant differences in the capillaroscopic findings ($p > 0.05$ for all). As a result of the correlation analyses, a statistically significant positive relationship was determined between the median number of dilated capillaries and both age (r = 0.228, p = 0.048) and disease duration (r = 0.252, p = 0.028) (Figure 2). There were not seen to be any other significant correlations between other capillaroscopic parameters and clinical or demographic variables, including BMI-SDS and tTG-IgA levels.

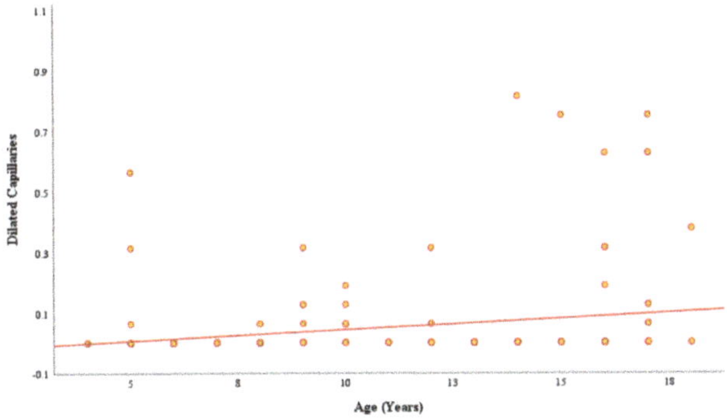

a)

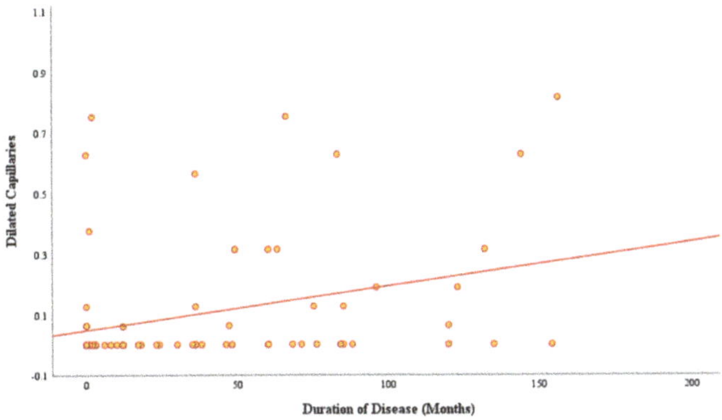

b)

Figure 2. The correlation between the number of dilated capillaries and both (**a**) age (r = 0.228, p = 0.048) and (**b**) disease duration (r = 0.252, p = 0.028).

3.2.3. The Effect of Adherence to a Gluten-Free Diet on Capillaroscopic Parameters

When the CD patients were grouped according to tTG-IgA levels and clinical symptoms, the median counts of dilated, tortuous, and crossing capillaries were seen to be significantly lower and capillary density was notably higher in the control group than in either of the CD subgroups.

The highest median number of capillaries with abnormal morphology was observed in patients from Group 1, significantly surpassing both the good-adherence group and the control group. Group 2 also displayed a higher frequency of abnormal capillary morphology compared to the control group. In terms of capillary density, dilated capillaries, crossing patterns, or tortuosity, there was seen to be no significant difference between Groups 1 and 2. These capillaroscopic findings are presented in detail in Table 3.

Table 3. Comparison of capillaroscopic parameters among patient subgroups and healthy controls.

Capillaroscopic Parameters (per mm)	Group 1 (*n*:44)	Group 2 (*n*:32)	HCs (*n*:76)	p^K Value	p^{1-2}	p^{1-3}	p^{2-3}
Capillary length (µm), median (IQR)	279.5 (242.5–325.5)	270 (249–302)	255 (230–290)	0.081	-	-	-
Capillary density, median (IQR)	6.93 (6.81–7.06)	7 (6.87–7)	7.06 (7–7.12)	<0.001	>0.999	<0.001	0.003
Dilated capillaries, median (IQR)	0 (0–0.12)	0 (0–0.03)	0 (0–0)	<0.001	0.33	<0.001	0.029
Capillaries with abnormal shape, median (IQR)	0.12 (0–0.18)	0 (0–0.18)	0 (0–0)	<0.001	0.022	<0.001	<0.001
Crossing capillaries, median (min–max)	0.18 (0–0.93)	0.12 (0–0.68)	0 (0–0.37)	<0.001	>0.999	<0.001	<0.001
Tortuous capillaries, median (min–max)	0.12 (0–0.93)	0.12 (0–0.62)	0 (0–0.03)	<0.001	>0.999	<0.001	0.001

Group 1 included patients without tTG-IgA normalization (>10 U/mL) and with symptoms suggestive of gluten exposure. Group 2 included those with normalized tTG-IgA (≤10 U/mL) and no symptoms. HCs: healthy controls, IQR: interquartile range. K Kruskal–Wallis H test, Dunn test, post hoc Bonferroni correction. The numbers used in the representation of post hoc analysis results are as follows: p^{1-2}: Comparison of Group 1 and Group 2; p^{1-3}: Comparison of Group 1 and HCs; p^{2-3}: Comparison of Group 2 and HCs.

3.2.4. Capillaroscopic Findings According to Antinuclear Antibody Status

Comparisons of the capillaroscopic parameters showed no significant differences between the ANA-negative (*n*:66) and ANA-positive (*n*:10) CD patients ($p > 0.05$ for all). Although the ANA-negative group exhibited a higher mean capillary length (284.9 ± 75.7 µm) compared to the ANA-positive group (249.9 ± 55.8 µm), the difference was not at a statistically significant level ($p = 0.057$). Other parameters, including capillary density, dilatation, abnormal shape, crossing, and tortuosity, were seen to be similar in both groups, and there was found to be no significant difference with respect to inflammatory markers such as ESR, CRP, PT, or INR ($p > 0.05$).

4. Discussion

Although NVC is commonly used to assess microvascular architecture in autoimmune conditions, its application in detecting comparable vascular alterations in children with CD remains largely unexplored in the literature. In this context, the current study can be considered to provide the first insights into NVC patterns observed in pediatric CD, addressing a gap that has not been previously explored. The observed reduction in capillary density, together with higher rates of dilated loops, microhemorrhages, and morphological abnormalities, suggests that possible microvascular alterations occur throughout the disease, even in the absence of clinically apparent vasculitis or systemic autoimmune involvement.

Specific NVC patterns are well characterized only in jSSc; however, nonspecific capillary abnormalities such as decreased density, dilated loops, and microhemorrhages have also been reported in pediatric SLE, JDM, and other connective tissue diseases [9,16–18]. Such microvascular alterations can emerge even when Raynaud's phenomenon is not clinically evident, suggesting that overlapping immune-related mechanisms may underlie various autoimmune disorders [19]. Consistent with this perspective, the current study findings revealed that children with CD exhibited a markedly increased frequency of these nonspecific capillary changes. We also observed a positive correlation between the number of dilated capillaries and both patient age and disease duration, indicating that microvascular changes may progress over time. Considering that pediatric CD has not been previously evaluated in this context, the only available evidence in adults comes from a cross-sectional study comparing newly diagnosed active celiac disease, remission cases, and HCs [12].

That study reported capillary abnormalities in 60% of active cases—most often capillary density loss, avascular areas, dilated capillaries, and occasionally microhemorrhages or tortuosity—without giant capillaries, disorganization, extravasation, or abnormal shapes. In contrast, we observed abnormal capillary shapes in our patient group, possibly related to the inclusion of individuals with longer disease duration, as well as reduced capillary density, dilated, tortuous, and crossing capillaries in the healthy control group, consistent with reports that such findings may also occur in healthy children [20]. Taken together, our results provide a detailed quantitative evaluation of NVC parameters in a pediatric population and offer novel insights into the potential microvascular involvement in celiac disease during childhood.

Another key finding of this study was the significant difference in abnormal capillary morphology according to dietary adherence. In CD, the absence of a gold standard method for assessing adherence to a GFD (gluten-free diet) presents a significant challenge, as patients must maintain lifelong gluten-free nutrition [15]. Currently, the best available non-invasive adherence marker is tTG-IgA; however, normalization of tTG serology may take more than a year, particularly in individuals with high initial titers or severe mucosal injury, limiting its sensitivity as an early adherence indicator [21]. In our cohort, participants without tTG-IgA normalization (>10 U/mL) exhibited the highest frequency of capillary morphological abnormalities, whereas even those with normalized tTG-IgA (≤10 U/mL) had higher counts than healthy peers. These findings may reflect ongoing gluten exposure and greater microvascular disruption, warranting further investigation. Previous study has demonstrated elevated serum levels of endothelial adhesion molecules (VCAM-1, ICAM-1, and E-selectin) in pediatric CD, with partial normalization following GFD compliance [22]. Although both biochemical markers and NVC alterations may reflect shared underlying endothelial involvement in CD, the cross-sectional design of the present study precludes establishing a direct cause-and-effect relationship. Longitudinal studies are needed to assess whether sustained GFD adherence leads to NVC normalization and if follow-up NVC, combined with tTG-IgA levels, could serve as an additional tool for monitoring adherence in clinical practice.

Since the capillary alterations identified in our study have also been described in other autoimmune conditions, they are not unique to celiac disease. Their presence supports the hypothesis that the autoimmune nature of the disease may predispose affected children to microvascular abnormalities. CD triggers a wide range of immune-mediated reactions. One hypothesized pathway is that exposure to gliadin impairs the intestinal barrier function, allowing immunologically active peptide fragments to enter the bloodstream. This process activates tissue transglutaminase 2 and initiates a Th1-driven immune response, leading to the generation of autoantibodies and immune complexes [23], which may contribute to microvascular damage. Given that CD is more frequently associated with other immune-mediated diseases, such as autoimmune thyroiditis, T1DM, SLE, and jSSc, than in the general population [1,24–26], the exclusion of any diagnosed connective tissue disease in our cohort is particularly noteworthy. Although systemic autoantibodies are known to contribute to vascular damage in connective tissue disorders such as SLE [27], our findings did not reveal significant differences in capillaroscopic features between ANA-positive and ANA-negative children with CD. ANA testing is widely used as an adjunctive tool in the evaluation of autoimmune diseases, especially SLE and other rheumatic disorders, with a negative result providing strong evidence against active autoimmunity [28]. While increased ANA positivity has been reported in CD [29], its clinical significance in the absence of coexisting autoimmune diseases remains unclear. In CD, ANA positivity may result from a genetic predisposition to autoimmunity (e.g., HLA-DQ2/DQ8), chronic mucosal inflammation with subsequent antigen spreading and nuclear antigen exposure in the gut, coexisting autoimmune disorders, or nonspecific polyclonal B cell activation during chronic immune stimulation [30]. Indeed, ANA positivity on its own is neither pathognomonic nor diagnostic for a specific autoimmune condition, as it may be present in up to 15% of children in the general population [31] and should always be interpreted within the broader clinical context. Taken together, these results suggest that the microvascular changes observed in CD are unlikely to be driven by systemic autoantibodies such as ANA.

Endothelial cells are central components of inflammation, acting both as targets and mediators [32]. Previous studies have shown elevated serum levels of several proinflammatory cytokines, which correlate with IgA anti-TG2 titers and villous atrophy, as well as increased endothelial adhesion molecules in pediatric CD patients [22,33], potentially indicating microvascular damage. Furthermore, CD-related autoantibodies, particularly anti-tTG, may impair endothelial function and inhibit angiogenesis, leading to vascular disorganization and immaturity in the small intestinal mucosa of untreated patients [34]. A recent study aiming to clarify the mechanisms of autoantibody formation in CD demonstrated that IgA-switched TG2-specific B cells are uniquely present in untreated patients and are distinct from those observed in autoimmune diseases—most notably SLE—and in particular chronic infectious diseases [35]. These findings support a gluten-driven pathway for organ-specific autoantibody production in CD, distinct from the mechanisms underlying autoimmune connective tissue diseases such as SLE. Collectively, these findings suggest that microvascular involvement in CD may arise through disease-specific pathways, highlighting important directions for future research.

NVC is a validated, easy-to-use, non-invasive technique for microvascular assessment in rheumatologic diseases. It provides immediate visual results during outpatient evaluation [9,16,17]. In pediatric rheumatology, NVC is a key imaging modality for jSSc, with diagnostic value in evaluating Raynaud's phenomenon as part of the jSSc criteria [16]. It has also proven useful in monitoring treatment response, particularly in JDM [9]. From a gastroenterology perspective, interest in NVC is limited but increasing in inflammatory bowel disease [11]. Our findings indicate that NVC could also be a valuable tool in CD, as it differentiated the capillary pattern from that of HCs. Further research is warranted to establish a cost-effective strategy for disease monitoring and for assessing adherence to GFD, potentially in combination with tTGA measurement. If confirmed in larger prospective studies, this approach could be integrated into routine follow-up to enable early detection of systemic changes, identify potential coexisting autoimmune diseases such as rheumatologic or endocrinologic disorders, and assess GFD adherence. This may help to optimize patient management and improve long-term outcomes in pediatric CD.

There were some limitations to this study, primarily the cross-sectional design, which prevented the assessment of the longitudinal progression or reversibility of NVC abnormalities following dietary intervention. A second limitation was that the relatively small number of participants may limit the extent to which these findings can be generalized to the broader pediatric CD population. Third, ethical constraints prevented the use of serological tests and intestinal biopsies in healthy control subjects, so the possibility of undetected subclinical CD in this group cannot be entirely ruled out. As this can be considered a pilot study, all NVC assessments were performed by a single evaluator, and inter- or intra-observer reliability could not be assessed. Future studies should incorporate independent evaluations by multiple observers to assess and improve measurement reliability. Additionally, although the presence of nonspecific NVC patterns was significantly more frequent in CD patients compared to healthy controls, their nonspecific nature limits the potential use of NVC as a diagnostic tool. Finally, the lack of long-term clinical and NVC follow-up restricts the ability to determine the prognostic value of capillaroscopic findings in predicting future autoimmune or vascular complications. Nevertheless, to the best of our knowledge, this is the first report to have evaluated NVC findings in pediatric CD patients. The findings obtained indicate the potential role of NVC as a non-invasive and cost-effective method for assessing microvascular involvement and for screening coexisting autoimmune conditions in children with CD.

5. Conclusions

This paper provides the first evidence of microvascular alterations in pediatric CD as assessed by NVC. The observed abnormalities, notably reduced capillary density and increased morphological changes, suggest potential microvascular involvement, possibly driven by disease-specific immune mechanisms. Associations between these microvascular changes and factors such as tTG-IgA levels, patient age, and disease duration indicate that both ongoing disease activity and long-term immune-mediated damage may contribute to their development. Although the study results indicate that NVC has potential as a practical, non-invasive approach in the detection of vascular alterations in children with celiac disease, the nonspecific abnormalities identified can also occur in various autoimmune and non-autoimmune conditions, and their clinical significance remains uncertain. There is a need for long-term follow-up studies to investigate whether the microvascular changes observed are reversible, the mechanisms driving them, and whether they can provide insight into the course or prognosis of the disease. In addition, future research using standardized semi-quantitative scoring systems could enhance the comparability of results across studies.

Author Contributions: Conceptualization: G.Ç., R.B.T.; supervision: G.Ç.; project administration: R.B.T.; methodology: G.Ç., R.B.T.; data curation: G.Ç.; formal analysis: G.Ç.; investigation: G.Ç.; visualization: G.Ç.; nailfold videocapillaroscopy assessment: R.B.T.; writing—original draft: R.B.T.; writing—review and editing: G.Ç., R.B.T. G.Ç. and R.B.T. contributed equally to this work. Final approval: All authors have read and agreed to the published version of the manuscript.

Funding: This research received no external funding.

Institutional Review Board Statement: This study was conducted in accordance with the Declaration of Helsinki, and approved by the Ethics Committee of Tepecik Training and Research Hospital (Decision No: 2025/01-16, approval date: 5 February 2025).

Informed Consent Statement: Informed consent was obtained from all subjects or legal guardian involved in this study and written informed consent has been obtained from the patients to publish this paper.

Data Availability Statement: All data generated or analyzed during this study are included in this published article. Additional information can be obtained from the corresponding author upon reasonable request. The data are not publicly available due to patient privacy concerns and institutional data protection policies.

Acknowledgments: We thank all patients and healthy donors for their participation in this study.

Conflicts of Interest: The authors declare no conflicts of interest.

References

1. Catassi, C.; Verdu, E.F.; Bai, J.C.; Lionetti, E. Coeliac disease. *Lancet* **2022**, *399*, 2413–2426. [CrossRef]
2. Wang, Y.; Chen, B.; Ciaccio, E.J.; Jneid, H.; Virani, S.S.; Lavie, C.J.; Lebovits, J.; Green, P.H.R.; Krittanawong, C. Celiac Disease and the Risk of Cardiovascular Diseases. *Int. J. Mol. Sci.* **2023**, *24*, 9974. [CrossRef]
3. Laurikka, P.; Kivelä, L.; Kurppa, K.; Kaukinen, K. Review article: Systemic consequences of coeliac disease. *Aliment. Pharmacol. Ther.* **2022**, *56*, 64–72. [CrossRef]
4. Keppeler, K.; Pesi, A.; Lange, S.; Helmstädter, J.; Strohm, L.; Ubbens, H.; Kuntić, M.; Kuntić, I.; Mihaliková, D.; Vujačić-Mirski, K.; et al. Vascular Dysfunction and Arterial Hypertension in Experimental Celiac Disease Are Mediated by Gut-Derived Inflammation and Oxidative Stress. *Redox Biol.* **2024**, *70*, 103071. [CrossRef]

5. Rohrer, T.R.; Wolf, J.; Liptay, S.; Zimmer, K.P.; Fröhlich-Reiterer, E.; Scheuing, N.; Marg, W.; Stern, M.; Kapellen, T.M.; Hauffa, B.P.; et al. Microvascular Complications in Childhood-Onset Type 1 Diabetes and Celiac Disease: A Multicenter Longitudinal Analysis of 56,514 Patients From the German-Austrian DPV Database. *Diabetes Care* **2015**, *38*, 801–807. [CrossRef]
6. Kıran Taşcı, E.; Taner, S.; Doğan, E.; Karakoyun, M.; Kaplan Bulut, İ.; Kabasakal, C. Evaluation of Vascular Involvement in Children with Celiac Disease. *J. Pediatr. Res.* **2023**, *10*, 167–172. [CrossRef]
7. Cutolo, M.; Sulli, A.; Secchi, M.E.; Olivieri, M.; Pizzorni, C. The Contribution of Capillaroscopy to the Differential Diagnosis of Connective Autoimmune Diseases. *Best. Pract. Res. Clin. Rheumatol.* **2007**, *21*, 1093–1108. [CrossRef]
8. Smith, V.; Ickinger, C.; Hysa, E.; Snow, M.; Frech, T.; Sulli, A.; Cutolo, M. Nailfold Capillaroscopy. *Best. Pract. Res. Clin. Rheumatol.* **2023**, *37*, 101849. [CrossRef] [PubMed]
9. Schonenberg-Meinema, D.; Cutolo, M.; Smith, V. Capillaroscopy in the Daily Clinic of the Pediatric Rheumatologist. *Best. Pract. Res. Clin. Rheumatol.* **2024**, *38*, 101978. [CrossRef]
10. Komai, M.; Takeno, D.; Fujii, C.; Nakano, J.; Ohsaki, Y.; Shirakawa, H. Nailfold Capillaroscopy: A Comprehensive Review on Its Usefulness in Both Clinical Diagnosis and Improving Unhealthy Dietary Lifestyles. *Nutrients* **2024**, *16*, 1914. [CrossRef]
11. Kurowski, J.A.; Patel, S.R.; Wechsler, J.B.; Izaguirre, M.R.; Morgan, G.A.; Pachman, L.M.; Brown, J.B. Nailfold Capillaroscopy as a Biomarker in the Evaluation of Pediatric Inflammatory Bowel Disease. *Crohns Colitis 360* **2021**, *3*, otab069. [CrossRef]
12. Okyar, B.; Yıldırım, A.E.; Barutçu, S. The Relationship Between Gluten Enteropathy and Nail Capillaroscopy Findings and Disease Activation. *Clin. Exp. Health Sci.* **2022**, *12*, 760–764. [CrossRef]
13. Husby, S.; Koletzko, S.; Korponay-Szabó, I.; Kurppa, K.; Mearin, M.L.; Ribes-Koninckx, C.; Shamir, R.; Troncone, R.; Auricchio, R.; Castillejo, G.; et al. European Society for Paediatric Gastroenterology, Hepatology and Nutrition Guidelines for Diagnosing Coeliac Disease 2020. *J. Pediatr. Gastroenterol. Nutr.* **2020**, *70*, 141–156. [CrossRef]
14. Marsh, M.N. Gluten, Major Histocompatibility Complex, and the Small Intestine: A Molecular and Immunobiologic Approach to the Spectrum of Gluten Sensitivity ("Celiac Sprue"). *Gastroenterology* **1992**, *102*, 330–354. [CrossRef]
15. Mearin, M.L.; Agardh, D.; Antunes, H.; Al-Toma, A.; Auricchio, R.; Castillejo, G.; Catassi, C.; Ciacci, C.; Discepolo, V.; Dolinsek, J.; et al. ESPGHAN Special Interest Group on Celiac Disease. ESPGHAN Position Paper on Management and Follow-up of Children and Adolescents With Celiac Disease. *J. Pediatr. Gastroenterol. Nutr.* **2022**, *75*, 369–386. [CrossRef]
16. Smith, V.; Herrick, A.L.; Ingegnoli, F.; Damjanov, N.; De Angelis, R.; Denton, C.P.; Distler, O.; Espejo, K.; Foeldvari, I.; Frech, T.; et al. Standardisation of Nailfold Capillaroscopy for the Assessment of Patients with Raynaud's Phenomenon and Systemic Sclerosis. *Autoimmun. Rev.* **2020**, *19*, 102458. [CrossRef]
17. Melsens, K.; Cutolo, M.; Schonenberg-Meinema, D.; Foeldvari, I.; Leone, M.C.; Mostmans, Y.; Badot, V.; Cimaz, R.; Dehoorne, J.; Deschepper, E.; et al. Standardized Nailfold Capillaroscopy in Children with Rheumatic Diseases: A Worldwide Study. *Rheumatology* **2023**, *62*, 1605–1615. [CrossRef]
18. Schonenberg-Meinema, D.; Bergkamp, S.C.; Nassar-Sheikh Rashid, A.; van der Aa, L.B.; de Bree, G.J.; Ten Cate, R.; Cutolo, M.; Hak, A.E.; Hissink Muller, P.C.; van Onna, M.; et al. Nailfold Capillary Abnormalities in Childhood-Onset Systemic Lupus Erythematosus: A Cross-Sectional Study Compared with Healthy Controls. *Lupus* **2021**, *30*, 818–827. [CrossRef]
19. Chanprapaph, K.; Fakprapai, W.; Limtong, P.; Suchonwanit, P. Nailfold Capillaroscopy with USB Digital Microscopy in Connective Tissue Diseases: A Comparative Study of 245 Patients and Healthy Controls. *Front. Med.* **2021**, *8*, 683900. [CrossRef]
20. Dundar, H.A.; Adrovic, A.; Demir, S.; Demir, F.; Cakmak, F.; Ayaz, N.A.; Sözeri, B.; Bilginer, Y.; Kasapçopur, O.; Unsal, E. Description of the characteristics of the nailfold capillary structure in healthy children: A multi-centric study. *Rheumatology* **2024**, *63*, SI152–SI159. [CrossRef]
21. Gidrewicz, D.; Trevenen, C.L.; Lyon, M.; Butzner, J.D. Normalization Time of Celiac Serology in Children on a Gluten-free Diet. *J. Pediatr. Gastroenterol. Nutr.* **2017**, *64*, 362–367. [CrossRef]
22. Comba, A.; Çaltepe, G.; Yank, K.; Gör, U.; Yüce, Ö.; Kalayc, A.G. Assessment of Endothelial Dysfunction With Adhesion Molecules in Patients With Celiac Disease. *J. Pediatr. Gastroenterol. Nutr.* **2016**, *63*, 247–252. [CrossRef]
23. Lupu, V.V.; Sasaran, M.O.; Jechel, E.; Starcea, I.M.; Ioniuc, I.; Mocanu, A.; Rosu, S.T.; Munteanu, V.; Nedelcu, A.H.; Danielescu, C.; et al. Celiac Disease—A Pluripathological Model in Pediatric Practice. *Front. Immunol.* **2024**, *15*, 1390755. [CrossRef]
24. Lupu, V.V.; Jechel, E.; Mihai, C.M.; Mitrofan, E.C.; Lupu, A.; Starcea, I.M.; Fotea, S.; Mocanu, A.; Ghica, D.C.; Mitrofan, C.; et al. Connection between Celiac Disease and Systemic Lupus Erythematosus in Children—A Development Model of Autoimmune Diseases Starting from What We Inherit to What We Eat. *Nutrients* **2023**, *15*, 2535. [CrossRef]
25. Bartoloni, E.; Bistoni, O.; Alunno, A.; Cavagna, L.; Nalotto, L.; Baldini, C.; Priori, R.; Fischetti, C.; Fredi, M.; Quartuccio, L.; et al. Celiac Disease Prevalence Is Increased in Primary Sjögren's Syndrome and Diffuse Systemic Sclerosis: Lessons from a Large Multi-Center Study. *J. Clin. Med.* **2019**, *8*, 540. [CrossRef] [PubMed]
26. Flores Monar, G.V.; Islam, H.; Puttagunta, S.M.; Islam, R.; Kundu, S.; Jha, S.B.; Rivera, A.P.; Sange, I. Association Between Type 1 Diabetes Mellitus and Celiac Disease: Autoimmune Disorders With a Shared Genetic Background. *Cureus* **2022**, *14*, e22912. [CrossRef]

27. Dai, X.; Fan, Y.; Zhao, X. Systemic lupus erythematosus: Updated insights on the pathogenesis, diagnosis, prevention and therapeutics. *Signal Transduct. Target. Ther.* **2025**, *10*, 102. [CrossRef]
28. Satoh, M.; Vázquez-Del Mercado, M.; Chan, E.K. Clinical interpretation of antinuclear antibody tests in systemic rheumatic diseases. *Mod. Rheumatol.* **2009**, *19*, 219–228. [CrossRef]
29. Almeida, R.M.; da Silva, Z.D.L.; Leite, F.B.; de Medeiros Nóbrega, Y.K. Antinuclear antibodies patterns in patients with celiac disease. *Biomed. J.* **2019**, *1*, 3. [CrossRef]
30. Dahan, S.; Shor, D.B.; Comaneshter, D.; Tekes-Manova, D.; Shovman, O.; Amital, H.; Cohen, A.D. All disease begins in the gut: Celiac disease co-existence with SLE. *Autoimmun. Rev.* **2016**, *15*, 848–853. [CrossRef]
31. Wananukul, S.; Voramethkul, W.; Kaewopas, Y.; Hanvivatvong, O. Prevalence of positive antinuclear antibodies in healthy children. *Asian Pac. J. Allergy Immunol.* **2005**, *23*, 153–157. [PubMed]
32. Xue, J.; Zhang, Z.; Sun, Y.; Jin, D.; Guo, L.; Li, X.; Zhao, D.; Feng, X.; Qi, W.; Zhu, H. Research Progress and Molecular Mechanisms of Endothelial Cells Inflammation in Vascular-Related Diseases. *J. Inflamm. Res.* **2023**, *16*, 3593–3617. [CrossRef]
33. Auricchio, R.; Calabrese, I.; Galatola, M.; Cielo, D.; Carbone, F.; Mancuso, M.; Matarese, G.; Troncone, R.; Auricchio, S.; Greco, L. Gluten consumption and inflammation affect the development of celiac disease in at-risk children. *Sci. Rep.* **2022**, *12*, 5396, Erratum in Sci. Rep. 2022, 12, 8157. https://doi.org/10.1038/s41598-022-12636-0. [CrossRef]
34. Fontana, G.; Ziberna, F.; Barbi, E.; Di Leo, G.; De Leo, L. Intestinal celiac disease-related autoantibodies. *Front. Immunol.* **2025**, *16*, 1567416. [CrossRef]
35. Lindeman, I.; Høydahl, L.S.; Christophersen, A.; Risnes, L.F.; Jahnsen, J.; Lundin, K.E.A.; Sollid, L.M.; Iversen, R. Generation of circulating autoreactive pre-plasma cells fueled by naive B cells in celiac disease. *Cell Rep.* **2024**, *43*, 114045. [CrossRef]

diagnostics

Review

Omphalocele and Associated Anomalies: Exploring Pulmonary Development and Genetic Correlations—A Literature Review

Dina Al Namat [1,2], Romulus Adrian Roșca [1,3], Razan Al Namat [1,*], Elena Hanganu [1,3], Andrei Ivan [1,2], Delia Hînganu [1], Ancuța Lupu [4] and Marius Valeriu Hînganu [1]

1 Faculty of Medicine, University of Medicine and Pharmacy "Grigore T. Popa", 700115 Iasi, Romania; dina.rosca-al.namat@umfiasi.ro (D.A.N.); adrianrosca82@yahoo.com (R.A.R.); dr.elenahanganu@gmail.com (E.H.); ivan.andrei89@gmail.com (A.I.); hinganu.delia@umfiasi.ro (D.H.); marius.hinganu@umfiasi.ro (M.V.H.)
2 Department of Surgery II-Pediatric Surgery, 700309 Iasi, Romania
3 "Saint Mary" Emergency Children Hospital, 700309 Iasi, Romania
4 Department of Mother and Child Medicine, University of Medicine and Pharmacy "Grigore T. Popa", 700115 Iasi, Romania; anca_ign@yahoo.com
* Correspondence: dr.razan_romania@yahoo.com

Abstract: Omphalocele is a rare congenital abdominal wall defect, occurring in approximately 3.38 per 10,000 pregnancies. It is characterized by the herniation of abdominal organs through the base of the umbilical cord, enclosed by a peritoneal sac. While omphalocele can occur as an isolated anomaly, it is more commonly associated with congenital syndromes and structural abnormalities. Among its most significant complications, pulmonary hypoplasia (PH) and pulmonary hypertension (PPH) have been shown to negatively impact neonatal prognosis. These conditions result from impaired pulmonary vascular development, leading to respiratory distress and hypoxemia. Unlike many congenital disorders, there is no universally accepted surgical approach for omphalocele repair. The choice of surgical strategy depends on multiple factors, including the size of the abdominal wall defect, presence of herniated solid organs, associated anomalies, and severity of pulmonary complications. Notably, giant omphaloceles are frequently linked to lung hypoplasia, as reduced intra-abdominal space restricts fetal lung expansion, leading to structural lung abnormalities and increased pulmonary vascular resistance. These factors contribute to a higher risk of respiratory morbidity and mortality in affected neonates. This literature review examines the prevalence, significance, and clinical implications of the association between omphalocele and pulmonary abnormalities. Through a systematic analysis of published studies, we evaluated 157 full-text articles along with available titles and abstracts. Our findings indicate that infants with omphalocele often exhibit respiratory complications detectable prenatally and at birth. Severe respiratory insufficiency, particularly due to pulmonary hypoplasia and pulmonary hypertension, significantly increases neonatal morbidity and mortality. While surgical correction may initially exacerbate respiratory challenges, most patients demonstrate short-term recovery with appropriate multidisciplinary management. This review highlights the importance of early diagnosis, comprehensive prenatal assessment, and tailored postnatal management to improve outcomes in newborns with omphalocele and associated pulmonary complications. Further research is needed to establish standardized treatment protocols and optimize long-term respiratory outcomes in these patients.

Keywords: omphalocele; pulmonary abnormalities; anterior abdominal wall; anatomy; exomphalos; pulmonary hypoplasia

 https://doi.org/10.3390/diagnostics15060675

1. Introduction

Omphalocele, also known as exomphalos, is a congenital abdominal wall defect characterized by the herniation of abdominal organs through a midline opening at the base of the umbilical cord. These organs remain enclosed within a three-layered protective membrane composed of peritoneum, Wharton's jelly, and amnion. The condition occurs in approximately 1 in 1100 pregnancies, but due to a high rate of spontaneous abortions, its incidence in live births is estimated between 1 in 4000 and 1 in 6000 [1]. Based on the extent of the defect and organ involvement, omphalocele can be classified into small, giant, and ruptured types [2]. Omphalocele is often associated with genetic abnormalities, with over 50% of affected infants presenting chromosomal anomalies such as trisomy 13, 18, and 21, as well as syndromic conditions like Beckwith–Wiedemann syndrome [3]. In addition to gastrointestinal complications, up to 24% of newborns with omphalocele exhibit extra-abdominal abnormalities, including cardiac defects and pulmonary hypoplasia [4].

In recent years, studies have highlighted the link between giant omphalocele and abnormalities in both pulmonary parenchyma and vasculature, leading to pulmonary hypoplasia and pulmonary hypertension (PH) [5,6]. The altered development of the thoracic cage further contributes to respiratory complications [7]. Several case reports and series have documented chronic pulmonary issues, including PH, in newborns with omphalocele [8–10]. The underlying causes of pulmonary hypertension in these infants are complex.

Pulmonary hypoplasia remains the most frequently reported cause, as demonstrated in post-mortem findings of 14 out of 27 infants with giant omphalocele [9]. Additionally, alveolar capillary dysplasia has been identified as a potential contributor in some cases. Other factors linked to pulmonary hypertension include structural anomalies of the pulmonary arteries, left-to-right cardiac shunts, and congenital heart disease [11,12]. It has been suggested that abnormal prenatal lung development in these infants results from an in utero deformation sequence, influenced by multiple factors [13–15]. The displacement of the liver affects thoracic cavity formation, leading to reduced intra-abdominal pressure. Consequently, the lower rib cage flattens inward during fetal breathing movements, further restricting lung development [14]. In many cases, the rectus abdominis muscles attach laterally rather than at the midline, exerting a downward force on the rib cage and contributing to a narrow thorax with slanted ribs [15,16].

Prenatal detection of pulmonary hypoplasia in fetuses with abdominal wall defects has become increasingly feasible through ultrasonographic and MRI assessments. Two-dimensional ultrasound (2D-US) can predict pulmonary hypoplasia by measuring the lung-to-thorax ratio, while the chest-to-trunk length ratio helps identify thoracic restriction [15–19]. More recently, fetal MRI imaging has been used to quantify total lung volumes, offering a more accurate assessment of lung development in fetuses with giant omphalocele [20].

2. Materials and Methods

Electronic Databases and Search Strategy

This review was conducted in accordance with the Preferred Reporting Items for Systematic Reviews and Meta-Analysis (PRISMA) Statement (available at http://www.prisma-statement.org/, accessed on 12 January 2024). PRISMA guidelines were followed throughout the review process to ensure transparency, rigor, and reproducibility in our methodology. The approach involved independent data extraction and quality assessment, which were performed by four researchers, each contributing to the accuracy and thoroughness of the review.

We employed three major electronic databases—PubMed, Web of Science, and EMBASE—to conduct an extensive literature search. These databases were chosen due to their broad coverage of medical and clinical studies, as well as their inclusion of both peer-reviewed articles and the gray literature, ensuring that the search would provide a comprehensive view of the topic. The search was focused on identifying studies that explored the association between omphalocele and pulmonary malformations or pulmonary hypoplasia, specifically examining any correlations between these conditions and their potential effects on lung function and overall respiratory health.

In order to ensure the inclusion of the most relevant and high-quality evidence, we defined a set of inclusion criteria. Initially, we focused on original studies published in English to minimize language bias and ensure accessibility to the broader scientific community. The review included systematic reviews, randomized controlled trials (RCTs), and observational studies, as well as case studies and case reports. These types of studies were selected because they provide a broad spectrum of data—ranging from large-scale quantitative analyses to detailed reports of individual patient experiences—allowing for a comprehensive exploration of the relationship between omphalocele and pulmonary abnormalities.

The time frame for the search spanned from the earliest published studies available up to January 2024, to ensure the inclusion of both foundational research and the latest findings in the field. The inclusion of both historical and recent studies allowed for an exploration of how the understanding of omphalocele and its associated pulmonary complications has evolved over time.

The search process involved the use of specific, well-defined keywords and MeSH (Medical Subject Headings) terms, including "omphalocele", "pulmonary malformations", "pulmonary hypoplasia", "congenital anomalies", and "lung function". Boolean operators were employed to refine the search results and ensure that only the most relevant articles were retrieved. After the initial search, the retrieved articles were carefully screened for eligibility based on predefined inclusion and exclusion criteria, focusing on studies that specifically addressed the association between omphalocele and pulmonary issues.

Data extraction was performed independently by each of the four researchers, and any discrepancies between their findings were resolved through discussion and consensus. Following data extraction, the quality of the included studies was assessed using established quality assessment tools appropriate for each study design, ensuring that the final analysis was based on reliable and robust evidence.

By adhering to these procedures, we aimed to provide a comprehensive, objective, and up-to-date synthesis of the literature on the association between omphalocele and pulmonary malformations, contributing valuable insights into this complex area of pediatric medicine.

3. Results

The initial PubMed search yielded a total of 6896 articles. To refine the selection, we applied filters to include only studies with available abstracts and free full-text access, reducing the number to 1426. We then used the Medical Subject Headings (MeSH) terms "pulmonary malformation" and "pulmonary hypoplasia" to narrow down the most relevant studies. This search identified 48 and 55 articles, respectively. After a thorough title and abstract screening, 41 studies were determined to be eligible for inclusion in our review. From the Web of Science database, we identified 2339 articles related to omphalocele. To ensure relevance, we conducted a focused search using the terms "omphalocele" AND "pulmonary malformation" and "omphalocele" AND "pulmonary hypoplasia", which resulted in 110 articles. To further refine our selection, we applied category filters related to Respiratory System, Pediatrics, Obstetrics and Gynecology, Genetics & Heredity, and

Surgery, leading to a final dataset of 90 studies for detailed analysis. Our EMBASE search retrieved 4623 articles on omphalocele. When we applied the terms "pulmonary malformation" OR "pulmonary hypoplasia", we identified 404 and 259 articles, respectively. After filtering for human studies and reviews, 36 and 24 articles met the inclusion criteria. Following duplicate removal and relevance screening, we selected 16 articles from EMBASE for our review. After merging and deduplicating results from all three databases, a total of 876 unique articles were initially considered. Following title and abstract screening, 2199 records underwent further review.

Based on predefined exclusion criteria, 729 studies were removed, including the following: 20 articles filtered out based on Web of Science category restrictions, 603 studies excluded for being non-human research or reviews, 44 duplicates and non-relevant studies removed, and 62 studies excluded after title and abstract assessment. Ultimately, 147 full-text articles were assessed for eligibility. An additional 10 studies were identified through reference screening, leading to a final inclusion of 157 studies in this review.

4. Literature Review

During the second step, we revised 147 papers, focusing on the titles, the abstracts, and the full texts in order to select significant data for our review. In total, 157 relevant studies with their citation were included in our reference list. The chest wall is made up of the intercostal muscles, rib cage, and abdominal wall. The only area of the abdominal compartment that can move freely is the ventral abdominal wall since the lateral and posterior abdomen are restricted in their mobility by the back, lower rib cage, pelvis, and iliac crests. The motion of the diaphragm in respect to the thorax provides crucial insight into the mechanics of the chest wall and respiratory pump. Changes in the properties of the abdominal wall influence total respiratory pump operation. Furthermore, congenital anomalies of the ventral abdominal wall may be linked to pulmonary hypoplasia and infant respiratory distress [19,21]. Numerous genes have been associated with the development of the ventral abdominal wall [22,23]. The amount of pulmonary hypoplasia present frequently determines the survival rate of live-born neonates with abdominal wall defects [21].

Abdominal wall abnormalities not only affect respiratory mechanics and diaphragm function postnatally but also impact prenatal lung and chest wall development. Pulmonary hypoplasia in enormous omphalocele may be caused by a variety of factors. Argyle hypothesized that pulmonary hypoplasia is the result of thoracic cage movement impairment, which includes the abdominal musculature and diaphragm [24]. A significant incidence of respiratory insufficiency has been reported to be associated with giant omphalocele. Pulmonary hypoplasia, diaphragmatic dysfunction, and an elongated, narrow thorax have been identified as contributing factors to respiratory issues [25].

4.1. *Embryology*

Embryological Theories of zOmphalocele Development

The precise embryological mechanisms leading to omphalocele remain uncertain, with multiple hypotheses attempting to explain its etiology [26]. Gross and Blodgett proposed that restricted body cavity expansion between the 8th and 12th weeks of gestation prevents the midgut from returning to the abdominal cavity after physiological herniation, resulting in omphalocele [27]. Margulies, on the other hand, suggested that the defect arises before the third week of gestation, due to either a failure of the mesodermal transverse septum to unite with its amniotic covering or inadequate proliferation of embryonal connective tissue in the transverse septum, both of which are crucial for the development of the supra-umbilical abdominal wall [28]. Gray and Skandalakis proposed that omphalocele results from a developmental arrest during the physiological herniation of intestines into the umbilical coelom, preventing their normal reintegration into the abdomen [29].

Role of the Diaphragm in Ventral Wall Development

Normal diaphragm development begins with the formation of the pleuroperitoneal fold, a lateral structure that connects dorsally to the mesonephric ridge and ventrally to the transverse septum. During early development, lung buds extend into the peritoneal cavity but do not yet reach the pleuroperitoneal canal. Meanwhile, closure of the pleuropericardial canal separates the pleural and pericardial cavities. At this stage, the developing lungs remain in close proximity to the liver on the right and to both the liver and stomach on the left. As the embryo grows, the pleural cavities expand, leading to a gradual reduction in the peritoneal portion of the lungs. By embryonic day (ED) 13, the posthepatic mesenchymal plate (PHMP) begins to form between the transverse septum, liver, and pleuroperitoneal fold. The PHMP rapidly expands in a laterodorsal direction, staying closely associated with the underlying abdominal organs. By ED 13.5, it forms a ridge that partially covers the liver, while the stomach shifts closer to it on the left side. This stage is also marked by the appearance of the phrenic nerve between the PHMP and the transverse septum. By ED 15, the pleural cavities remain small and cubic, positioned dorsally to both the peritoneal and pericardial cavities. At this stage, the transverse septum has formed the pericardial floor, while the pleuroperitoneal canals remain widely open, with the left canal being larger and more horizontally oval and the right smaller and vertically oriented. The PHMP continues its ventral expansion, interacting with adjacent abdominal organs and gradually closing the pleuroperitoneal canals. The right canal seals approximately six hours before the left, and by ED 17, both are fully closed. As this occurs, the pleural cavities expand rapidly, shifting from a dorsal to a lateroventral position around the pericardial cavity.

Molecular and Mechanical Factors in Ventral Body Wall Formation

Transcription Factor AP-2α has been identified as a key regulator of cell migration, differentiation, and apoptosis—processes critical to ventral body wall formation. Disruptions in these pathways may contribute to defects like omphalocele. The link between abdominal wall defects and lung development is complex. Lung growth requires adequate intrathoracic space, and studies on Mek1flox/flox; Mek2−/−; and Dermo1+/Cre mutants suggest that kyphosis and omphalocele can impose physical constraints on lung expansion, compromising respiratory function and neonatal survival [30]. Additionally, normal lung development relies on amniotic fluid inhalation, which expands airways and promotes alveolarization. Fetal breathing movements in the third trimester further stimulate distal airway and capillary growth [31]. Altered amniotic fluid dynamics in utero may lead to pulmonary capillary remodeling, increasing vascular reactivity and contributing to reduced lung volumes [11].

4.2. Epidemiology

A study conducted by the National Birth Defects Prevention Network in the United States analyzed 2308 cases of omphalocele recorded across twelve state population-based registries from 1995 to 2005. The findings indicated an increased likelihood of omphalocele occurrence among infants born to mothers aged 35 and older and those younger than 20 [26].

Additionally, data from the New York State Congenital Malformations Registry (1992–1999) revealed that Black infants had a 70% higher risk of being born with an omphalocele compared to White infants [26]. Maternal obesity, particularly a BMI over 30, has also been identified as a contributing risk factor [26].

Trisomy 18 is the most frequently associated chromosomal abnormality, with 80–90% of affected individuals presenting with an omphalocele [26]. Prenatal ultrasound can detect this condition as early as 13 weeks of gestation, often in conjunction with elevated maternal serum alpha-fetoprotein levels [31]. The incidence of omphalocele ranges between 1 in 4000 and 1 in 10,000 live births, with a female-to-male ratio of 1:1.9 [32,33]. More than half of omphalocele cases involve structural or chromosomal anomalies, with the prevalence potentially reaching 80% [34].

4.3. *Omphalocele Patients with Pulmonary Abnormalities*

The abdominal wall plays a decisive role during inspiration, exhalation, and airway clearance through coughing. The abdominal wall's compliance plays a crucial role in determining the diaphragmatic motion during inspiration [35]. Similar to what occurs after a large meal, a non-compliant abdominal compartment will restrict diaphragmatic descent, and a non-compliant abdominal wall will impede lower rib cage expansion. However, it is important to note that patients with Prune Belly Syndrome may have a highly compliant abdominal wall. This condition can cause changes in the relationship between the rib cage and abdominal wall, as well as diaphragmatic function, which are corrected when the subjects lie in a supine position [36].

Ewig et al. hypothesized that the extremely flexible abdominal wall prevented the lower rib cage from expanding and allowed the diaphragm muscle fibers to shorten excessively by removing the fulcrum impact of the stomach contents on the lower rib cage. These mechanical drawbacks ultimately led to abdominal paradox—the inward migration of the abdominal wall during inspiration—functional diaphragmatic weakening, and the requirement to recruit auxiliary muscles of inspiration [36]. When the identical subjects were examined in a supine position, all of these findings vanished. Additionally, when the diaphragm was subjected to supine gravity, abdominal viscera exerted cephalad pressure, which improved length–tension relationships and increased area of apposition. Primary closure of the defect in infants with gastroschisis or omphalocele may lead to respiratory compromise, particularly if the abdominal compartment has experienced area loss and there is a significant viscera–abdominal disproportion. It has been postulated that the act of relocating organs to the abdominal compartment leads to inflated intra-abdominal pressures, accompanied by cephalic diaphragmatic displacement and motion restriction [37].

4.3.1. Pulmonary Hypoplasia

Griscom and Driscoll examined the radiographs of a number of stillborn babies and babies who passed away soon after birth. They observed that almost all omphalocele fetuses had noticeably smaller chests [38]. Hershenson et al. similarly observed that within a year, newborns with giant omphaloceles gradually reverted to a normal chest structure [25]. To further, Argyle et al. observed that children with omphalocele who had any large abdominal wall abnormalities in addition to narrow thoracic cages were at a higher risk of developing pulmonary hypoplasia and experiencing respiratory distress [24]. Prenatal ultrasound indicators of pulmonary hypoplasia include a reduced lung-to-thorax transverse area ratio and an elevated chest-to-trunk length ratio [19,39].

In another study, total lung volumes (TLVs) in omphalocele were determined using fetal MRI [20,40]. Infants with giant omphaloceles with less than 50% O/E TLV had poorer Apgar scores at birth, they needed more ventilatory assistance, and they had longer hospital admissions than those with more than 50% [20,41].

4.3.2. Pulmonary Hypertension

Omphalocele has also been associated with the development of pulmonary hypertension. It is often diagnosed with an echocardiography, which uses conventional criteria such as higher right ventricular systolic pressures and septal flattening [42,43]. Partridge et al. found that individuals with giant omphalocele often need pulmonary vasodilator treatment, such as nitric oxide or continuous sildenafil [42].

Patients with omphalocele are more likely to have chronic respiratory issues beyond the first prenatal respiratory distress [43] compared to patients without pulmonary hypertension. Multiple studies have reported cases of left lung collapse and/or narrowing of the left mainstem bronchus in patients with giant omphalocele. Lung collapse, which is occasionally found in this group, could be caused by physical deformation of the bronchus due to increased pressure caused by omphalocele reduction [8,44].

4.3.3. Post-Surgical Respiratory Issues

The primary challenge in repairing this anomaly is of respiratory nature, associated with abdominal hypertension. Circulatory disorders may be evidently linked to the reintegration process [45]. The respiratory impact during management is of particular significance due to the frequent association with pulmonary hypoplasia, which may result in respiratory failure [46,47].

Patients with GO have a reduced abdominal cavity. Therefore, the early closure of the abdominal wall can lead to an abrupt surge in intra-abdominal pressure and to respiratory failure because of the reduced lung capacity. There is a special concern in the case of patients with GO, as they also typically manifest pulmonary hypoplasia, which could result in respiratory failure [48,49]. However, the following factors lead to the impossibility of early surgical treatment: the abdominal–visceral disproportion in neonates, the large diameter of the abdominal wall defect, the presence of large liver tissue in the sac, and other organ anomalies that coexist in infants [50,51].

According to a study conducted by Dimitriou et al., newborns with abdominal wall abnormalities showed a temporary reduction in lung compliance following surgical repair; however, by the third postoperative day, this impact had improved. Nakayama et al. investigated the impact of the closure of abdominal wall abnormalities using pulmonary function testing before and after surgery [52,53].

4.3.4. Diaphragmatic Hernia

Anomalies associated with congenital diaphragmatic hernia (CDH) have been reported in 30–40% of patients [54,55]. Omphalocele, also known as exomphalos, is a congenital anomaly characterized by a midline defect in the abdominal wall that allows abdominal organs, mainly the liver and intestines, to herniate, although they remain covered by a protective membrane. The clinical presentation of omphalocele patients frequently includes pulmonary hypoplasia and/or pulmonary hypertension [40,42,56].

The literature on congenital diaphragmatic hernia (CDH) with an accompanying omphalocele is primarily limited to case reports [57,58], with most of the documented cases being of the anterior or antero-lateral type [59–62]. In isolated CDH, pulmonary hypoplasia and pulmonary hypertension are the leading factors contributing to higher morbidity and mortality [63–70]. Additionally, pulmonary hypoplasia [20,48] and/or pulmonary hypertension have been identified as independent predictors of survival in cases of isolated omphalocele [6,71]—a finding that is quite unexpected.

The coexistence of these two conditions in the developing fetus is likely to result in a more pronounced degree of pulmonary hypoplasia and/or pulmonary hypertension, which in turn may significantly worsen respiratory insufficiency after birth. This explains why many of these newborns experience a rapid decline in their condition immediately postnatally [72].

According to Harmath et al., Sweed, and Puri, there were approximately 3–4% of CDH cases characterized by an associated abdominal wall defect with an omphalocele (4 out of 100 and 4 out of 116 CDH cases, respectively) [73]. The incidence of CDH associated with an omphalocele was 0.077%, as concluded in a 10-year review of autopsy cases conducted by Borys and Taxy [74]. The clinical management challenges are presented by this uncommon combination of CDH and omphalocele due to the scarcity of literature reviews on their perinatal management. It has been reported that the combination of CDH and omphalocele represented a component of syndromes, including Fryns syndrome and pentalogy of Cantrell [75]. The literature has also documented chromosomal abnormalities, including trisomy 13 [76] and trisomy 18 [73].

The timing of surgical treatment is vital in cases involving both CDH and omphalocele [61]. There was a report that documented CDH resulting in severe respiratory distress or circulatory instability following the closure of the abdominal wall defect [65].

5. Chromosomal Abnormalities and Syndromes

Isolated omphalocele is an uncommon congenital defect, occurring in approximately 2–3 per 10,000 live births [77]. These abnormalities are relatively rare, and about 56% of affected individuals exhibit chromosomal abnormalities, including trisomies 13, 15, 16, and 18, as well as Beckwith–Wiedemann syndrome [78–80]. Symbrachydactyly, a deformity of the right upper limb, was first identified by Blauth and Gekeler in 1973. This condition is considered a transverse deficit caused by bone dysplasia, with severity categorized into four groups [81,82]. The clinical features are typically consistent, and some cases are associated with pectoralis muscle abnormalities, as seen in Poland syndrome [83]. The frequency of skeletal dysplasia is 2.14 per 10,000 births [84].

Other associated phenotypic features include pulmonary hypoplasia, cardiovascular defects, craniofacial dysmorphism (such as trigonocephaly and forehead prominence), midfacial abnormalities (such as anteverted nares and a long philtrum), gonadal dysgenesis with sex reversal, cryptorchidism, hypospadias, and malformed genitalia, among others. However, the exact correlations between genotype and phenotype remain unclear due to significant variation in phenotypic presentation [82].

Chromosomal abnormalities are commonly associated with fetal growth restriction (FGR), a condition that can be observed as early as the first trimester. Advances in three-dimensional (3D) ultrasound have enabled precise measurements of fetal head and trunk volume, offering significant insights into growth patterns in chromosomally abnormal fetuses. A study conducted on fetuses between 11 + 0 and 13 + 6 weeks of gestation revealed that in trisomy 21 and Turner syndrome, the crown–rump length (CRL) appeared normal, but the head and trunk volume were reduced by 10–15%. In contrast, trisomy 18, trisomy 13, and triploidy exhibited a more significant reduction in trunk volume (about 45%), while CRL remained largely unaffected (under 15%). These findings suggest that chromosomal abnormalities result in generalized growth disturbances, with organ development being more severely affected than skeletal growth [85].

The ability to evaluate the head-to-trunk volume ratio has revealed notable patterns in early-onset FGR for chromosomally abnormal fetuses. The study confirmed that triploidy and trisomies 18 and 13, which are associated with high rates of intrauterine lethality, typically present with severe, early-onset asymmetrical FGR. In contrast, trisomy 21 and Turner syndrome, which have better survival outcomes, display milder, symmetrical growth restriction. These differences in growth patterns are likely due to the variation in fetal and placental development, with different degrees of impairment in both systems [85].

When considering omphalocele in the context of chromosomal abnormalities, particularly in trisomy 13 and trisomy 18, the growth disturbances associated with these conditions have a direct impact on organ development, including the lungs. In these conditions, impaired development of the abdominal wall and lungs can lead to significant pulmonary hypoplasia, making it difficult for the lungs to develop properly. This underscores the importance of early-onset FGR and the interconnectedness of fetal growth and organ development in chromosomally abnormal fetuses. The severe early-onset FGR observed in trisomy 13 and 18 likely exacerbates pulmonary underdevelopment, contributing to the high mortality rates seen in these conditions. Furthermore, the abnormal placental development in these fetuses could also play a role in the reduced fetal circulation and impaired oxygenation, further complicating the growth of the abdominal organs and lungs.

5.1. PAGOD Syndrome

PAGOD syndrome is a rare disorder of unknown cause that presents with multiple congenital anomalies and a poor prognosis. It is defined by a combination of malformations—including pulmonary hypoplasia, agonadism (sex reversal), omphalocele, and a diaphragmatic defect—that reflects abnormalities in the pulmonary artery and lung [86]. In most cases, the pulmonary hypoplasia in PAGOD syndrome manifests as a hypoplastic right lung accompanied by a small right pulmonary artery. Additionally, muscular defects in the right hemidiaphragm are frequently observed along with hypogenetic right lung abnormalities [87].

5.2. Edward's Syndrome

Edwards syndrome, also known as trisomy 18, is a chromosomal disorder marked by a wide spectrum of clinical manifestations, multiple congenital malformations, and a high mortality rate. It occurs in approximately 1 in 3000–8000 live births [88,89]. Characteristic features include low birth weight; craniofacial dysmorphism such as microcephaly, micrognathia, and low-set ears; as well as skeletal, renal, and cardiac anomalies. Studies have shown that females with trisomy 18 tend to have a better survival rate compared to males, and survival is also relatively higher among Black infants. The syndrome presents with a variety of phenotypic abnormalities affecting the nervous system, growth, and the structures of the cranium, face, thorax, abdomen, limbs, genitalia, skin, its appendages, and internal organs [90,91].

An abdominal wall defect is observed in fewer than 10% of patients with Edwards syndrome [86,90]. Only about 30% of affected infants survive the neonatal period, and merely 5–10% reach their first birthday [92,93]. Acute cardiopulmonary failure—primarily due to associated cardiac malformations present in 70–100% of cases—is the most common cause of death [94].

Omphalocele is frequently observed in fetuses with trisomy 18. A study by Snijders et al. [95] reported that 31% of fetuses diagnosed with trisomy 18 (n = 137) also had omphalocele. Similarly, research by Chen [77] found that 24.1% of fetuses with prenatally detected omphalocele (277 out of 1,148 cases) were affected by trisomy 18. In an analysis of first-trimester ultrasound findings in trisomy 18 cases, Sepulveda et al. [96] identified several common structural anomalies. Among these, 21% of cases presented with omphalocele, while other abnormalities included abnormal hand positioning (6%), megacystis (4%), and anomalies in the four-chamber heart view (4%).

5.3. Patau Syndrome (Trisomy 13)

In the United States, Patau syndrome affects approximately 1 in every 12,000 births, with a survival rate of only 10% and a median survival of 7–10 days [77,83,96–99]. The condition is generally fatal within the first year of life. Key features of Patau syndrome include severe intellectual disability, microphthalmia, cutis aplasia, polycystic kidney disease, holoprosencephaly, cleft lip and palate, low-set ears, polydactyly, congenital heart defects, rocker-bottom feet, and omphalocele [100]. In addition, the disorder impacts multiple systems, including the genitourinary tract, digestive tract, pancreas, liver, kidneys, and lungs [101]. Due to facial deformities, affected infants frequently require postnatal respiratory support—such as oxygenation and ventilation—with many necessitating intubation or tracheostomy [102]. Ultrasound performed after 17 weeks of gestation is the most effective way to identify abnormalities associated with Patau syndrome [103]. Among chromosomal disorders linked to omphalocele, the most frequently observed are trisomy 18 and trisomy 13 [95]. The association between omphalocele and Patau syndrome is particularly significant due to its implications for prenatal diagnosis, genetic counseling, and clinical management.

5.4. *Pentalogy of Cantrell*

A group of anomalies involving the midline abdominal wall, lower sternum, anterior diaphragm, diaphragmatic pericardium, and an intracardiac defect is termed the Pentalogy of Cantrell [104]. Coleman et al. evaluated a range of disorders arising from the faulty closure of the lateral and craniocaudal embryonic folds, which encompasses conditions such as the Pentalogy of Cantrell, OEIS (omphalocele, exstrophy, imperforate anus, and spina bifida), and LBWC (limb–body wall complex). Their case series demonstrated that the severity of pulmonary hypoplasia proved to be a more reliable prognostic factor than any specific classification system, largely due to the extensive overlap in clinical features among these syndromes [105]. In line with Cantrell's original observations, common cardiac abnormalities include a ventricular septal defect (100%), atrial septal defect (53%), left ventricular diverticulum (20%), pulmonary stenosis or atresia (33%), and tetralogy of Fallot (20%) [106].

5.5. *Prune Belly Syndrome (Eagle–Barrett Syndrome)*

In 1895, Osler coined the term "Prune Belly Syndrome (PBS)", even though Frolich had earlier reported a case of congenital absence of abdominal wall musculature in 1839. The condition, also known as triad syndrome or abdominal musculature deficiency syndrome [107], is a rare congenital anomaly occurring at rates of 3.8 per 100,000 live births in males and 1.1 per 100,000 in females [108,109]. PBS is classically defined by a triad consisting of urinary tract malformations, bilateral cryptorchidism, and absence of the anterior abdominal wall muscles, although the specific abnormalities in the abdominal wall and urinary tract can vary in affected females [110].

The characteristic prune-like, wrinkled appearance of the abdominal wall results from either a deficiency or complete absence of its muscular components [111]. In a rare case reported by Gyawali S. et al., an infant presented with a distended abdomen and an omphalocele due to an abdominal wall muscle defect; a mass was noted protruding through the umbilical region. This infant also exhibited bilateral cryptorchidism, but his vital signs and other clinical findings were normal, and no significant facial deformities were observed. Initial laboratory tests showed mild hyponatremia, mild hyperkalemia, and an elevated C-reactive protein level (see Table 1). Blood cultures isolated Enterococcus species, prompting treatment with intravenous Amikacin and Ampicillin based on sensitivity profiles. Additionally, abdominal and pelvic ultrasonography revealed congenital absence of the left kidney. Echocardiography demonstrated mild anterior tricuspid leaflet prolapse with moderate tricuspid regurgitation (gradient of 22 mm Hg), a patent foramen ovale with a left-to-right shunt, and normal biventricular function with a left ventricular ejection fraction of 69% [112].

Table 1. Congenital syndromes linked to omphalocele and their effects on pulmonary function.

Congenital Anomalies	Association with Omphalocele	Impact on Pulmonary Function
Pentalogy of Cantrell	Multiple congenital defects, including omphalocele, diaphragmatic hernia, ectopia cordis, and sternum defects.	• Diaphragmatic hernia can severely impede lung development (pulmonary hypoplasia), causing respiratory issues. • Ectopia cordis and chest wall defects might impair the thoracic cavity, resulting in limited lung expansion.
Patau Syndrome (Trisomy 13)	Often feature omphalocele as part of a spectrum of abnormalities.	• Pulmonary hypoplasia that may result in chronic respiratory distress. • Associated congenital cardiac abnormalities may further impair pulmonary function.
Prune Belly Syndrome (Eagle–Barrett Syndrome)	Some cases of Prune Belly Syndrome may present omphalocele.	• The deficiency of abdominal musculature might hinder efficient breathing mechanics, complicating lung expansion. • Pulmonary hypoplasia may also arise from the underdevelopment of the thoracic cavity, especially in cases of oligohydramnios during gestation.
PAGOD Syndrome	Multiple congenital defects, including omphalocele, diaphragmatic defects, pulmonary hypoplasia, gastrointestinal defects, and agonadism.	• Pulmonary hypoplasia is a key characteristic of PAGOD. • Omphalocele and diaphragmatic anomalies (common in PAGOD)
Edward's Syndrome (Trisomy 18)	Omphalocele is a common congenital defect in Edward's syndrome (30–50%).	• Mechanical compression following surgical repair. • Pulmonary hypoplasia frequently occurs in newborns with omphalocele and Edwards syndrome. • Diaphragm displacement. • Hypotonia. • Congenital heart defects.

6. Genetic Features

Omphalocele is linked to an increased rate of aneuploidy [113], with trisomy 18 being the most frequently observed chromosomal abnormality [114]. This indicates that when omphalocele occurs alongside other systemic malformations, chromosomal anomalies are significantly more common. Therefore, a prenatal ultrasound that detects an omphalocele should prompt comprehensive structural screening and genetic testing to identify any associated chromosomal issues [115]. Chromosomal microarray analysis (CMA) offers a genome-wide approach capable of detecting imbalanced rearrangements, including small deletions and duplications [116].

Following CMA, whole exome sequencing (WES) can further improve diagnostic yield by approximately 8–10% in fetuses with structural defects [117]. For instance, in one proband, WES identified a heterozygous, potentially pathogenic mutation inherited from the father; such mutations in the COL2A1 gene are frequently associated with various skeletal abnormalities, including dwarfism [118]. Additionally, WES detected a mutation in the SDHB gene inherited from the mother, which is associated with hereditary paraganglioma–pheochromocytoma syndromes (PGL/PCC syndromes, OMIM 115310). Although omphalocele is not commonly linked to SDHB mutations in the literature, the presence of an omphalocele on prenatal ultrasound suggests that the c.725G>A (p.R242H) mutation might contribute to its development [115].

Given the increased risk of fetal aneuploidy in cases of prenatal omphalocele—especially when other ultrasound abnormalities are present [115]—it is advisable to perform routine karyotyping along with CMA testing. If both the karyotype and CMA results are normal, WES should be considered, and if these tests are inconclusive, further molecular methods may be employed to exclude phenotypes such as Beckwith–Wiedemann syndrome (BWS). When the fetal karyotype is normal and no additional anomalies are identified, fetuses with omphalocele generally have a better survival outlook, and elective termination without clear indications is not recommended [115].

Moreover, if a perinatal evaluation reveals holoprosencephaly (HPE), polydactyly, and omphalocele, the possibility of fetal trisomy 13 should be considered. Quantitative fluorescent PCR (QF-PCR) is effective for rapidly confirming trisomy 13 and determining its paternal origin, particularly when cell culture fails, and it provides crucial information for genetic counseling [119]. Chen reported that trisomy 18 was present in 24.1% (277/1148) of fetuses with prenatally diagnosed omphalocele [83]. Furthermore, Sepulveda et al. found that the most common structural defects observed by ultrasound in trisomy 18 were omphalocele (21%), abnormal hand posture (6%), megacystis (4%), and an abnormal four-chamber cardiac view [104].

7. Management

The ultimate goal of surgical intervention for omphalocele is to prevent a dangerous rise in intra-abdominal pressure while achieving complete coverage of the fascial and skin layers. Treatment strategies fall into three categories: (1) immediate (primary) repair; (2) staged repair with delayed primary closure; and (3) delayed repair using the "paint and wait" technique.

During the process of reducing the herniated viscera, it is crucial to continuously monitor intra-abdominal pressure. This vigilance helps avoid the development of abdominal compartment syndrome (ACS) along with its associated complications—such as reduced cardiac output, splanchnic hypoperfusion, lactic acidosis, renal failure, intestinal ischemia, and hypoventilation—which can be fatal [120]. Historically, non-surgical management of omphalocele was first described by Ahlfeld in 1899, who used alcohol for its antiseptic and escharotic properties [9]. Later, in 1967, Schuster introduced a staged closure technique employing two Teflon® sheets, a method that paved the way for the "silo" approach. In 1969, Allen and Wrenn refined this technique by using a single, circular Dacron-reinforced silastic sheet attached to the abdominal defect [9].

Although a one-stage, primary closure is ideal because it is associated with favorable survival and morbidity outcomes, it is not always technically feasible—especially in cases where the defect is large and the abdominal domain is insufficient to allow a secure fascial closure [121]. For giant omphaloceles featuring an externalized liver or significant viscero-abdominal disproportion, or in cases accompanied by marked pulmonary hypoplasia and hypertension, the "paint and wait" method is generally preferred [54].

In addition to primary closure, several alternative techniques have been explored over the past three decades, including amnion inversion, the application of prosthetic silos, vacuum-assisted closure, tissue expansion, and the use of various mesh materials, as well as non-surgical escharotic therapy or delayed repair. Despite these advances, no single procedure has emerged as the definitive treatment option [122]. The optimal timing for surgical repair in neonates with giant omphalocele (GO) remains a topic of debate, with limited published guidance available. Delayed closure techniques, such as the Gross procedure—which involves creating skin flaps to cover the sac without incising it—and gradual visceral reduction using a prosthetic silo, have been developed to minimize complications associated with early surgical intervention. Topical treatments like sulfadiazine cream and povidone–iodine, known as the "paint and wait" approach, are also used [123].

For infants with large omphaloceles, a tailored, shared decision-making process with parents is essential. This process should consider factors such as defect size, gestational age, and cardiorespiratory status, as well as the potential need to address other malformations (e.g., diaphragmatic hernia, esophageal or intestinal atresia, congenital heart defects) and appropriate antibiotic prophylaxis. Moreover, the overall care plan should reflect the anticipated trajectory of treatment—such as a palliative approach in cases with trisomy 13 or 18—and take into account the parents' preferences regarding a more aggressive surgical strategy for earlier closure versus a conservative approach that may involve a prolonged course of dressing changes, frequent outpatient visits, a higher risk of sepsis, and delayed abdominal wall reconstruction [52,124].

The management of GO aims to reduce the herniated contents and close the abdominal defect once the patient is medically stable and adequately supported. However, early closure in patients with small abdominal cavities and trunks can lead to a sudden rise in intra-abdominal pressure and respiratory compromise due to reduced diaphragmatic movement. This concern is particularly significant in patients with GO, who often present with pulmonary hypoplasia and cardiac anomalies that further predispose them to respiratory insufficiency [8,20,124–126]. Topical agents, such as povidone–iodine, have shown promise in minimizing pulmonary complications, allowing for hospital discharge under close parental supervision with plans for definitive closure at a later date [126].

The COVID-19 pandemic has adversely impacted many aspects of healthcare, including a decline in the early diagnosis of conditions such as antenatal abdominal wall defects. Social, educational, and financial challenges during the pandemic have also led to delays in seeking timely medical care for the closure of these defects.

8. Conclusions

In summary, individuals with omphalocele often exhibit various respiratory complications that can be identified during prenatal assessments and become evident shortly after birth. Severe respiratory failure, particularly due to pulmonary hypoplasia and pulmonary hypertension, substantially increases both morbidity and mortality in these patients [42]. Although surgical repair of the omphalocele may temporarily worsen respiratory function, patients generally experience a short-term recovery.

Author Contributions: Conceptualization, M.V.H. and D.A.N.; methodology, A.I. and D.A.N.; software, R.A.R.; validation, M.V.H., D.H. and D.A.N.; formal analysis, R.A.R.; investigation, R.A.N., D.H. and A.L.; resources, D.A.N.; data curation, D.H.; writing—original draft preparation, M.V.H. and D.A.N.; writing—review and editing, D.A.N. and A.L.; visualization, M.V.H. and E.H.; supervision, A.I. and M.V.H.; project administration, D.H. and E.H. All authors have read and agreed to the published version of the manuscript.

Funding: This research received no external funding.

Institutional Review Board Statement: Not applicable.

Informed Consent Statement: Not applicable.

Conflicts of Interest: The authors declare no conflicts of interest.

References

1. Mansfield, S.A.; Jancelewicz, T. Ventral Abdominal Wall Defects. *Pediatr. Rev.* **2019**, *40*, 627–635. [CrossRef] [PubMed]
2. Gonzalez, K.W.; Chandler, N.M. Ruptured omphalocele: Diagnosis and management. *Semin. Pediatr. Surg.* **2019**, *28*, 101–105. [CrossRef]
3. Frolov, P.; Alali, J.; Klein, M.D. Clinical risk factors for gastroschisis and omphalocele in humans: A review of the literature. *Pediatr. Surg. Int.* **2010**, *26*, 1135–1148. [CrossRef] [PubMed]
4. Arnold, M.A.; Chang, D.C.; Nabaweesi, R.; Colombani, P.M.; Bathurst, M.A.; Mon, K.S.; Hosmane, S.; Abdullah, F. Risk stratification of 4344 patients with gastroschisis into simple and complex categories. *J. Pediatr. Surg.* **2007**, *42*, 1520–1525. [CrossRef] [PubMed]
5. Gerrits, L.C.; De Mol, A.C.; Bulten, J.; Van der Staak, F.H.; Van Heijst, A.F. Omphalocele and alveolar capillary dysplasia: A new association. *Pediatr. Crit. Care Med.* **2010**, *11*, e36–e37. [CrossRef]
6. Hutson, S.; Baerg, J.; Deming, D.; St Peter, S.D.; Hopper, A.; Goff, D.A. High prevalence of pulmonary hypertension complicates the care of infants with omphalocele. *Neonatology* **2017**, *112*, 281–286. [CrossRef]
7. Liu, T.X.; Du, L.Z.; Ma, X.L.; Chen, Z.; Shi, L.P. Giant omphalocele associated pulmonary hypertension: A retrospective study. *Front. Pediatr.* **2022**, *10*, 940289. [CrossRef] [PubMed] [PubMed Central]
8. Edwards, E.A.; Broome, S.; Green, S.; Douglas, C.; McCall, E.; Nuthall, G.; Nixon, G.M. Long-term respiratory support in children with giant omphalocele. *Anaesth Intensive Care* **2007**, *35*, 94–98, Erratum in *Anaesth Intensive Care* **2007**, *35*, 316. [CrossRef] [PubMed]
9. Tarcă, E.; Aprodu, S. Past and present in omphalocele treatment in Romania. *Chirurgia* **2014**, *109*, 507–513. [PubMed]
10. Miller, O.I.; Gaynor, J.W.; Macrae, D.J.; Tasker, R.C. Inhaled nitric oxide for pulmonary hypertension after repair of exomphalos. *Arch. Dis. Child.* **1993**, *69*, 518–520. [CrossRef]
11. Gibbin, C.; Touch, S.; Broth, R.E.; Berghella, V. Abdominal wall defects and congenital heart disease. *Ultrasound Obstet. Gynecol.* **2003**, *21*, 334–337. [CrossRef]
12. Corey, K.M.; Hornik, C.P.; Laughon, M.M.; McHutchison, K.; Clark, R.H.; Smith, P.B. Frequency of anomalies and hospital outcomes in infants with gastroschisis and omphalocele. *Early Hum. Dev.* **2014**, *90*, 421–424. [CrossRef] [PubMed] [PubMed Central]
13. Bielicki, I.N.; Somme, S.; Frongia, G.; Holland-Cunz, S.G.; Vuille-dit-Bille, R.N. Abdominal Wall Defects—Current Treatments. *Children* **2021**, *8*, 170. [CrossRef]
14. Teillet, B.; Boukhris, M.R.; Sfeir, R.; Mur, S.; Cailliau, E.; Sharma, D.; Vaast, P.; Storme, L.; Le Duc, K. Systemic Inflammation Is Associated with Pulmonary Hypertension in Isolated Giant Omphalocele: A Population-Based Study. *Healthcare* **2022**, *10*, 1998. [CrossRef] [PubMed] [PubMed Central]
15. Panitch, H.B. Pulmonary complications of abdominal wall defects. *Paediatr. Respir. Rev.* **2015**, *16*, 11–17. [CrossRef] [PubMed]
16. Puvabanditsin, S.; Burger, R.; Puthenpura, V.; Walzer, L.; Madubuko, A.; Minerowicz, C.; Mehta, R. A Giant Gastroschisis Associated with Pulmonary Hypoplasia and Spinal Anomaly: A Case Report and a Literature Review. *Case Rep. Pathol.* **2018**, *2018*, 8378769. [CrossRef] [PubMed] [PubMed Central]
17. Feldkamp, M.L.; Carey, J.C.; Sadler, T.W. Development of gastroschisis: Review of hypotheses, a novel hypothesis, and implications for research. *Am. J. Med. Genet.* **2007**, *143A*, 639–652. [CrossRef] [PubMed]
18. Prendergast, M.; Rafferty, G.F.; Davenport, M.; Persico, N.; Jani, J.; Nicolaides, K.; Greenough, A. Three-dimensional ultrasound fetal lung volumes and infant respiratory outcome: A prospective observational study. *BJOG* **2011**, *118*, 608–614. [CrossRef] [PubMed]
19. Kamata, S.; Usui, N.; Sawai, T.; Nose, K.; Fukuzawa, M. Prenatal detection of pulmonary hypoplasia in giant omphalocele. *Pediatr. Surg. Int.* **2008**, *24*, 107–111. [CrossRef] [PubMed]
20. Danzer, E.; Victoria, T.; Bebbington, M.W.; Siegle, J.; Rintoul, N.E.; Johnson, M.P.; Flake, A.W.; Adzick, N.S.; Hedrick, H.L. Fetal MRI-calculated total lung volumes in the prediction of short-term outcome in giant omphalocele: Preliminary findings. *Fetal Diagn Ther.* **2012**, *31*, 248–253. [CrossRef] [PubMed]
21. Ein, S.H.; Langer, J.C. Delayed management of giant omphalocele using silver sulfadiazine cream: An 18-year experience. *J. Pediatr. Surg.* **2012**, *47*, 494–500. [CrossRef] [PubMed]
22. Dauve, V.; McLin, V.A. Recent advances in the molecular and genetic understanding of congenital gastrointestinal malformations. *J. Pediatr. Gastroenterol. Nutr.* **2013**, *57*, 4–13. [CrossRef] [PubMed]
23. Wilson, R.D.; Johnson, M.P. Congenital abdominal wall defects: An update. *Fetal Diagn. Ther.* **2004**, *19*, 385–398. [CrossRef]
24. Argyle, J.C. Pulmonary hypoplasia in infants with giant abdominal wall defects. *Pediatr. Pathol.* **1989**, *9*, 43–55. [CrossRef]
25. Hershenson, M.B.; Brouillette, R.T.; Klemka, L.; Raffensperger, J.D.; Poznanski, A.K.; Hunt, C.E. Respiratory insufficiency in newborns with abdominal wall defects. *J. Pediatr. Surg.* **1985**, *20*, 348–353. [CrossRef] [PubMed]
26. Khan, F.A.; Hashmi, A.; Islam, S. Insights into embryology and development of omphalocele. Semin. *Pediatr. Surg.* **2019**, *28*, 80–83. [CrossRef] [PubMed]

27. Gross, R.E.; Blodgett, J.B. Omphalocele (umbilical eventration) in the newly born. *Surg. Gynec. Obst.* **1940**, *71*, 520–527.
28. Margulies, L. Omphalocele (amniocele): Its anatomy and etiology in relation to hernias of umbilicus and the umbilical cord. *Am. J. Obstet. Gynecol.* **1945**, *49*, 695–699. [CrossRef]
29. Gray, S.W.; Skandalakis, J.E. *Embryology for Surgeons: The Embryological Basis for the Treatment of Congenital Defects*; WB Saunders Company: Philadelphia, PA, USA, 1972.
30. Boucherat, O.; Landry-Truchon, K.; Aoidi, R.; Houde, N.; Nadeau, V.; Charron, J.; Jeannotte, L. Lung development requires an active ERK/MAPK pathway in the lung mesenchyme. *Dev. Dyn.* **2017**, *246*, 72–82. [CrossRef] [PubMed]
31. Tunell, W.P. Anterior Abdominal Wall Defects. In *Pediatric Gastrointestinal Disease: Pathophysiology, Diagnosis, Management*, 2nd ed.; Wyllie, R., Hyams, J.S., Eds.; W.B. Saunders Co.: Philadelphia, PA, USA, 1999; pp. 515–522.
32. Marshall, J.; Salemi, J.L.; Tanner, J.P.; Ramakrishnan, R.; Feldkamp, M.L.; Marengo, L.K.; Meyer, R.E.; Druschel, C.M.; Rickard, R.; Kirby, R.S.; et al. Prevalence, Correlates, and Outcomes of Omphalocele in the United States, 1995–2005. *Obstet Gynecol.* **2015**, *126*, 284–293. [CrossRef] [PubMed]
33. Ayub, S.S.; Taylor, J.A. Cardiac anomalies associated with omphalocele. *Semin. Pediatr. Surg.* **2019**, *28*, 111–114. [CrossRef] [PubMed]
34. Christison-Lagay, E.R.; Kelleher, C.M.; Langer, J.C. Neonatal abdominal wall defects. *Semin. Fetal Neonatal Med.* **2011**, *16*, 164–172. [CrossRef]
35. De Troyer, A.; Loring, S. Action of the respiratory muscles. In *Handbook of Physiology*; Macklem, P.T., Mead, J., Eds.; American Physiological Society: Bethesda, MD, USA, 1986; pp. 443–461.
36. Ewig, J.M.; Griscom, N.T.; Wohl, M.E. The effect of the absence of abdominal muscles on pulmonary function and exercise. *Am. J. Respir. Crit. Care Med.* **1996**, *153*, 1314–1321. [CrossRef]
37. Ein, S.H.; Rubin, S.Z. Gastroschisis: Primary closure or Silon pouch. *J. Pediatr. Surg.* **1980**, *15*, 549–552. [CrossRef] [PubMed]
38. Griscom, N.T.; Driscoll, S.G. Radiography of stillborn fetuses and infants dying at birth. *Am. J. Roentgenol.* **1980**, *134*, 485–489. [CrossRef] [PubMed]
39. Yang, S.S.; Huang, W.C.; Wang, P.; Gong, F.Q.; Liu, T.X.; Tou, J.F.; Lai, D.M. Echocardiographic measurements of left ventricular dimensions and function in newborns with omphalocele and pulmonary. *BMC Pediatr.* **2023**, *23*, 585. [CrossRef] [PubMed] [PubMed Central]
40. Akinkuotu, A.C.; Sheikh, F.; Cass, D.L.; Zamora, I.J.; Lee, T.C.; Cassady, C.I.; Mehollin-Ray, A.R.; Williams, J.L.; Ruano, R.; Welty, S.E.; et al. Are all pulmonary hypoplasias the same? A comparison of pulmonary outcomes in neonates with congenital diaphragmatic hernia, omphalocele and congenital lung malformation. *J. Pediatr. Surg.* **2015**, *50*, 55–59. [CrossRef] [PubMed]
41. Duggan, E.; Puligandla, P.S. Respiratory disorders in patients with omphalocele. *Semin. Pediatr. Surg.* **2019**, *28*, 115–117. [CrossRef] [PubMed]
42. Partridge, E.A.; Hanna, B.D.; Panitch, H.B.; Rintoul, N.E.; Peranteau, W.H.; Flake, A.W.; Scott Adzick, N.; Hedrick, H.L. Pulmonary hypertension in giant omphalocele infants. *J. Pediatr. Surg.* **2014**, *49*, 1767–1770. [CrossRef] [PubMed]
43. Baerg, J.E.; Thirumoorthi, A.; Carlton, W.; Haug, S.; Hopper, A.O.; Goff, D.; Ramlogan, S.; Peter, S.D. Late onset of pulmonary hypertension and sepsis in omphalocele infants. *J. Pediatr. Surg. Case Rep.* **2016**, *15*, 14–18. [CrossRef]
44. Headley, B.M.; McDougall, P.N.; Stokes, K.B.; Dewan, P.A.; Dargaville, P.A. Left-lung-collapse bronchial deformation in giant omphalocele. *J. Pediatr. Surg.* **2001**, *36*, 846–850. [CrossRef]
45. Binet, A.; Gelas, T.; Jochault-Ritz, S.; Noizet, O.; Bory, J.P.; Lefebvre, F.; Belouadah, M.; James-Robert, I.; Aubert, D.; Bouche-Pillon Persyn, M.A.; et al. VAC® therapy a therapeutic alternative in giant omphalocele treatment: A multicenter study. *J. Plast. Reconstr. Aesthet. Surg.* **2013**, *66*, e373–e375. [CrossRef] [PubMed]
46. Gamba, P.; Midrio, P. Abdominal wall defects: Prenatal diagnosis, newborn management, and long-term outcomes. *Semin. Pediatr. Surg.* **2014**, *23*, 283–290. [CrossRef] [PubMed]
47. Binet, A.; Scalabre, A.; Amar, S.; Alzahrani, K.; Boureau, C.; Bastard, F.; Lefebvre, F.; Koffi, M.; Moufidath, S.; Nasser, D.; et al. Operative versus conservative treatment for giant omphalocele: Study of French and Ivorian management. *Ann. Chir. Plast. Esthétique* **2020**, *65*, 147–153. [CrossRef] [PubMed]
48. Skarsgard, E.D. Immediate versus staged repair of omphaloceles. *Semin. Pediatr. Surg.* **2019**, *28*, 89–94. [CrossRef] [PubMed]
49. Malhotra, R.; Malhotra, B.; Ramteke, H. Enhancing Omphalocele Care: Navigating Complications and Innovative Treatment Approaches. *Cureus* **2023**, *15*, e47638. [CrossRef] [PubMed] [PubMed Central]
50. Dingemann, C.; Sonne, M.; Ure, B.; Bohnhorst, B.; von Kaisenberg, C.; Pirr, S. Impact of maternal education on the outcome of newborns requiring surgery for congenital malformations. *PLoS ONE* **2019**, *14*, 214967. [CrossRef]
51. Chakhunashvili, D.G.; Lomidze, N.; Karalashvili, L.; Kikalishvili, L.; Chakhunashvili, K.; Kakabadze, Z. Challenges and management of congenital abdominal wall defects (Review). *Georgian Med. News* **2018**, *276*, 24–33.
52. Dimitriou, G.; Greenough, A.; Giffin, F.; Davenport, M.; Nicolaides, K.H. Temporary impairment of lung function in infants with anterior abdominal wall defects who have undergone surgery. *J. Pediatr. Surg.* **1996**, *31*, 670–672. [CrossRef]

53. Nakayama, D.K.; Motoyama, E.K.; Tagge, E.M. Effect of preoperative stabilization on respiratory system compliance and outcome in newborn infants with congenital diaphragmatic hernia. *J. Pediatr.* **1991**, *118*, 793–799. [CrossRef]
54. Pober, B.R. Overview of epidemiology, genetics, birth defects, and chromosome abnormalities associated with CDH. *Am. J. Med. Genet. C Semin. Med. Genet.* **2007**, *145C*, 158–171. [CrossRef] [PubMed]
55. Skari, H.; Bjornland, K.; Haugen, G.; Egeland, T.; Emblem, R. Congenital diaphragmatic hernia: A meta-analysis of mortality factors. *J. Pediatr. Surg.* **2000**, *35*, 1187–1197. [CrossRef] [PubMed]
56. Baerg, J.E.; Thorpe, D.L.; Sharp, N.E.; Ramlogan, S.R.; Hutson, S.M.; Goff, D.A.; Hopper, A.O.; St Peter, S.D. Pulmonary hypertension predicts mortality in infants with omphalocele. *J. Neonatal Perinat. Med.* **2015**, *8*, 333–338. [CrossRef] [PubMed]
57. Chee, Y.Y.; Wong, S.C.M.; Wong, M.S.R. Rare combination of left-sided congenital diaphragmatic hernia and omphalocele. *BMJ Case Rep.* **2017**, *2017*, bcr-2017-220696. [CrossRef]
58. Nonaka, A.; Hidaka, N.; Kido, S.; Fukushima, K.; Kato, K. Prenatal imaging of a fetus with the rare combination of a right congenital diaphragmatic hernia and a giant omphalocele. *Congenit. Anom.* **2014**, *54*, 246–249. [CrossRef] [PubMed]
59. Zhang, G.; Liu, D.; Wang, G.; Chen, X.; Tian, J. Congenital intrapericardial diaphragmatic hernia with omphalocele. *Hernia* **2014**, *18*, 423–425. [CrossRef] [PubMed]
60. Scahill, M.D.; Maak, P.; Kunder, C.; Halamek, L.P. Anterolateral congenital diaphragmatic hernia with omphalocele: A case report and literature review. *Am. J. Med. Genet. A* **2013**, *161A*, 585–588. [CrossRef] [PubMed]
61. Chen, C.P. Omphalocele and congenital diaphragmatic hernia associated with fetal trisomy 18. *Prenat. Diagn.* **2005**, *25*, 421–423. [CrossRef] [PubMed]
62. Nishimura, M.; Taniguchi, A.; Imanaka, H.; Taenaka, N. Hypoplastic left heart syndrome associated with congenital right-sided diaphragmatic hernia and omphalocele. *Chest* **1992**, *101*, 263–264. [CrossRef] [PubMed]
63. Waag, K.L.; Loff, S.; Zahn, K.; Ali, M.; Hien, S.; Kratz, M.; Neff, W.; Schaffelder, R.; Schaible, T. Congenital diaphragmatic hernia: A modern day approach. *Semin. Pediatr. Surg.* **2008**, *17*, 244–254. [CrossRef] [PubMed]
64. Hartnett, K.S. Congenital diaphragmatic hernia: Advanced physiology and care concepts. *Adv. Neonatal Care* **2008**, *8*, 107–115. [CrossRef] [PubMed]
65. Chiu, P.; Hedrick, H.L. Postnatal management and long-term outcome for survivors with congenital diaphragmatic hernia. *Prenat. Diagn.* **2008**, *28*, 592–603. [CrossRef] [PubMed]
66. Mohseni-Bod, H.; Bohn, D. Pulmonary hypertension in congenital diaphragmatic hernia. *Semin. Pediatr. Surg.* **2007**, *16*, 126–133. [CrossRef]
67. Logan, J.W.; Rice, H.E.; Goldberg, R.N.; Cotten, C.M. Congenital diaphragmatic hernia: A systematic review and summary of best-evidence practice strategies. *J. Perinatol.* **2007**, *27*, 535–549. [CrossRef] [PubMed]
68. Putnam, L.R.; Harting, M.T.; Tsao, K.; Morini, F.; Yoder, B.A.; Luco, M.; Lally, P.A.; Lally, K.P.; Congenital Diaphragmatic Hernia Study Group. Congenital Diaphragmatic Hernia Defect Size and Infant Morbidity at Discharge. *Pediatrics* **2016**, *138*, e20162043. [CrossRef] [PubMed]
69. Congenital Diaphragmatic Hernia Study Group; Congenital diaphragmatic hernia: Defect size correlates with developmental defect. *J. Pediatr. Surg.* **2013**, *48*, 1177–1182. [CrossRef]
70. Congenital Diaphragmatic Hernia Study Group; Lally, K.P.; Lally, P.A.; Lasky, R.E.; Tibboel, D.; Jaksic, T.; Wilson, J.M.; Frenckner, B.; Van Meurs, K.P.; Bohn, D.J.; et al. Defect size determines survival in infants with congenital diaphragmatic hernia. *Pediatrics* **2007**, *120*, e651–e657. [CrossRef] [PubMed]
71. Tsakayannis, D.E.; Zurakowski, D.; Lillehei, C.W. Respiratory insufficiency at birth: A predictor of mortality for infants with omphalocele. *J. Pediatr. Surg.* **1996**, *31*, 1088–1090, discussion 1090–1081. [CrossRef]
72. Burgos, C.M.; Frenckner, B.; Harting, M.T.; Lally, P.A.; Lally, K.P. Congenital diaphragmatic hernia and associated omphalocele: A study from the CDHSG registry. *J. Pediatr. Surg.* **2019**, *55*, 2099–2104. [CrossRef]
73. Harmath, A.; Hajdú, J.; Csaba, A.; Hauzman, E.; Pete, B.; Görbe, E.; Beke, A.; Papp, Z. Associated malformations in congenital diaphragmatic hernia cases in the last 15 years in a tertiary referral institute. *Am. J. Med. Genet. A* **2006**, *140*, 2298–2304. [CrossRef] [PubMed]
74. Borys, D.; Taxy, J.B. Congenital diaphragmatic hernia and chromosomal anomalies: Autopsy study. *Pediatr. Dev. Pathol.* **2004**, *7*, 35–38. [CrossRef] [PubMed]
75. Holder, A.M.; Klaassens, M.; Tibboel, D.; de Klein, A.; Lee, B.; Scott, D.A. Genetic factors in congenital diaphragmatic hernia. *Am. J. Hum. Genet.* **2007**, *80*, 825–845. [CrossRef] [PubMed] [PubMed Central]
76. Inoue, S.; Odaka, A.; Muta, Y.; Beck, Y.; Sobajima, H.; Tamura, M. Coexistence of congenital diaphragmatic hernia and abdominal wall closure defect with chromosomal abnormality: Two case reports. *J. Med. Case Rep.* **2016**, *10*, 19. [CrossRef] [PubMed] [PubMed Central]
77. Chen, C.P. Chromosomal abnormalities associated with omphalocele. *Taiwan J. Obstet. Gynecol.* **2007**, *46*, 1–8. [CrossRef]
78. Nyberg, D.A.; Fitzsimmons, J.; Mack, L.A.; Hughes, M.; Pretorius, D.H.; Hickok, D.; Shepard, T.H. Chromosomal abnormalities in fetuses with omphalocele. Significance of omphalocele contents. *J. Ultrasound Med.* **1989**, *8*, 299–308. [CrossRef] [PubMed]

79. Lakasing, L.; Cicero, S.; Davenport, M.; Patel, S.; Nicolaides, K.H. Current outcome of antenatally diagnosed exomphalos: An 11 year review. *J. Pediatr. Surg.* **2006**, *41*, 1403–1406. [CrossRef] [PubMed]
80. Chen, C.P.; Su, Y.N.; Chen, S.U.; Chang, T.Y.; Wu, P.C.; Chern, S.R.; Wu, P.S.; Kuo, Y.L.; Wang, W. Prenatal diagnosis of hypomethylation at KvDMR1 and Beckwith-Wiedemann syndrome in a pregnancy conceived by intracytoplasmic sperm injection and in vitro fertilization and embryo transfer. *Taiwan J. Obstet. Gynecol.* **2014**, *53*, 90–94. [CrossRef] [PubMed]
81. Ogino, T. Clinical features and teratogenic mechanisms of congenital absence of digits. *Dev. Growth Differ.* **2007**, *49*, 523–531. [CrossRef]
82. Hou, W.C.; Chen, C.P.; Hwang, K.S.; Chen, Y.C.; Lai, Y.J.; Tien, C.Y.; Su, H.Y. Prenatal diagnosis of a de novo 9p terminal chromosomal deletion in a fetus with major congenital anomalies. *Taiwan J. Obstet. Gynecol.* **2014**, *53*, 602–605. [CrossRef] [PubMed]
83. Ferraro, G.A.; Perrotta, A.; Rossano, F.; D'Andrea, F. Poland syndrome: Description of an atypical variant. *Aesthetic Plast. Surg.* **2005**, *29*, 32–33. [CrossRef]
84. Rasmussen, S.A.; Bieber, F.R.; Benacerraf, B.R.; Lachman, R.S.; Rimoin, D.L.; Holmes, L.B. Epidemiology of osteochondrodysplasias: Changing trends due to advances in prenatal diagnosis. *Am. J. Med. Genet.* **1996**, *61*, 49–58. [CrossRef]
85. Falcon, O.; Cavoretto, P.; Peralta, C.F.; Csapo, B.; Nicolaides, K.H. Fetal head-to-trunk volume ratio in chromosomally abnormal fetuses at 11 + 0 to 13 + 6 weeks of gestation. *Ultrasound Obstet Gynecol.* **2005**, *26*, 755–760. [CrossRef] [PubMed]
86. Kinoshita, M.; Nakamura, Y.; Nakano, R.; Morimatsu, M.; Fukuda, S.; Nishimi, Y.; Hashimoto, T. Thirty-one autopsy cases of trisomy 18: Clinical features and pathological findings. *Pediatr. Pathol.* **1989**, *9*, 445–457. [CrossRef]
87. Maaswinkel-Jooij, P.D.; Stovis-Brantsma, W.H. Phenotypically normal girl with male pseudohermaphroditism, hypoplastic left ventricle, lung aplasia, horseshoe kidney and diaphragmatic hernia. *Am. J. Med. Genet.* **1992**, *42*, 647–648. [CrossRef] [PubMed]
88. Rosa, R.F.; Rosa, R.C.; Lorenzen, M.B.; de Moraes, F.N.; Graziadio, C.; Zen, P.R.; Paskulin, G.A. Trisomy 18: Experience of a reference hospital from the south of Brazil. *Am. J. Med. Genet. A* **2011**, *155A*, 1529–1535. [CrossRef] [PubMed]
89. Rosa, R.F.; Rosa, R.C.; Lorenzen, M.B.; de Oliveira, C.A.; Graziadio, C.; Zen, P.R.; Paskulin, G.A. Trisomy 18: Frequency, types, and prognosis of congenital heart defects in a Brazilian cohort. *Am. J. Med. Genet. A* **2012**, *158A*, 2358–2361. [CrossRef]
90. Rosa, R.F.M.; Rosa, R.C.M.; Lorenzen, M.B.; Zen, P.R.G.; Oliveira, C.A.V.; Graziadio, C.; Paskulin, G.A. Trisomy 18 (Edwards syndrome) and major gastrointestinal malformations. *Sao Paulo Med. J.* **2013**, *131*, 133–134. [CrossRef]
91. Ţarcă, E.; Plămădeală, P.; Savu, B. Plurimalformative syndrome associating trisomy 18 and omphalocele. Case report and review of the literature. *Rom. J. Morphol. Embryol.* **2014**, *55*, 209–213. [PubMed]
92. Wu, J.; Springett, A.; Morris, J.K. Survival of trisomy 18 (Edwards syndrome) and trisomy 13 (Patau syndrome) in England and Wales: 2004–2011. *Am. J. Med. Genet. A* **2013**, *161*, 2512–2518. [CrossRef]
93. Rasmussen, S.A.; Wong, L.Y.; Yang, Q.; May, K.M.; Friedman, J.M. Population-based analyses of mortality in trisomy 13 and trisomy 18. *Pediatrics* **2003**, *111 Pt 1*, 777–784. [CrossRef]
94. Goc, B.; Walencka, Z.; Włoch, A.; Wojciechowska, E.; WiecekWłodarska, D.; Krzystolik-Ładzińska, J.; Bober, K.; Swietliński, J. Trisomy 18 in neonates: Prenatal diagnosis, clinical features, therapeutic dilemmas and outcome. *J. Appl. Genet.* **2006**, *47*, 165–170. [CrossRef]
95. Snijders, R.J.; Sebire, N.J.; Souka, A.; Santiago, C.; Nicolaides, K.H. Fetal exomphalos and chromosomal defects: Relationship to maternal age and gestation. *Ultrasound Obstet. Gynecol. Off. J. Int. Soc. Ultrasound Obstet. Gynecol.* **1995**, *6*, 250–255. [CrossRef]
96. Sepulveda, W.; Wong, A.E.; Dezerega, V. First-trimester sonographic findings in trisomy 18: A review of 53 cases. *Prenat Diagn* **2010**, *30*, 256e9. [CrossRef] [PubMed]
97. Snijders, R.J.M.; Farrias, M.; von Kaisenberg, C.; Nicolaides, K.H. Fetal abnormalities. In *Ultrasound Markers for Fetal Chromosomal Defects*; Snijders, R.J.M., Nicolaides, K.H., Eds.; Parthenon Publishing Group: New York, NY, USA, 1996; p. 1e62.
98. Wyllie, J.P.; Wright, M.J.; Burn, J.; Hunter, S. Natural history of trisomy 13. *Arch. Dis. Child.* **1994**, *71*, 343–345. [CrossRef]
99. Peroos, S.; Forsythe, E.; Pugh, J.H.; Arthur-Farraj, P.; Hodes, D. Longevity and Patau syndrome: What determines survival? *BMJ Case Rep.* **2012**, *2012*, bcr0620114381. [CrossRef]
100. Patau, K.; Smith, D.; Therman, E.; Inhorn, S.; Wagner, H. Multiple congenital anomaly caused by an extra autosome. *Lancet* **1960**, *275*, 790–793. [CrossRef] [PubMed]
101. Khan, U.; Hussain, A.; Usman, M.; Abiddin, Z.U. An infant with patau syndrome associated with congenital heart defects. *Ann. Med. Surg.* **2022**, *80*, 104100. [CrossRef] [PubMed]
102. Williams, G.M.; Brady, R. *Patau Syndrome*; StatPearls: Treasure Island, FL, USA, 2019.
103. Watson, W.J.; Miller, R.C.; Wax, J.R.; Hansen, W.F.; Yamamura, Y.; Polzin, W.J. Sonographic detection of trisomy 13 in the first and second trimesters of pregnancy. *J. Ultrasound Med.* **2007**, *26*, 1209–1214. [CrossRef]
104. Kheir, A.E.; Bakhiet, E.A.; Elhag, S.M.; Karrar, M.Z. Pentalogy of Cantrell: Case report and review of the literature. *Sudan J. Paediatr.* **2014**, *14*, 85–88. [PubMed] [PubMed Central]
105. Coleman, P.W.; Marine, M.B.; Weida, J.N.; Gray, B.W.; Billmire, D.F.; Brown, B.P. Fetal MRI in the Identification of a Fetal Ventral Wall Defect Spectrum. *AJP Rep.* **2018**, *8*, e264–e276. [CrossRef] [PubMed] [PubMed Central]

106. Cantrell, J.R.; Haller, J.A.; Ravitch, M.M. A syndrome of congenital defects involving the abdominal wall, sternum, diaphragm, pericardium, and heart. *Surg. Gynecol. Obstet.* **1958**, *107*, 602–614. [PubMed]
107. Hassett, S.; Smith, G.H.; Holland, A.J. Prune belly syndrome. *Pediatr. Surg. Int.* **2012**, *28*, 219–228. [CrossRef] [PubMed]
108. Routh, J.C.; Huang, L.; Retik, A.B.; Nelson, C.P. Contemporary epidemiology and characterization of newborn males with prune belly syndrome. *Urology* **2010**, *76*, 44–48. [CrossRef]
109. Druschel, C.M. A descriptive study of prune belly in New York State, 1983 to 1989. *Arch. Pediatr. Adolesc. Med.* **1995**, *149*, 70–76. [CrossRef] [PubMed]
110. Rabinowitz, R.; Schillinger, J.F. Prune belly syndrome in the female subject. *J. Urol.* **1977**, *118*, 454–456. [CrossRef]
111. Pomajzl, A.J.; Sankararaman, S. *Prune Belly Syndrome*; StatPearls: Treasure Island, FL, USA, 2023.
112. Gyawali, S.; Gyawali, B.; Ghimire, B.; Shrestha, B.; Khanal, P.; Dahal, G.R.; Koirala, D.P. Prune belly syndrome: A rare case report. *Clin. Case Rep.* **2024**, *12*, e8922. [CrossRef] [PubMed] [PubMed Central]
113. Shi, X.; Tang, H.; Lu, J.; Yang, X.; Ding, H.; Wu, J. Prenatal genetic diagnosis of omphalocele by karyotyping, chromosomal microarray analysis and exome sequencing. *Ann. Med.* **2021**, *53*, 1286–1292. [CrossRef]
114. Khalil, A.; Arnaoutoglou, C.; Pacilli, M.; Szabo, A.; David, A.L.; Pandya, P. Outcome of fetal exomphalos diagnosed at 11–14 weeks of gestation: Exomphalos at 11–14 weeks. *Ultrasound Obstet. Gynecol.* **2012**, *39*, 401–406. [CrossRef]
115. Que, Y.; Cai, M.; Yang, F.; Ji, Q.; Zhang, S.; Huang, W.; Gao, Y.; Zhou, B.; Huang, H.; Cao, H.; et al. Ultrasonographic characteristics, genetic features, and maternal and fetal outcomes in fetuses with omphalocele in China: A single tertiary center study. *BMC Pregnancy Childbirth* **2023**, *23*, 679. [CrossRef] [PubMed] [PubMed Central]
116. Brady, P.D.; Vermeesch, J.R. Genomic microarrays: A technology overview. *Prenat. Diagn.* **2012**, *32*, 336–343. [CrossRef]
117. Monaghan, K.G.; Leach, N.T.; Pekarek, D.; Prasad, P.; Rose, N.C.; ACMG Professional Practice and Guidelines Committee. The use of fetal exome sequencing in prenatal diagnosis: A points to consider document of the American College of Medical Genetics and Genomics (ACMG). *Genet. Med. Off. J. Am. Coll. Med. Genet.* **2020**, *22*, 675–680. [CrossRef] [PubMed]
118. Zhang, B.; Zhang, Y.; Wu, N.; Li, J.; Liu, H.; Wang, J. Integrated analysis of COL2A1 variant data and classification of type II collagenopathies. *Clin. Genet.* **2020**, *97*, 383–395. [CrossRef]
119. Chen, C.P. Rapid diagnosis of maternal origin of fetal trisomy 13 by quantitative fluorescent polymerase chain reaction in a pregnancy associated with young maternal age and omphalocele on prenatal ultrasound. *Taiwan J. Obstet. Gynecol.* **2024**, *63*, 108–110. [CrossRef] [PubMed]
120. Divarci, E.; Karapinar, B.; Yalaz, M.; Ergun, O.; Celik, A. Incidence and prognosis of intraabdominal hypertension and abdominal compartment syndrome in children. *J. Pediatr. Surg.* **2016**, *51*, 503–507. [CrossRef]
121. Fawley, J.A.; Peterson, E.L.; Christensen, M.A.; Rein, L.; Wagner, A.J. Can omphalocele ratio predict postnatal outcomes? *J. Pediatr. Surg.* **2016**, *51*, 62–66. [CrossRef] [PubMed]
122. Barrios Sanjuanelo, A.; Abelló Munarriz, C.; Cardona-Arias, J.A. Systematic review of mortality associated with neonatal primary staged closure of giant omphalocele. *J. Pediatr. Surg.* **2021**, *56*, 678–685. [CrossRef] [PubMed]
123. Akinkuotu, A.C.; Sheikh, F.; Olutoye, O.O.; Lee, T.C.; Fernandes, C.J.; Welty, S.E.; Ayres, N.A.; Cass, D.L. Giant omphaloceles: Surgical management and perinatal outcomes. *J. Surg. Res.* **2015**, *198*, 388–392. [CrossRef] [PubMed]
124. Ţarcă, E.; Cojocaru, E.; Trandafir, L.M.; Luca, A.C.; Tiutiucă, R.C.; Butnariu, L.I.; Costea, C.F.; Radu, I.; Moscalu, M.; Ţarcă, V. Current Challenges in the Treatment of the Omphalocele—Experience of a Tertiary Center from Romania. *J. Clin. Med.* **2022**, *11*, 5711. [CrossRef] [PubMed] [PubMed Central]
125. Ţarcă, E.; Al Namat, D.; Luca, A.C.; Lupu, V.V.; Al Namat, R.; Lupu, A.; Bălănescu, L.; Bernic, J.; Butnariu, L.I.; Moscalu, M.; et al. Omphalocele and Cardiac Abnormalities—The Importance of the Association. *Diagnostics* **2023**, *13*, 1413. [CrossRef] [PubMed] [PubMed Central]
126. Widatella, H.; Abd Elwahab, S.; Penny, Z.; Paran, S.T. A case series of successfully managing exomphalos major with awake graduated compression dressing and early enteral feeding. *Ir. J. Med. Sci.* **2024**, *193*, 1453–1459. [CrossRef] [PubMed] [PubMed Central]

diagnostics

MDPI

Correction

Correction: Al Namat et al. Omphalocele and Associated Anomalies: Exploring Pulmonary Development and Genetic Correlations—A Literature Review. *Diagnostics* 2025, *15*, 675

Dina Al Namat [1,2], Romulus Adrian Roșca [1,3], Razan Al Namat [1,*], Elena Hanganu [1,3], Andrei Ivan [1,2], Delia Hînganu [1], Ancuța Lupu [4] and Marius Valeriu Hînganu [1]

1 Faculty of Medicine, University of Medicine and Pharmacy "Grigore T. Popa", 700115 Iasi, Romania; dina.rosca-al.namat@umfiasi.ro (D.A.N.); adrianrosca82@yahoo.com (R.A.R.); dr.elenahanganu@gmail.com (E.H.); ivan.andrei89@gmail.com (A.I.); hinganu.delia@umfiasi.ro (D.H.); marius.hinganu@umfiasi.ro (M.V.H.)

2 Department of Surgery II-Pediatric Surgery, 700309 Iasi, Romania

3 "Saint Mary" Emergency Children Hospital, 700309 Iasi, Romania

4 Department of Mother and Child Medicine, University of Medicine and Pharmacy "Grigore T. Popa", 700115 Iasi, Romania; anca_ign@yahoo.com

* Correspondence: dr.razan_romania@yahoo.com

In the original publication [1], the author Andrei Ivan's contributions are incomplete. The updated author contributions are as follows: methodology, A.I. and D.A.N.

The mention of "funding acquisition" in the Author Contributions section was an error. This study did not receive any external funding. We removed "funding acquisition, R.A.R. and R.A.N.".

Two of the cited works (References [124,128]) are irrelevant and off-topic and should be removed. With this correction, the order of some references has been adjusted accordingly.

The authors state that the scientific conclusions are unaffected. This correction was approved by the Academic Editor. The original publication has also been updated.

Reference

1. Al Namat, D.; Roșca, R.A.; Al Namat, R.; Hanganu, E.; Ivan, A.; Hînganu, D.; Lupu, A.; Hînganu, M.V. Omphalocele and Associated Anomalies: Exploring Pulmonary Development and Genetic Correlations—A Literature Review. *Diagnostics* **2025**, *15*, 675. [CrossRef] [PubMed]

diagnostics

MDPI

Review

From Genes to Treatment: Literature Review and Perspectives on Acid Sphingomyelinase Deficiency in Children

Raluca Maria Vlad [1,2], Ruxandra Dobritoiu [1,2,*] and Daniela Pacurar [1,2]

1 Department of Paediatrics, "Carol Davila" University of Medicine and Pharmacy, 020021 Bucharest, Romania; raluca.vlad@umfcd.ro (R.M.V.); daniela.pacurar@umfcd.ro (D.P.)
2 "Grigore Alexandrescu" Emergency Children's Hospital, Bld. Iancu de Hunedoara 30-32 Bucharest, 011743 Bucharest, Romania
* Correspondence: ruxandra.darie@drd.umfcd.ro

Abstract: Background: Acid sphingomyelinase deficiency (ASMD), most commonly known as Niemann–Pick disease (NPD), is a rare progressive genetic disorder regarding lipid storage. Subtypes A and B are inherited in an autosomal recessive fashion and consist of a genetic defect which affects the sphingomyelin phosphodiesterase 1 gene, leading to residual or lack of enzymatic activity of acid sphingomyelinase (ASM). **Materials and Methods:** This paper provides a brief history and overview to date of the disease and a comprehensive review of the current literature on ASMD in children, conducted on published papers from the past 10 years. **Results:** We identified 19 original publications (16 individual case reports and three series of cases—30 patients). The male/female ratio was 1.4. The youngest patient at disease onset was a female newborn with NPD-A. The youngest patient was diagnosed at 4 months. The longest timeframe between onset symptoms and diagnostic moment was 5 years 3 months. A total of nine patients exhibited red cherry macular spots. A total of 13 children exhibited associated lung disease, and four NPD-A patients with pulmonary disease died due to respiratory complications. A total of 11 children exhibited associated growth impairment. Genetic assays were performed in 25 cases (15 homozygous; 9 heterozygous). A total of four children (13.3%) received enzyme replacement therapy (ERT). Therapy outcomes included decreased liver and spleen volumes, improved platelet and leukocytes counts, and body mass index and stature improvement. **Conclusions:** Sometimes, a small child with a big belly hides a huge dilemma; inherited metabolic disorders are here to challenge clinicians and set the record straight, and genetics is the way of the future in terms of diagnosis and novel treatments. NPD must be considered children with persistent and progressive hepatosplenomegaly and growth failure. Diagnosis requires good clinical skills and access to genetic assays. Since 2022, the FDA has given a green light to a revolutionary enzymatic replacement therapy with human recombinant ASM called Olipudase-alfa. Clinical trial outcomes support its reliability and efficacy in the pediatric population.

Keywords: Niemann–Pick; acid sphingomyelinase deficiency; metabolic disorder; sphingomyelin; enzyme replacement therapy

1. History and Overview of Acid Sphingomyelinase Deficiency

Lysosomal storage disorders (LSDs) are a rare group of heterogenous genetic disorders with multisystem involvement. More than 50 LSDs have been described. Ages of onset vary from the perinatal period to adulthood, and the spectrum of clinical features depends on the most affected organ or system. These diseases most commonly cause liver damage, whether it is asymptomatic hepatomegaly or advance cirrhosis. Splenomegaly, coarse facial features, and neurological impairment accompany the clinical picture of LSD. The combined prevalence of LSD is 1 to 7000 live births, which might come across as a high number, but keep in mind that these pathologies are seen as scarce among the general population [1–5].

Lysosomes are intracellular organelles considered recycling centers, where large, potentially harmful substances are broken-down to be reused by the body. They undertake a vital job: catabolism of a wide range of macromolecules. Each of these are bound to a particular molecule and are essential for its degradation. When enzymes are missing or there is a defect in their activity, specific materials will accumulate in the lysosomes, leading to cellular impairment [3–5].

To understand a concept, weather is a political idea, an engine car, or a groundbreaking treatment, one must dig into the past. Figure 1 displays the "founding fathers" of Niemann–Pick Disease, each playing an essential role in describing and explaining the disease.

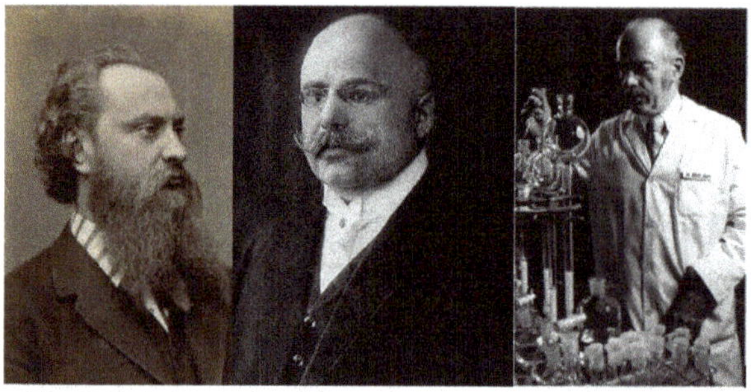

Figure 1. Illustrious figures in the history of Niemann–Pick disease [6].

The history of Niemann–Pick disease goes way back into the 20th century, particularly to 1914, when German pediatrician Albert Niemann described a young child with jaundice, hepatosplenomegaly, and nervous system impairment, completing a report of "Irene D". The patient died at 18 months of age. At autopsy, fatty large vacuolated cells had replaced the normal liver and spleen structure. Doctor Niemann believed these cells were fairly similar to those found in Gaucher disease [6,7].

Later, in 1926, German pathologist Dr. Ludwig Pick accurately described the pathology of NPD in a series of papers. He identified the "Pick cell", a type of foamy cell found in the spleen and bone marrow of NPD patients. In 1934, Klenk identified the lipids accumulating in NPD as sphingomyelins (sphingosine, choline, a fatty acid, and a phosphoric acid). That was an early suggestion that this disease was due to the lack of an enzyme that catalyzed degradation of sphingomyelin. So, it was an entirely different lipid storage disease [6,7].

In 1961, Allan Crocker and Sidney Farber divided NPD into four subcategories (A→D), depending on the patient's phenotype, the specific symptoms expressed, and the presence of unique "foam cells". In 1965, Roscoe Brady demonstrated a profound decrease in acid sphingomyelinase activity in affected cells (from rat liver) for NPD types A and B, but not for types C and D. In 1966, Dr. Brady and his co-workers described a sphingomyelin-cleaving enzyme from rat liver. After that, they identified this enzyme deficiency in tissue samples obtained from infants with NPD parents. One year later, Brady characterized acid sphyngomyelinase activity in peripheral blood leukocytes, thus defining NPD-A and NPD-B types. But the journey went on, and Dr. Brady found another group of patients with similar features to ASMD types A and B, but who associated severe neurological impairment; he distinguished this group as NPD type C. In the late 1980s, an investigator identified a defect in the cholesterol metabolism of NPD-C patients, clearly discriminating them from types A and B. The first reliable diagnostic tests applicable to cultured skin fibroblasts for ASMD types A and B [6,7] were brought forward in 1988.

The quest for a cure kept going. In 2022, an exogenous source of ASM to prevent lysosomal accumulation of sphingomyelin in body tissues, called Olipudase-alfa, was put on the market. This molecule was developed for the treatment of non-neurological ASMD and was first approved by the FDA in August 2022. Since then, it has proved its efficacy and safety, both in pediatric and adult populations [8–11].

Acid sphingomyelinase deficiency (ASMD) is a rare lysosomal storage disorder. Subtypes A and B, most commonly known as Niemann–Pick disease type A (NPD-A) and type B (NPD-B) are rare genetically inherited conditions, with a prevalence between 0.4 and 0.6 to 100.000 live births. The incidence of NPD-A is 1 in 250,000 in the general population, but higher in Ashkenazi Jews (1 in 40,000) [1,2,4,5,12,13]. Niemann–Pick disease type C is a completely different genetic disease, the metabolic defect resulting in cholesterol esterification issues, and this condition is not the subject of this paper.

Both A and B types consist of a genetic defect which affects the sphingomyelin phosphodiesterase 1 (SMPD1) gene, leading to residual or lack of enzymatic activity, and so lysosomes are unable to break-down a fat called sphingomyelin. This fat is included in the membrane of many different cells. When body cells get old, they are eaten by macrophages. The immune system cells contain lysosomes, which crack-down sphingomyelin by using an enzyme called acid sphingomyelinase [1–5]. Mutations in the SMPD1 gene lead to complete absence of sphingomyelinase activity, as in NPD-A, while NPD-B has some residual enzymatic activity remaining (5–20%) [14–17]. In this way, sphingomyelin primarily accumulates in lysosomes of macrophages, cells that travel throughout the body and cause damage in multiple organs and tissues. Macrophages develop a specific lipid-laden microscopic appearance, becoming the histological hallmark of this pathology; they are called "Niemann–Pick cells" or "foam cells" (Figure 2) [1,2,4,18,19].

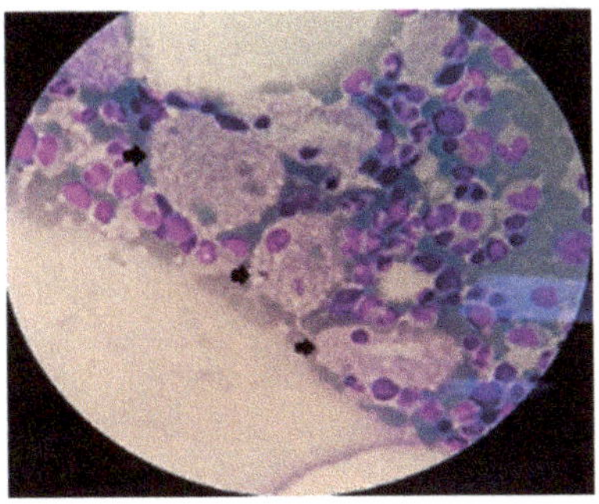

Figure 2. Bone marrow biopsy in ASMD—arrows show "foam cells" [18].

NPD-A onset is in early infancy, and the disease course is marked by a rapid progression to systemic manifestations and neurological degeneration. These children rarely make it over 3 years of age, death usually occurring from extrahepatic involvement (terminal liver disease is not common in type A). On the other hand, NPD-B patients are considered to be "favored"; chronic visceral ASMD has a slow, progressive course, mainly affecting the liver, with a variable onset from infancy to adulthood, and a lack of neurological symptoms. Most patients survive into adulthood. Death in visceral ASMD occurs later in life from recurrent respiratory infections, advanced cirrhosis, massive hemorrhage by spleen rupture, or neuronal degeneration. In addition, there are patients who fall somewhere between type A and B [1,4,5,20]. Chronic neurovisceral ASM deficiency is an intermediate NPD-A/NPD-

B phenotype defined by later onset and slowed neurological/visceral disease progression, also known as NPD type A/B (NPD-A/B) [21,22]. The main features of NPD-A and -B are shown in Table 1 [1,4,5,20].

Table 1. Main features of NPD type A, B, and A/B [1,4,5,20].

	NPD Type A	NPD Type B	NPD Type A/B
Onset	Early infancy	Any time in life	Infancy to childhood
Signs and Symptoms	Hepatosplenomegaly Jaundice Red cherry macular spot Loss of reflexes, muscle tone Feeding difficulties Growth delay Rapid neurodegeneration Interstitial lung disease Atherogenic lipid profile	Splenomegaly Liver enlargement Red cherry macular spot Slow neurodegeneration Growth delay Interstitial lung disease Thrombocytopenia Anemia Low white blood cells Atherogenic lipid profile	Slower progression Variable multiorgan manifestations Neurodegeneration
Severity	Life-threatening	Slowly progressive	Slow neurologic degeneration
Life expectancy	2 to 3 years	Childhood to late adulthood	Childhood to mid-adulthood

A differential diagnosis of ASMD types A and B should include Gaucher disease and Niemann–Pick Disease type C. Patients with type 1 non-neuronopathic Gaucher disease present with splenomegaly, anemia, and low platelet numbers, which leads to nosebleeds or easily induced bruises. They may also exhibit enlarged liver, bone pain, or pathologic fractures. Type 2 Gaucher disease debuts at birth or in early infancy, and alongside organomegaly, it presents with seizures and increased muscle tone. Children with chronic neuronopathic type 3 Gaucher disease have progressive neurological impairment from infancy. Diagnosis of Gaucher disease is confirmed through measurement of glucocerebrosidase activity in leukocytes and analysis of the GBA1 gene [23,24]. NPD type C patients are unable to transport cholesterol and other fatty substances inside cells, so lipids accumulate in various body tissues, including the brain. Onset of NPD-C is highly variable, from the neonatal period to isolated cases diagnosed in late adulthood. Neurological impairment is a constant sign of the disease. Diagnosis is confirmed by molecular gene sequencing of NPC1 and NPC2 genes [25–27].

Because NPD types A and B are inherited in an autosomal recessive fashion, genetic counselling is crucial for future parents. Keeping in mind the Mendelian pattern, if both parents are known to be heterozygous for a pathogenic SMPD1 variant, they will have a 25% chance of conceiving an affected child. We must also remember that ERT has not been studied in pregnant women. Thus, affected individuals must clearly know their genetic status before thinking of having off-spring [8,10,11,27].

In terms of diagnostic methods, ASM deficiency requires a high suspicion index due to its heterogenic phenotype. Clinical examinations showing liver and spleen enlargement, laboratory investigations displaying low white blood cell numbers and thrombocytopenia, low/absent enzymatic activity of ASM in cell or tissue extracts, imaging investigations showing alterations in liver/spleen/lungs/brain, and eye examinations describing red-cherry spots on the macula must lead to one diagnosis: Niemann–Pick disease [28–31].

Subtypes A and B are distinguished through laboratory assessment, by measuring low ASM activity and elevated levels of the biomarker lyso-sphingomyelin, which is also used to monitor efficacy of treatment [10,29]. But heterozygote detection is not reliable by enzyme assay and requires molecular study [17,32]. In other words, genetic testing for pathogenic mutations is the gold-standard diagnostic method for ASMD, even more so with the full-length cDNA and genomic sequence encoding ASM being isolated and defined [15–17]. Prenatal diagnosis is also available through enzymatic or molecular assay from amniocytes and chorionic villi [17,33].

The liver volume should be obtained every 3 to 6 months in order to assess disease progression. Liver morphology exhibits vacuoles in Kupffer cells because of sphingomyelin and cholesterol build-ups, which react strongly positive with Sudan black B and oil red O but negatively or weakly positive with PAS stain. Electron-opaque, concentrically laminated inclusions within the macrophage cytoplasm are observed using electronic microscopy [1,4,32,34]. Liver fibrosis remains a hallmark of NPD, so fibro-scan measurements are required for clear assessment of these patients [4,12,28]. Spleen assessment includes routine volume measurements from imaging studies and platelet counts because even in NPD-B patients with the mild-kind, slow-progressive disease, there have been reported early sudden deaths after massive hemorrhages from spleen ruptures [12,28,35].

Figure 3 depicts the clinical and Figure 4 the imagistic natural course of ASMD in two male patients diagnosed by the authors (images from personal archive).

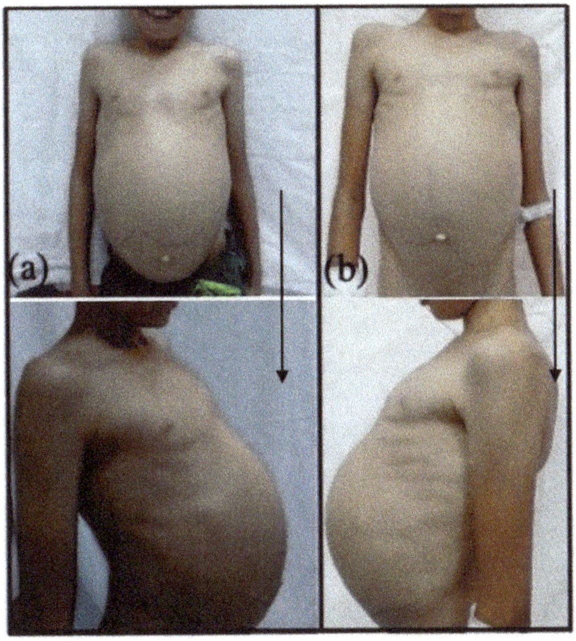

Figure 3. Clinical evolution of organomegaly in a NPD-A/B male. (**a**) At age 9 (BMI = 12.1 kg/m^2; −3.44 SD), the patient had an abdominal circumference of 70 cm, lower liver edge 10 cm under costal rim, and lower spleen edge 9 cm under costal rim. (**b**) At age 14 (BMI = 15.2 kg/m^2; −2.74 SD), the abdominal circumference increased by 9 cm, lower liver edge 12 cm under costal rim, lower spleen below the iliac spine (images from authors' personal archive).

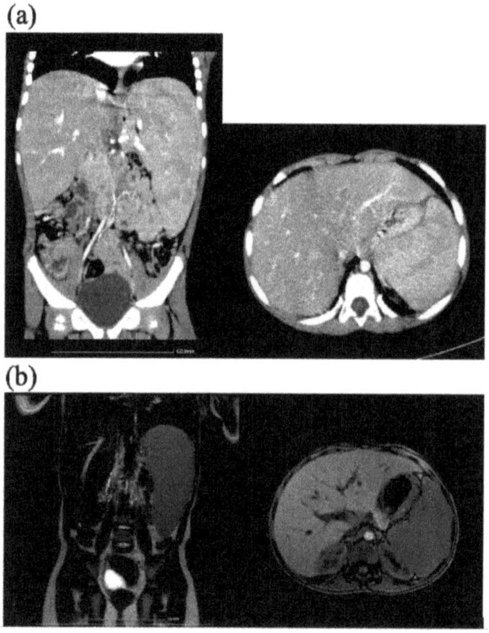

Figure 4. Hepatic and splenic volume evolution in NPD-A/B male: (**a**) abdominal CT scan at 4 years 7 months—liver volume 737.7 cm^3, spleen volume 339.13 cm^3; (**b**) abdominal MRI scan at 6 years 5 months—liver volume 892.66 cm^3, spleen 486.11 cm^3 (images from author's personal archive).

Respiratory complications may occur in both types of Niemann–Pick Disease, type B being the most common. In ASMD type A, pulmonary involvement is rare, and if it emerges, it mainly consists of recurrent respiratory infections, interstitial lung disease, or aspiration pneumonia. Death in children with NPD-A typically happens due to respiratory failure by the age of 3 [14,32,34,36]. NPD-B patients exhibit specific pulmonary symptoms, such as interstitial lung disease (ILD), pulmonary hypertension, alveolar hypoventilation, upper airway obstruction (with or without obstructive sleep apnea syndrome), and recurrent airway infections caused by mucosal membrane swelling. Infants with ASMD type B may develop progressive respiratory symptoms and experience frequent respiratory infections due to aspiration, which can lead to severe respiratory failure, one of the main early causes of death in NPD-B patients [2,12,36–38]. The lung pathogenic process in ASMD involves accumulation of Niemann–Pick cells ("foam cells") in the alveolar septum, bronchial walls, and pleura, causing a restrictive pattern. Histological examination shows intense blue staining with the May Grunwald–Giemsa and the Schmorl reaction—"sea-blue histiocytes". These cells are large, multivacuolated and contain fine and coarse granules. Bronchoscopy detects the presence of Niemann–Pick cells in the bronchoalveolar lavage fluid and lung biopsy specimens [2,4,18,38].

The clinical clue to chronic pulmonary disease is the presence of clubbing fingers and toes (Figure 5a). X-rays may serve as a diagnostic tool in NPD type B, describing micronodular interstitial infiltrate. HRCT scans reveal basal interstitial lung disease (ILD) in most of the cases, with a thickened interlobular septum, which are primarily seen in lower lung zones and ground-glass opacities (Figure 5b), which are described often in the upper lung regions because alveoli are filled with Niemann–Pick cells. Pulmonary function tests usually show normal lung volumes with reduced diffusion capacity for carbon monoxide (DL_{CO}) (Figure 5c) [4,32,38].

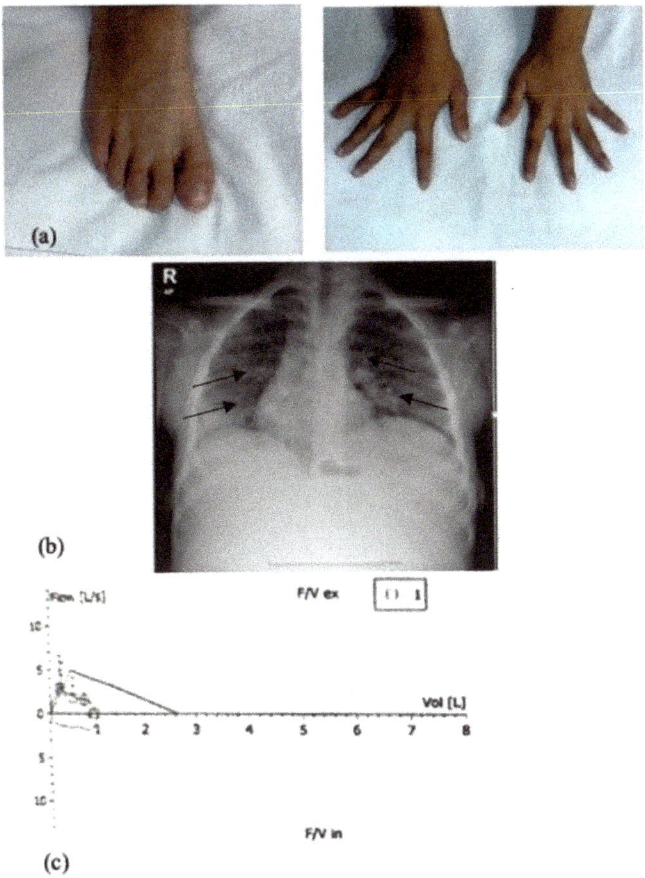

Figure 5. Respiratory findings in a 9 years old NPD-A/B male with (**a**) nail clubbing; (**b**) interstitial lung disease on thoracic X-ray; (**c**) pulmonary interstitial disease with reduced DL_{CO} (images from author's personal archive).

Echocardiography and catheter angiography are useful in NPD-B patients because they develop pulmonary hypertension with multiple arterio-venous fistulas [38].

Eye examination is important in ASMD patients. "Red cherry spot" refers to a red-tinted region in the center of the macula surrounded by retinal opacification. The peri-macular tissue of the retina becomes less transparent, while the fovea maintains its normal color, thus resulting in a red cherry spot appearance. In type A, the macular red cherry spot (Figure 6) is present in half of children at diagnosis moment, and by one year of age, all of them will exhibit this trait. On the other hand, only 1/3 of NPD-B patients display this sign [1,18,39].

NPD-A always presents with neurological manifestations such as seizures, hypotonia, and loss of muscle reflexes, while NPD-B patients have normal neurological development. Typical findings in brain imaging are cerebral atrophy or leukodystrophy, but usually scans come out negative. This, however, does not rule out later neurological impairment due to disease heterogeneity [2,4,5,18,31].

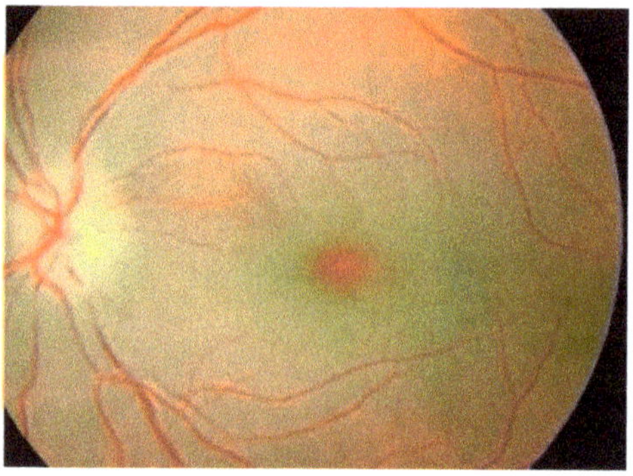

Figure 6. Red cherry macular spot on eye fundus examination [39].

In July 2022, the Food and Drug Administration (FDA) approved a new and revolutionary drug for pediatric and adult populations with non-central nervous system ASMD, called Olipudase-alfa. This molecule is a recombinant human acid sphingomyelinase that reduces lipid build-up in organs and tissues of ASMD-affected patients and is intended as a lifelong enzyme replacement treatment (ERT) [8,40,41]. Efficacy of Olipudase-alfa was determined in three clinical studies: the ASCEND study for the adult population—a multicenter, randomized, double-blind, placebo-controlled phase II/III study [11]; ASCEND-Peds, which included young children and adolescents—a multicentric, open, phase I/II study [11,40,42]; and an extension study for both children over 5 years and adults [11].

Olipudase-alfa comes in 20 mg powder vials for intravenous infusion [11]. Patients receive progressively increased dosages via infusion pump every two weeks, until reaching a maintenance dose. Liver enzymes must be monitored throughout dosage escalation [11,40–42]. Treatment with Olipudase-alfa consists of two phases: first, a dosage escalation phase, which patients must undergo for at least 16 weeks in the pediatric population, and a maintenance phase, when the dosage has reached 3 mg/kg (Table 2) [11,41]. This type of administration is required because rapid, massive degeneration of sphingomyelin by ERT leads to large amounts of waste products with proinflammatory effects that can cause severe, immediate adverse reactions or increases in liver enzymes [11,41].

Table 2. Olipudase-alfa dosage escalation protocol in pediatric population [11].

Dosage Escalation									Maintanance Dosing
Start	**Week 2**	**Week 4**	**Week 6**	**Week 8**	**Week 10**	**Week 12**	**Week 14**	**Week 16**	**Every 2 Weeks**
0.03 mg/kg	0.1 mg/kg	0.3 mg/kg	0.3 mg/kg	0.6 mg/kg	0.6 mg/kg	1.0 mg/kg	2.0 mg/kg	3.0 mg/kg	3.0 mg/kg

Olipudase-alfa has proved its efficacy in lung function. In the ASCEND-Peds open label trial, at week 52 compared with week 26 of treatment, there was a 33% mean increase in DL_{CO} from baseline ($p = 0.0053$) [42]. Regarding spleen and liver measurements, at 52 weeks compared to 26 weeks of Olipudase-alfa infusion, Diaz et al. observed a 49.2% mean decrease in spleen volume from baseline ($p < 0.0001$) and a 40.6% mean decrease in liver volume from baseline ($p < 0.0001$) [42]. ERT also exhibited great outcomes regarding height growth in children with ASMD. Mean height Z-scores improved from baseline after 1 year: +0.56, $p < 0.0001$ (N = 20) [9,40,42].

All outcomes showed further improvement with Olipudase-alfa treatment after 2 years (in ASCEND and ASCEND-Peds/LTS, also for lipid profile, liver enzymes, and platelet counts) or 6.5 years (in Phase 1b/LTS, also for lipid profile, liver enzymes). Olipudase-alfa continued to be well tolerated, and there were no new safety signals [8–10,21,35,40–43].

Solid organ transplantation is another open treatment possibility for NPD patients. However, getting rid of a damaged organ does not prevent recurrence of disease in the transplanted one, nor progression of disease in other organs or tissues [38,44–47]. Lung transplantation should be considered in NPD-B patients with severe respiratory impairment [38,45,46]. Liver transplantation might be a viable therapeutic option for both ASMD type A and B, keeping in mind that hepatic failure is one of the leading causes of death in Niemann–Pick disease. Organ replacement should be performed when the liver becomes cirrhotic and complications emerge, such as portal hypertension, ascites, esophageal varices, and hepatic encephalopathy [38,44,47]. Bone marrow transplantation may alleviate hepato-splenomegaly and improve blood count, but possible complications (graft rejection, renal failure, etc.) make this therapy option highly unrecommended [38].

The ultimate treatment-step is gene therapy, though its efficacy and safety have not yet been demonstrated in humans [38].

2. Review of the Published ASMD Cases in the Literature and Case Data from the Authors' Personal Experience

Published literature is scarce regarding ASMD cases, so the authors aimed to add to the existing data a comprehensive review of the data published in the last 10 years and details from their personal experience with the diagnosis of two patients with NPD-A/B and their enzyme replacement treatment.

This literature review is based on PubMed papers published in the last 10 years (from 2014 to January 2025) regarding Niemann–Pick disease type A and B characteristics, from genetic status to therapy options, with a primary interest in the pediatric field. The following particular search terms in different combinations with filters for case reports, clinical trials, and reviewed articles were used in order to find the most suitable papers for this review: "Niemann–Pick disease", "acid-sphingomyelinase deficiency", "genetic traits in NPD-A and NPD-B", "enzyme replacement therapy", "olipudase-alfa", "metabolic disorder" or "sphingomyelin". Inclusion criteria were a definite diagnosis of Niemann–Pick disease type A, B, or A/B; confirmation of diagnosis by biopsy, enzyme activity level, or molecular assay; and proper evaluation of main affected organs/tissues (liver, spleen, lungs, central nervous system). Exclusion criteria were non-ASMD lysosomal storage disorders, incomplete patient history or diagnostic work-up, non-English published papers, and adult patients with NPD-A, B, A/B, or NPD-C.

All papers concerning Niemann–Pick disease type A and B in children were reviewed (which were published since 2014). A total of 26 of the 62 publications cited in this paper included data regarding children, whether they were case reports, series of cases, or enzyme replacement therapy outcomes. Two papers detailed case reports describing children with NPD type C. One publication outlined a prospective study regarding causes of death in chronic visceral and chronic neurovisceral ASMD but included both children and adults. In the 19 publications detailing case reports (16) and series of cases (3), we assessed number of patients, gender distribution, type of ASMD, symptoms and diagnosis onset age, organ involvement, type of diagnosis, gene mutation, vital status, enzyme replacement therapy, and its outcome.

According to the current reviewed literature, acid sphingomyelinase deficiency types A and B are a rare disease among the pediatric population; from 2014 to January 2025 we identified 30 cases. Table 3 comprises all ASMD cases published in the last decade.

The male/female ratio was 1.4 (one case without gender information). The youngest patient at disease onset was a female newborn with NPD-A. The lowest diagnosis age was

4 months. The longest timeframe between onset symptoms and diagnostic moment was 5 years and 3 months (onset age at 9 months to diagnosis at 6 years); it was a case of chronic visceral non-CNS ASMD.

Sphingomyelin and other lipids accumulate in hepatocytes, monocytes, and macrophages, which leads to organ damage and dysfunction. Therefore, liver and spleen functions and volumes should become part of routine assessment of NPD children, in order to observe disease progression [2,4]. McGovern et al. state that in children, the mean liver volume was 2.2 ± 0.7 MN at baseline, 2.1 ± 0.7 at 1 year, and 1.7 ± 0.4 at the final visit [31]. Moderate to severe hepatomegaly was observed in 96% at baseline, 97% at 1 year, and 88% at the final visit [31]. McGovern et al. concluded that individuals with significant splenomegaly were at higher chance of death than those with smaller or intact spleens (odds ratio = 10.29, 95% CI: 1.7, 62.7) [31].

Both our NPD patients exhibited enlarged liver and spleen, with dimensions progressively increasing over the years. The older NPD-A/B patient had massive hepatomegaly and splenomegaly, starting from an abdominal perimeter of 70 cm at 9 years of age, with lower liver edge at 10 cm and lower spleen edge at 9 cm under the costal rib; by age 14, the abdominal perimeter went up 9 cm (Figure 3). This patient's CT scan showed massive organomegaly, with a spleen volume of 2201 cm^3 and liver volume of 2213 cm^3. Spleen and liver volumes significantly increased over the course of two years in the younger NPD-A/B boy as well, the liver volume from 737.7 cm^3 to 892.66 cm^3 and spleen volume from 339.13 cm^3 to 486.11 cm^3 (Figure 4).

Laboratory findings in both types of ASMD may include lipid abnormalities such as reduced HDL cholesterol, hypertriglyceridemia, and elevated LDL cholesterol (which contributes to cardiac disease), also liver cytolysis and cholestasis [18,32,38,48–51]. Kavcic et al. reported on NPD-A in an 11-month-old boy with increased total cholesterol (5.2 mmol/L), decreased HDL-cholesterol (0.6 mmol/L), and high LDL and triglyceride levels [34]. Velarde-Felix et al. reported on a 16-year-old Mexican girl with NPD-B and persistently low levels of HLD-cholesterol [52].

Platelet count must also be included, especially in NPD-B patients who exhibit frequent mild to severe thrombocytopenia and subsequent bleeding [12,28]. Ceron-Rodriguez et al. reported on a 6-year-old girl with NPD-B epistaxis episodes occurring once a month on average [53], and Sideris et al. found easy bruising or nasal bleeding in an 8-year-old girl with NPD-B [37]. Regarding the 19 publications reviewed, all patients, whether they were diagnosed with NPD-A or NPD-B, displayed hepatic and spleen involvement, the marked enlargement of the liver and spleen, and altered laboratory findings (cytolysis, dyslipidemia, low platelet number) [13,14,18,19,21,22,32,34,35,37,43,52–59]. This is also true for our 14-year-old patient with NPD-A/B. Despite significant hepatosplenomegaly as presented, the 6-year-old NPD-A/B patient had normal liver enzymes and hematologic counts.

Table 3. Literature cases published on ASMD types A, B, and A/B (2014–2024).

Article by Type and Year	Subject Age/Gender	Type of ASMD	Onset Age	Diagnosis Age	Organ Involvement	Type of Diagnosis	Gene Involved	Vital Status	ERT	ERT Outcome
Sideris et al., 2016 [37] Case report	8 years Female	NPD-B	9 month	6 years	Lungs Liver Spleen	Genetic	Homozygous c.C947A	Alive	NO	/
Van Baelen A. et al., 2024 [35] Case report	1 yr 10 month Male	NPD-B	7 month	3 years	Liver Spleen	Enzyme activity Genetic	Homozygous (deletion) c.1829_1831	Alive	Since 4 years 7 month; 16 weeks dose escala-tion	No AR No hepatomegaly Mild splenomegaly Growth failure recovered No heart/lung involvement
Ngoenmak T. et al., 2023 [32] Case report	7 month Female	NPD-A	2 month	7 month	Lungs Liver Spleen Red cherry spot Developmental delay	Liver biopsy Enzyme activity Genetic	Homozygous c.1214T>C	Died at 4 years (respiratory failure and neurological deterioration)	NO	/
Ota S. et al., 2020 [14] Case report	4 month Female	NPD-A	4 month	4 month	Lungs Liver Spleen Red cherry spot Developmental delay	Enzyme activity Genetic	p.C133Y	Died at 3 years 1 month (liver and respiratory failure)	NO	/
Gul F. et al., 2024 [13] Case report	11 month Male	NPD-A	5 month	11 month	Lungs Liver Spleen Growth failure Developmental delay Hypotonia	Liver biopsy NO genetic NO enzyme activity	/	Alive (1 yr 7 month)	NO	/
Kavcic A. et al., 2022 [34] Case report	11 month Male	NPD-A	3 month	10 month	Lungs Liver Spleen Growth failure Developmental delay Hypotonia	Liver biopsy Enzyme activity Genetic	Compound Heterozygous (both pathogenic variants) C573delT (from monthther) c.1267C>T (from father)	Alive	NO	/
Velez Pinos P.J. et al., 2022 [18] Case report	4 years 3 month Male	NPD-A/B	2 month	4 years 3 month	Lungs Liver Spleen Growth failure NO neurological findings	Live biopsy Bone marrow biopsy Enzyme activity Genetic	Compound Heterozygous (both pathogenic variants) c.28C>7 c.362T>C	Alive	NO	/
Dalal P.G. et al., 2024 [54] Case report	1 yr 2 month Gender unknown	NPD-A	/	/	Liver Spleen Growth failure Developmental delay Hypotonia	Enzyme activity Genetic	Compound Heterozygous (both pathogenic variants) c.573delT c.1783_1784delCT	Alive	NO	/

Table 3. *Cont.*

Article by Type and Year	Subject Age/Gender	Type of ASMD	Onset Age	Diagnosis Age	Organ Involvement	Type of Diagnosis	Gene Involved	Vital Status	ERT	ERT Outcome
Mirani E. et al., 2021 [55] Case report	1 yr 6 month Male	NPD-A	6–7 month	1 yr 6 month	Liver Spleen Lungs Growth delay Developmental delay	Bone marrow biopsy Enzyme activity	/	Alive	NO	/
Deodato F. et al., 2024 [43] Case report	8 month Male	NPD-A/B	4 month	6 month	Liver Spleen Red cherry spot NO neurological findings	Enzyme activity Genetic	Homozygous c.739G>A	Alive	Since 8 month; 16 weeks dose escalation	Transient IgG-AMA AR: fever Improved lipid profile AST, ALT normalized Growth failure recovered Height from P25 to P75 Developed neurological impairment at 22 month
Hashemian S. et al., 2019 [56] Prospective study 2012->2016	Male	NPD-A	/	6 month	Liver Spleen Red cherry spot Developmental delay	Genetic	c.740delG	Died at 6 month	NO	/
	Male	NPD-A	/	5 month	Liver Spleen Developmental delay	Genetic	c.740delG	Died at 2 years 6 month	NO	/
	Female	NPD-B	/	6 month	Liver Spleen Developmental delay	Genetic	c.108delG	Died at 3 years	NO	/
	Male	NPD-B	/	6 month	Liver Spleen Developmental delay	Genetic	/	Died at 4 years 6 month	NO	/
	Female	NPD-B	/	6 month	Liver Spleen Developmental delay	Genetic	c.1110delT	Died at 3 years	NO	/
	Male	NPD-B	/	7 month	Liver Spleen Developmental delay	Genetic	c.573delT	Died at 1 yr 6 month	NO	/
	1 yr 6 month Male	NPD-B	/	/	Liver Spleen Red cherry spot Developmental delay	Genetic	c.1390G>T	Alive	NO	/
	2 years 4 month Female	NPD-B	/	/	Liver Spleen Developmental delay	Genetic	c.1524G>A	Alive	NO	/

Table 3. *Cont.*

Article by Type and Year	Subject Age/Gender	Type of ASMD	Onset Age	Diagnosis Age	Organ Involvement	Type of Diagnosis	Gene Involved	Vital Status	ERT	ERT Outcome
Pan Y.W. et al., 2023 [21] Case series	Male	NPD-A/B	< 3 years	3 years 2 month	Liver Spleen Lungs Red cherry spot Growth failure Developmental delay	Genetic	Compound Heterozygous c.1486+5G>C (from father) c.1497_1498delGTinsAC (from monthther)	Alive	Since 5 years 8 month	No severe AR IgG-AMA Reduced liver and spleen volume Lipid profile normalized Improved lung function (improved "ground-glass" aspect) WBC number improved Weight improved Height still under limit
	Male	NPD-A/B	< 1 yr	1 yr 11 month	Liver Spleen Lungs Red cherry spot Growth failure Developmental delay	Genetic	Compound Heterozygous c.1486+5G>C (from father) c.1498T>C (from monthther)	Alive	Since 2 years 6 month	No severe AR Transient elevation AST, ALT Reduced liver and spleen volume Lipid profile normalized Improved lung function (improved "ground-glass" aspect) WBC number improved Weight improved Height still under limit
Tangde A. et al., 2017 [19] Case report	1 yr 6 month Male	NPD-A	2 month	1 yr 6 month	Lungs Liver Spleen Developmental delay	Bone marrow biopsy Spleen aspiration Liver biopsy	/	?	NO	/
Taha I. et al., 2023 [22] Case report	13 years Male	NPD-A/B	/	13 years	Liver Spleen NO neurological findings	Enzyme activity Genetic	Heterozygous c.739G>A c.1829_1831del	Alive	Awaiting ERT	/
Aghamandi F. et al., 2022 [57] Case report	1 yr Male	NPD-A	9 month	1 yr	Liver Spleen Red cherry spot Developmental delay Hypotonia Seizures	Enzyme activity Genetic	Homozygous c.682T>G	Alive	NO	/
Sunil Mohan M. et al., 2014 [58] Case report	11 month Female	NPD-A	/	11 month	Liver Spleen Lungs Growth failure Developmental delay	Bone marrow biopsy Enzyme activity	/	Died at 1 yr 1 month (respiratory failure)	NO	/

Table 3. *Cont.*

Article by Type and Year	Subject Age/Gender	Type of ASMD	Onset Age	Diagnosis Age	Organ Involvement	Type of Diagnosis	Gene Involved	Vital Status	ERT	ERT Outcome
Ceron-Rodriguez M. et al., 2018 [53] Case series	1 yr 3 month Female	NPD-A	neonatal	1 yr 3 month	Liver Spleen Lungs Growth failure Developmental delay	Enzyme activity Genetic	Homozygous c.1343A>G	Died at 1 yr 5 month (pneumonia)	NO	/
	5 years Female	NPD-B	3 years	5 years	Liver Spleen Growth failure	Enzyme activity Genetic	Compound Heterozygous c.1343A>G c.1829_1831delGCC	Alive	NO	/
	7 years Female	NPD-B	2 years	7 years	Liver Spleen Lungs Growth failure	Liver biopsy Enzyme activity Genetic	Compound Heterozygous c.1547A>G c.1805G<A	Alive	NO	/
	6 years Female	NPD-B	2 years	6 years	Liver Spleen	Enzyme activity Genetic	Homozygous c.1263+8C>T	Alive	NO	/
Velarde-Felix J.S. et al., 2016 [52] Case report	16 years Female	NPD-B	/	/	Liver Spleen NO neurological findings	Bone marrow biopsy Genetic	Heterozygous (missense) c.1343A>G c.1426C>7			
Shubhankar M. et al., 2014 [59] Case report	9 month Male	NPD-A	6 month	9 month	Liver Spleen Red cherry sport	Liver biopsy	/	?	NO	/

"NO"—patient has not received enzyme replacement treatment. "?"—patients status (alive or dead) is unknown.

The literature data describe macular red cherry spots in all children with NPD-A by the age of 1 year and only in 1/3 of those with NPD-B [18]. Nine patients out of thirty showed this sign upon fundus eye examination (five of them were diagnosed with NPD-A, three with NPD-A/B, and only one had NPD-B). In their 5-year prospective study, Hashemian et al. reported only eight ASMD patients; two of them exhibited red cherry spots, a 6-month-old boy with NPD-A and 1.5-year-old male with NPD-B [56]. Both our patients exhibited this ophthalmologic sign.

The pulmonary pathogenic process in NPD involves the accumulation of "foam cells" in the alveolar septum, bronchial walls, and pleura, causing a restrictive pattern [2,4,18]. In NPD-A, lung involvement consists of recurrent respiratory infections that constitute the main cause of death (respiratory failure) by the age of three [14,32,34,36]. NPD-B patients primarily exhibit interstitial lung disease [2,38], as did our older patient since the age of 5. A total of 13 children exhibited associated lung disease (8 with NPD-A, 2 with NPD-B, 3 with NPD-A/B). A total of four out of eight patients with ASMD type A and pulmonary disease died due to respiratory complications. Those with chronic visceral and chronic neurovisceral ASMD are still alive, despite pulmonary issues such as dependency on supplemental oxygen and recurrent chest infections.

A total of 11 children exhibited associated growth impairment: 6 with NPD-A, 3 with NPD-A/B, and 2 with NPD-B. Gul et al. reported on an 11-month-old boy with NPD-A at 68 cm in height and 5.3 kg, both below the 3rd percentile in WHO growth charts [13]. Ceron-Rodriguez et al. outlined two cases of NPD-B (5 years and 7 years, both females) with stature and body weight below the 3rd percentile for their age [53]. Both our patients have low stature, below the 3rd percentile for their age.

NPD-A can be distinguished by NPD-B by measuring low ASM activity in designated cells [29]. In 15 cases, enzyme levels were used as a diagnostic tool, but never alone; genetic assay and liver/spleen/bone marrow biopsy were associated in order to establish an unquestionable diagnosis.

Genetic testing for pathogenic mutations remains the gold-standard diagnostic tool for NPD [15,17]. ASM deficiency has been defined in the Online Mendelian Inheritance in Men (OMIM) database [7]. Both NPD-A and NPD-B are caused by a homozygous or compound heterozygous mutation in the SPMD1 gene on the chromosome 11p15 (Figure 7a) [15,16]. Genotyping in the authors' two patients revealed a homozygous state for (p.(Trp393Gly)), a known missense mutation that confirmed NPD type A/B (Figure 7b).

The SMPD1 gene encodes an enzyme called acid sphingomyelinase, which breaks down sphingomyelin into ceramide and phosphocholine [16]. Type A is always inherited in an autosomal recessive fashion and is marked by small deletions or nonsense mutations that produce a cut-short version of ASM peptides, but also missense mutations that generate a non-catalytic enzyme [38]. Type B is not always an autosomal recessive disorder, although this is the main mode of inheritance. Some individuals are carriers, which means they are heterozygous for the mutation but can still present with milder forms of disease. NPD-B is mainly caused by missense mutations that result in a residual enzymatic catalytic activity [17,38].

More than 100 mutations in the SMPD1 gene are cited in the Human Gene Mutation Database (HGMD) for ASMD type A and B [16]. Over 60% are missense mutations, and 19% are frameshift mutations [38]. R496L, L302P, and fsP330 represent over 90% of the Ashkenazi mutant alleles and are linked to ASMD type A [17]. The most frequent mutation reported worldwide is a deletion associated with a mild form of NPD-B disease [38]. "Neuroprotective" status results from residual activity of ASM due to a common mutation of the SMPD1 gene found in type B patients, R608 [17].

Location	Phenotype	Inheritance	Gene/Locus	Gene/Locus MIM number
11p15.4	Niemann-Pick disease type A	AR	SMPD1	607608
11p15.4	Niemann-Pick disease type B	AR	SMPD1	607608

(a)

Result:

The following mutation was detected in homozygous state:

c.1177T>G (p.(Trp393Gly))

Interpretation:

Two mutations were detected: the homozygous p.Trp393Gly is a known missense mutation (ClinVar-ID: 2991) and confirms Niemann-Pick A/B disease (ASMD).

Result:

The following mutation was detected in homozygous state:

c.1177T>G (p.(Trp393Gly))

Interpretation:

(b)

Two mutations were detected: the homozygous p.Trp393Gly is a known missense mutation (ClinVar-ID: 2991) and confirms Niemann-Pick A/B disease (ASMD).

Figure 7. (**a**) Genotype–Phenotype relationship of NPD-A and NPD-B in the OMIM system [7]; (**b**) genotypes of the authors' cases: NPD-A/B.

In 25 out of 30 cases, a genetic assay was performed (15 were homozygous; in Hashemian et al.'s study, one child with NPD-B had no information regarding genetic status; nine were heterozygous [56]). Gul et al. established NPD-A diagnosis in an 11-month-old boy only on the basis of liver biopsy [13]. Mirani et al. proved NPD-A in a 1.5-year-old male by measuring ASM activity and performing a bone marrow biopsy [55]. Tangde et al. indicated NPD-A in a 1-year-6-month-old boy on the basis of liver, spleen, and bone marrow biopsies [19]. Sunil Mohan et al. described NPD-A in an 11-month-old girl by measuring ASM levels and performing bone marrow aspiration [58]. Shubhankar et al. established an NPD-A diagnosis in a 9-month-old boy only after liver biopsy [59]. All five cases without genetic assessment have one thing in common: they are all cases of ASMD type A, which embraces a high index of clinical suspicion in an infant with developmental delay, growth impairment, and hepatosplenomegaly. All this, alongside a low enzymatic activity and the presence of "foamy cells" at microscopy, leads to NPD-A diagnosis.

The Department of Health and Human Services in the U.S. developed a list called "The recommended universal screening panel", or RUSP, which identifies various genetic disorders, but Niemann–Pick disease is not included [33]. Currently in America, only two States—Illinois and New Jersey—offer newborn screening for ASMD [33]. Geberhiwot et al. elaborated two consensus clinical management guidelines for NPD-A, NPD-B, NPD-A/B, and NPD-C, papers published in the Orphanet Journal of Rare Diseases back in 2018 and 2023, which clearly state the steps of correct diagnosis for these types of ASMD [27,30]. As for Romania, a statement paper was recently published in the Romanian Journal of Pediatrics presenting a screening program developed in the Department of Pediatrics of "Grigore Alexandrescu" Emergency Children's Hospital, Bucharest, for those patients with a high index of clinical suspicion [60].

Since Olipudase-alfa was approved for pediatric and adult populations with non-central nervous system ASMD, ERT via intravenous infusion every two weeks has emerged as a treatment. Dosages are progressively scaled-up for at least 14 weeks (for children) and 16 weeks (for adults), until a maintenance dose is reached (3 milligrams per body kilogram) [8,11,41].

Four children received Olipudase-alfa (one with NPD-B, three with NPD-A/B) [21,35,43]. A 13-year-old boy with NPD-A/B was awaiting therapy back in 2023 (Taha et al.) [20]. Van Baelen et al. reported on NPD-B in a boy, diagnosed at 3 years of age, who started ERT at 4 years 7 months of age [35]. Deodato et al. presented NPD-A/B in a boy, diagnosed at 6 months of age, who began ERT two months after diagnosis [43]. Pan Y.W. et al. described two cases of NPD-A/B in boys diagnosed at 3 years 2 months and 1 year 11 months, respectively, who were treated starting at 5 years 8 months and 2.5 years, respectively [21]. In two cases, Olipudase-alfa dosages were escalated over a period of 16 weeks.

The authors included two patients in the treatment protocol in the last year (a 15-year-old male with NPD-A/B and a 6-year-old male with NPD-A/B). Figure 8 exhibits the evolution of liver and spleen volumes after six doses of Olipudase-alfa in the 15-year-old male with NPD-A/B. No side effects were noted so far.

Volume/Time	Before treatment	Dose 6 of Olipudase-alfa
Liver volume	2213 cmc	1856.3 cmc
Spleen volume	2201 cmc	1403.71 cmc

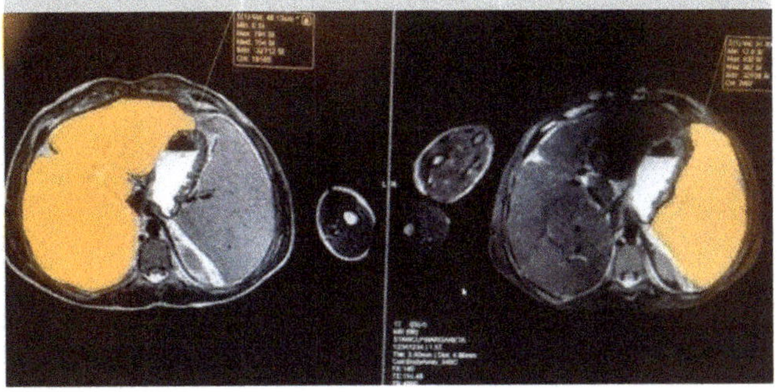

Figure 8. Evolution of liver and spleen volumes in NPD-A/B male after six doses of Olipudase-alfa (images from authors' personal archive).

Regarding intravenous-infusion-like adverse reactions, the pediatric population takes the leading spot. Children may exhibit mild symptoms from fever, nausea, vomiting, or headaches to a severe phenomenon like anaphylaxis. The main medication-like adverse reaction is an increase in liver enzymes, which is why ASMD disease monitoring requires routine check-ups of transaminase levels. After a few weeks of replacement therapy, anti-medication antibodies (AMAs) may emerge [8,11,41,61]. In the ASCEND-Peds study, 65% of children became AMA positive, but only five of them maintained that immunological status [11].

Van Baelen et al. reported no adverse reactions (ARs), no liver enlargement, and mild splenomegaly. Growth failure recovered, and no heart or lung involvement was described [35]. Deodato et al. reported fever after ERT infusions and transient anti-medication antibodies (AMAs). In this case, the lipid profile improved, and liver cytolysis disappeared.

The child recovered his growth status, with his height reaching the 75th percentile (at the beginning, his stature was in the 25th percentile). Unfortunately, he developed neurological impairment after 14 months of ERT [43]. Pan Y.W. et al. reported two children who received ERT; at first, they did not exhibit severe ARs but developed IgG-AMA; liver and spleen volume decreased, lipid profile normalized, lung function improved, WBC number enhanced, body weight picked-up, but stature stayed below the limit-line [21]. The second child had a transient elevation of liver enzymes, but liver and spleen volume went down; the lipid profile normalized, the pulmonary "ground-glass" pattern improved, body weight went up, but stature was not exceeded [21].

3. Conclusions

ASMD presents with significant variability in its clinical manifestation, ranging from the severe, early-onset neurodegeneration seen in NPD-A to the more slowly progressive visceral involvement without neurological deterioration in NPD-B. The intermediate NPD-A/B phenotype shows a slower progression, with both visceral and neurological features. The diversity in age of onset, organ involvement, and disease severity highlights the need for precise genetic testing and tailored clinical management for each. Early diagnosis and understanding of the subtype are crucial for proper prognostic counseling and treatment planning.

The literature is scarce on this subject, thus making the discovery of new cases harder. However, ASMD should be takin into consideration when confronted with a child with liver and spleen enlargement. A rapid laboratory assessment of WBC and platelet number alongside a basic abdominal ultrasound should provide sufficient information to raise clinical suspicion of the disease. Given the complex nature of ASMD, early and accurate diagnosis is essential for providing appropriate medical care. This involves not only genetic and enzymatic testing but also regular monitoring of organ function (e.g., liver, spleen, and lungs) and neurological status. A multidisciplinary approach is vital, including genetic counseling, symptom management, and consideration of advanced treatments like ERT. Moreover, new therapies such as gene therapy and organ transplantation are still being explored, emphasizing the importance of ongoing research and clinical trials to address the limitations of current treatments.

Olipudase-alfa is showing promising results in treating non-neurological forms of ASMD. It has been particularly effective in reducing organomegaly (liver and spleen volumes), improving lung function, and promoting growth in pediatric patients. ERT represents a significant advancement in managing the visceral symptoms of NPD-B and the intermediate NPD-A/B phenotype. However, it is important to note that ERT has not been proven effective for neurological involvement, which remains a challenge for patients with NPD-A and some with NPD-A/B.

In conclusion, while significant progress has been made in the understanding and treatment of ASMD, ongoing research, early diagnosis, and personalized care remain essential to improving outcomes and quality of life of affected individuals. And as with any rare disease, each new case provides the medical community with valuable information needed to achieve these goals.

Author Contributions: Conceptualization, R.M.V.; methodology, R.M.V., R.D. and D.P.; software, R.M.V. and R.D.; validation, R.M.V., R.D. and D.P.; formal analysis, R.M.V. and R.D.; investigation, R.M.V. and R.D.; resources, R.M.V. and R.D.; data curation, R.M.V., R.D. and D.P.; writing—original draft preparation, R.M.V. and R.D.; writing—review and editing, R.M.V. and D.P.; visualization, R.M.V., R.D. and D.P.; supervision, R.M.V. and D.P.; project administration, R.M.V. All authors have read and agreed to the published version of the manuscript.

Funding: This research received no external funding.

Data Availability Statement: Data are contained within the article.

Acknowledgments: Publication of this paper was supported by the University of Medicine and Pharmacy Carol Davila, through the institutional program Publish not Perish.

Conflicts of Interest: The authors declare no conflicts of interest.

References

1. Sen Sarma, M.; Tripathi, P.R. Natural history and management of liver dysfunction in lysosomal storage disorders. *World J. Hepatol.* **2022**, *14*, 1844–1861. [CrossRef] [PubMed] [PubMed Central]
2. Schuchman, E.H.; Desnick, R.J. Types A and B Niemann-Pick disease. *Mol. Genet Metab.* **2017**, *120*, 27–33. [CrossRef] [PubMed] [PubMed Central]
3. Torres, S.; Balboa, E.; Zanlungo, S.; Enrich, C.; Garcia-Ruiz, C.; Fernandez-Checa, J.C. Lysosomal and Mitochondrial Liaisons in Niemann-Pick Disease. *Front. Physiol.* **2017**, *8*, 982.
4. Patel, J.M.; Rohena, L.O. Sphingomyelinase Deficiency. 2024. Available online: https://emedicine.medscape.com/article/951564-overview (accessed on 14 February 2025).
5. Nascimbeni, F.; Dionisi Vici, C.; Vespasiani Gentilucci, U.; Angelico, F.; Nobili, V.; Petta, S.; Valenti, L.; AISF Rare Diseases Committee. AISF update on the diagnosis and management of adult-onset lysosomal storage diseases with hepatic involvement. *Dig. Liver Dis.* **2020**, *52*, 359–367. [CrossRef] [PubMed]
6. Dipharma. Niemann Pick C. Available online: https://www.dipharma.ch/science-innovation/metabolic-diseases/niemann-pick-c/ (accessed on 14 February 2025).
7. OMIM®. Available online: https://omim.org/ (accessed on 14 February 2025).
8. Penon-Portmann, M.; Poskanzer, S.A.; Ganesh, J.; Chang, I. Olipudase alfa approved for pediatric and adult patients with acid sphingomyelinase deficiency (ASMD): A therapeutics bulletin of the American College of Medical Genetics and Genomics (ACMG). *Genet. Med. Open* **2023**, *1*, 100780. [CrossRef] [PubMed] [PubMed Central]
9. Wasserstein, M.P.; Jones, S.A.; Soran, H.; Diaz, G.A.; Lippa, N.; Thurberg, B.L.; Culm-Merdek, K.; Shamiyeh, E.; Inguilizian, H.; Cox, G.F.; et al. Successful within-patient dose escalation of olipudase alfa in acid sphingomyelinase deficiency. *Mol. Genet. Metab.* **2015**, *116*, 88–97. [CrossRef] [PubMed] [PubMed Central]
10. Garside, B.; Ho, J.H.; Kwok, S.; Liu, Y.; Dhage, S.; Donn, R.; Iqbal, Z.; Jones, S.A.; Soran, H. Changes in PCSK 9 and apolipoprotein B100 in Niemann-Pick disease after enzyme replacement therapy with olipudase alfa. *Orphanet J. Rare Dis.* **2021**, *16*, 107.
11. Anexa I Rezumatul Caracteristicilor Produsului. Available online: https://ec.europa.eu/health/documents/community-register/2022/20220624156071/anx_156071_ro.pdf (accessed on 14 February 2025).
12. Cassiman, D.; Packman, S.; Bembi, B.; Turkia, H.B.; Al-Sayed, M.; Schiff, M.; Imrie, J.; Mabe, P.; Takahashi, T.; Mengel, K.E.; et al. Cause of death in patients with chronic visceral and chronic neurovisceral acid sphingomyelinase deficiency (Niemann-Pick disease type B and B variant): Literature review and report of new cases. *Mol. Genet. Metab.* **2016**, *118*, 206–213, Erratum in *Mol. Genet. Metab.* **2018**, *125*, 360. [CrossRef] [PubMed]
13. Gul, F.; Begum, S.; Rasool, P.; Shah, S.; Waqar, M. A Rare Case of Niemann-Pick Disease Type-A. *Cureus* **2024**, *16*, e59427. [CrossRef] [PubMed] [PubMed Central]
14. Ota, S.; Noguchi, A.; Kondo, D.; Nakajima, Y.; Ito, T.; Arai, H.; Takahashi, T. An Early-Onset Neuronopathic Form of Acid Sphingomyelinase Deficiency: A SMPD1 p.C133Y Mutation in the Saposin Domain of Acid Sphingomyelinase. *Tohoku J. Exp. Med.* **2020**, *250*, 5–11. [CrossRef] [PubMed]
15. Zampieri, S.; Filocamo, M.; Pianta, A.; Lualdi, S.; Gort, L.; Coll, M.J.; Sinnott, R.; Geberhiwot, T.; Bembi, B.; Dardis, A. SMPD1 Mutation Update: Database and Comprehensive Analysis of Published and Novel Variants. *Hum. Mutat.* **2016**, *37*, 139–147. [CrossRef] [PubMed]
16. Schuchman, E.H.; Desnick, R.J. Niemann-Pick Disease Types A and B: Acid Sphingomyelinase Deficiencies. In *The Online Metabolic and Molecular Bases of Inherited Disease*; Valle, D.L., Antonarakis, S., Ballabio, A., Beaudet, A.L., Mitchell, G.A., Eds.; McGraw-Hill Education: New York, NY, USA, 2019. Available online: https://ommbid.mhmedical.com/content.aspx?bookid=2709&sectionid=225545671 (accessed on 9 January 2025).
17. Tirelli, C.; Rondinone, O.; Italia, M.; Mira, S.; Belmonte, L.A.; De Grassi, M.; Guido, G.; Maggioni, S.; Mondoni, M.; Miozzo, M.R.; et al. The Genetic Basis, Lung Involvement, and Therapeutic Options in Niemann-Pick Disease: A Comprehensive Review. *Biomolecules* **2024**, *14*, 211. [CrossRef] [PubMed] [PubMed Central]
18. Vélez Pinos, P.J.; Saavedra Palacios, M.S.; Colina Arteaga, P.A.; Arevalo Cordova, T.D. Niemann-Pick Disease: A Case Report and Literature Review. *Cureus* **2023**, *15*, e33534. [CrossRef] [PubMed] [PubMed Central]

19. Tangde, A.; Pore, S.; Kulkarni, A.; Joshi, A.; Bindu, R. Niemann-pick disease type A—A case report. *Int. J. Res. Med. Sci.* **2017**, *6*, 366–369. [CrossRef]
20. Lidove, O.; Sedel, F.; Charlotte, F.; Froissart, R.; Vanier, M.T. Cirrhosis and liver failure: Expanding phenotype of Acid sphingomyelinase-deficient niemann-pick disease in adulthood. *JIMD Rep.* **2015**, *15*, 117–121. [CrossRef] [PubMed] [PubMed Central]
21. Pan, Y.W.; Tsai, M.C.; Yang, C.Y.; Yu, W.H.; Wang, B.; Yang, Y.J.; Chou, Y.Y. Enzyme replacement therapy for children with acid sphingomyelinase deficiency in the real world: A single center experience in Taiwan. *Mol. Genet. Metab. Rep.* **2023**, *34*, 100957. [CrossRef] [PubMed] [PubMed Central]
22. Taha, I.; Tadmori, I.; Hida, M. Niemann-Pick A/B Disease in a 13-Year-Old Child and Review of the Literature. *Open J. Pediatr.* **2023**, *13*, 907–913. [CrossRef]
23. Giacomarra, M.; Colomba, P.; Francofonte, D.; Zora, M.; Caocci, G.; Diomede, D.; Giuffrida, G.; Fiori, L.; Montanari, C.; Sapuppo, A.; et al. Gaucher disease or acid sphingomyelinase deficiency? The importance of differential diagnosis. *J. Clin. Med.* **2024**, *13*, 1487. [CrossRef] [PubMed] [PubMed Central]
24. Cappellini, M.D.; Motta, I.; Barbato, A.; Giuffrida, G.; Manna, R.; Carubbi, F.; Giona, F. Similarities and differences between Gaucher disease and acid sphingomyelinase deficiency: An algorithm to support the diagnosis. *Eur. J. Intern. Med.* **2023**, *108*, 81–84. [CrossRef] [PubMed]
25. Chen, F.; Guo, S.; Li, X.; Liu, S.; Wang, L.; Zhang, V.W.; Xu, H.; Huang, Z.; Ying, Y.; Shu, S. Case Report: Be Aware of "New" Features of Niemann-Pick Disease: Insights from Two Pediatric Cases. *Front. Genet.* **2022**, *13*, 845246. [CrossRef] [PubMed] [PubMed Central]
26. Sreekantam, S.; Rizvi, H.; Brown, R.; Santra, S.; Raiman, J.; Vijay, S.; Mckiernan, P.J.; Gupte, G.L. An uncommon cause of early infantile liver disease and raised chitotriosidase. *JIMD Rep.* **2020**, *54*, 22–24. [CrossRef] [PubMed] [PubMed Central]
27. Geberhiwot, T.; Moro, A.; Dardis, A.; Ramaswami, U.; Sirrs, S.; Marfa, M.P.; Vanier, M.T.; Walterfang, M.; Bolton, S.; Dawson, C.; et al. Consensus clinical management guidelines for Niemann-Pick disease type C. *Orphanet J. Rare Dis.* **2018**, *13*, 50. [CrossRef] [PubMed] [PubMed Central]
28. McGovern, M.M.; Dionisi-Vici, C.; Giugliani, R.; Hwu, P.; Lidove, O.; Lukacs, Z.; Mengel, E.; Mistry, P.K.; Schuchman, E.H.; Wasserstein, M.P. Consensus recommendation for K. a diagnostic guideline for acid sphingomyelinase deficiency. *Genet. Med.* **2017**, *19*, 967–974. [CrossRef] [PubMed] [PubMed Central]
29. Breilyn, M.S.; Zhang, W.; Yu, C.; Wasserstein, M.P. Plasmalyso-sphingomyelin levels are positively associated with clinical severity in acid sphingomyelinase deficiency. *Mol. Genet. Metab. Rep.* **2021**, *28*, 100780. [CrossRef]
30. Geberhiwot, T.; Wasserstein, M.; Wanninayake, S.; Bolton, S.C.; Dardis, A.; Lehman, A.; Lidove, O.; Dawson, C.; Giugliani, R.; Imrie, J.; et al. Consensus clinical management guidelines for acid sphingomyelinase deficiency (Niemann-pick disease types A, B and A/B). *Orphanet. J. Rare Dis.* **2023**, *18*, 85. [CrossRef] [PubMed] [PubMed Central]
31. McGovern, M.M.; Avetisyan, R.; Sanson, B.J.; Lidove, O. Disease manifestations and burden of illness in patients with acid sphingomyelinase deficiency (ASMD). *Orphanet J. Rare Dis.* **2017**, *12*, 41.
32. Ngoenmak, T.; Somran, J.; Foonoi, M.; Srisingh, K.; Singpan, N.; Tim-Aroon, T. Case report of a novel variant in SMPD1 of Niemann-Pick disease type A with a liver histology from Thailand. *Glob. Pediatr.* **2024**, *7*, 100096. [CrossRef]
33. NNPDF. The Importance of Newborn Screening for Niemann-Pick Disease. Available online: https://nnpdf.org/the-importance-of-newborn-screening-for-niemann-pick-disease/ (accessed on 14 February 2025).
34. Kavčič, A.; Homan, M.; Živanović, M.; Debeljak, M.; Butenko, T.; Drole Torkar, A.; Žerjav Tanšek, M.; Bertok, S.; Battelino, T.; Groselj, U. Compound Heterozygote Mutation in the SMPD1 Gene Leading to Nieman-Pick Disease Type, A. *Am. J. Case Rep.* **2022**, *23*, e937220. [CrossRef] [PubMed] [PubMed Central]
35. Van Baelen, A.; Verhulst, S.; Eyskens, F. Unexplained splenomegaly as a diagnostic marker for a rare but severe disease with an innovative and highly effective new treatment option: A case report. *Mol. Genet. Metab. Rep.* **2024**, *41*, 101144. [CrossRef] [PubMed] [PubMed Central]
36. Mauhin, W.; Borie, R.; Dalbies, F.; Douillard, C.; Guffon, N.; Lavigne, C.; Lidove, O.; Brassier, A. Acid Sphingomyelinase Deficiency: Sharing Experience of Disease Monitoring and Severity in France. *J. Clin. Med.* **2022**, *11*, 920. [CrossRef] [PubMed] [PubMed Central]
37. Sideris, G.A.; Josephson, M. Pulmonary alveolar proteinosis and Niemann Pick disease type B: An unexpected combination. *Respir. Med. Case Rep.* **2016**, *19*, 37–39. [CrossRef] [PubMed] [PubMed Central]
38. Kingma, S.D.; Bodamer, O.A.; Wijburg, F.A. Epidemiology and diagnosis of lysosomal storage disorders; challenges of screening. *Best. Pract. Res. Clin. Endocrinol. Metab.* **2015**, *29*, 145–157. [CrossRef] [PubMed]
39. EyeWiki. Cherry-Red Spot. Available online: https://eyewiki.org/Cherry-Red_Spot (accessed on 14 February 2025).
40. Diaz, G.A.; Giugliani, R.; Guffon, N.; Jones, S.A.; Mengel, E.; Scarpa, M.; Witters, P.; Yarramaneni, A.; Li, J.; Armstrong, N.M.; et al. Long-term safety and clinical outcomes of olipudase alfa enzyme replacement therapy in pediatric patients with acid sphingomyelinase deficiency: Two-year results. *Orphanet J. Rare Dis.* **2022**, *17*, 437, Erratum in *Orphanet J. Rare Dis.* **2023**, *18*, 55. [CrossRef] [PubMed] [PubMed Central]

41. Syed, Y.Y. Olipudase Alfa in Non-CNS Manifestations of Acid Sphingomyelinase Deficiency: A Profile of Its Use. *Clin. Drug Investig.* **2023**, *43*, 369–377, Erratum in *Clin. Drug Investig.* **2023**, *43*, 667. [CrossRef] [PubMed] [PubMed Central]
42. Diaz, G.A.; Jones, S.A.; Scarpa, M.; Mengel, K.E.; Giugliani, R.; Guffon, N.; Batsu, I.; Fraser, P.A.; Li, J.; Zhang, Q.; et al. One-year results of a clinical trial of olipudase alfa enzyme replacement therapy in pediatric patients with acid sphingomyelinase deficiency. *Genet. Med.* **2021**, *23*, 1543–1550, Erratum in *Genet Med.* **2022**, *24*, 2209. [CrossRef] [PubMed] [PubMed Central]
43. Deodato, F.; Boenzi, S.; Greco, B.; Graziosi, A.; Dionisi-Vici, C. Case Report: Two years of compassionate use with Olipudase-alfa in a child with neurovisceral acid sphingomyelinase deficiency. *Front. Pediatr.* **2025**, *12*, 1518344. Available online: https://www.frontiersin.org/journals/pediatrics/articles/10.3389/fped.2024.1518344 (accessed on 14 February 2025). [CrossRef]
44. Coelho, G.R.; Praciano, A.M.; Rodrigues, J.P.; Viana, C.F.; Brandão, K.P.; Valenca, J.T., Jr.; Garcia, J.H. Liver Transplantation in Patients With Niemann-Pick Disease—Single-Center Experience. *Transplant. Proc.* **2015**, *47*, 2929–2931. [CrossRef] [PubMed]
45. Tirelli, C.; Arbustini, E.; Meloni, F. Bilateral Cystic Bronchiectasis as Novel Phenotype of Niemann-Pick Disease Type B Successfully Treated with Double Lung Transplantation. *Chest* **2021**, *159*, e293–e297. [CrossRef]
46. Ding, F.; Mehta, A.C.; Arrossi, A.V. Successful lung transplantation in a patient with Niemann-Pick disease. *J. Heart Lung Transplant.* **2019**, *38*, 582–583. [CrossRef]
47. Liu, Y.; Luo, Y.; Xia, L.; Qiu, B.; Zhou, T.; Feng, M.; Xue, F.; Chen, X.; Han, L.; Xia, Q.; et al. The Effects of Liver Transplantation in Children with Niemann-Pick Disease Type, B. *Liver Transpl.* **2019**, *25*, 1233–1240. [CrossRef]
48. Constantin, A.T.; Streata, I.; Covăcescu, M.S.; Riza, A.L.; Roșca, I.; Delia, C.; Tudor, L.M.; Dorobanțu, Ș.; Dragoș, A.; Ristea, D.; et al. Genetic Testing for Familial Hypercholesterolemia in a Pediatric Group: A Romanian Showcase. *Diagnostics* **2023**, *13*, 1988. [CrossRef] [PubMed]
49. Constantin, A.T.; Delia, C.; Tudor, L.M.; Rosca, I.; Irimie, A.D.; Năstase, L.; Gherghina, I. Dyslipidemia in Pediatric Patients: A Cross-Sectional Study. *Medicina* **2023**, *59*, 1434. [CrossRef] [PubMed]
50. Jugulete, G.; Iacob, S.; Merisescu, M.; Luminos, M. Lipd Metabolism Abnormalities in Children and Adolescents with HIV/AIDS Treated with Protease Inhibitors. *Rev. Chim.* **2017**, *68*, 2467–2470. [CrossRef]
51. Vlad, R.M.; Albu, A.I.; Nicolaescu, I.D.; Dobritoiu, R.; Carsote, M.; Sandru, F.; Albu, D.; Păcurar, D. An Approach to Traumatic Brain Injury-Related Hypopituitarism: Overcoming the Pediatric Challenges. *Diagnostics* **2023**, *13*, 212. [CrossRef]
52. Velarde-Félix, J.S.; Osuna-Ramos, J.F.; Sánchez-Leyva, M.G.; Ríos Burguenõ, E.R.; Monroy Arellano, L.M. Pathogenic compound heterozygous mutations in a Mexican mestizo patient with Niemann Pick Disease Type, B. *Genet. Couns.* **2016**, *27*, 211–217.
53. Cerón-Rodríguez, M.; Vázquez-Martínez, E.R.; García-Delgado, C.; Ortega-Vázquez, A.; Valencia-Mayoral, P.; Ramírez-Devars, L.; Arias-Villegas, C.; Monroy-Muñoz, I.E.; López, M.; Cervantes, A.; et al. Niemann-Pick disease A or B in four pediatric patients and SMPD1 mutation carrier frequency in the Mexican population. *Ann. Hepatol.* **2019**, *18*, 613–619. [CrossRef] [PubMed]
54. Dalal, P.G.; Coleman, M.; Horst, M.; Rocourt, D.; Ladda, R.L.; Janicki, P.K. Case Report: Genetic analysis and anesthetic management of a child with Niemann-Pick disease Type, A. *F1000Research* **2015**, *4*, 1423. [CrossRef] [PubMed] [PubMed Central]
55. Mirani, E.; Pratiwi, R.; Widyastiti, N.S.; Ekowati, L.; Mexitalia, M. Niemann-Pick disease type A: A case report. Medica Hospitalia. *J. Clin. Med.* **2021**, *8*, 129–132. Available online: https://medicahospitalia.rskariadi.co.id/index.php/mh/article/view/577 (accessed on 14 February 2025).
56. Hashemian, S.; Eshraghi, P.; Dilaver, N.; Galehdari, H.; Shalbafan, B.; Vakili, R.; Ghaemi, N.; Ahangari, N.; Rezazadeh Varaghchi, J.; Zeighami, J.; et al. Niemann-Pick Diseases: The Largest Iranian Cohort with Genetic Analysis. *Iran. J. Child. Neurol.* **2019**, *13*, 155–162. [PubMed] [PubMed Central]
57. Aghamahdi, F.; Nirouei, M.; Savad, S. Niemann-Pick type A disease with new mutation: A case report. *J. Med. Case Rep.* **2022**, *16*, 288. [CrossRef] [PubMed] [PubMed Central]
58. Sunil Mohan, M.; Mohinuddin Siddique, A.; Somaiah, G.; Suresh Babu, M.; Kishore Babu, S.P.V.; Siva Rama Krishna, K. Case Report of Niemann-Pick Disease: Type-A. *Sch. J. Medica Case Rep.* **2014**, *2*, 52–53. [CrossRef]
59. Shubhankar, M.; Sunil, K.A.; Bikash, R.P.; Shantanu, K.M. Niemann Pick disease type A in an Infant: A case report. *Sch. Acad. J. Biosci.* **2014**, *2*, 728–730.
60. Vlad, R.M. Targeted screening for acid sphingomyelinase deficiency—a short guide to early diagnosis of a rare metabolic disease with available treatment. *Rom. J. Pediatr.* **2024**, *73*, 278–285. [CrossRef]
61. Cox, G.F.; Clarke, L.A.; Giugliani, R.; McGovern, M.M. Burden of illness in acid sphingomyelinase deficiency: A retrospective chart review of 100 patients. *JIMD Rep.* **2018**, *41*, 119–129.

diagnostics

MDPI

Case Report

Monosomy 18p with Unbalanced Translocation Between 13 and 18 Chromosomes: First Reported Case in Serbia

Bojana Marković [1,2], Marina Gazdić Janković [3,*], Zoran Igrutinović [1,2], Raša Medović [1,2], Nevena Stojadinović [1,4] and Biljana Ljujić [3]

1 Pediatric Clinic, University Clinical Centre Kragujevac, Zmaj Jovina 30, 34000 Kragujevac, Serbia; bojana.kovacevic96@gmail.com (B.M.); igzor@medf.kg.ac.rs (Z.I.); rasamedovic@gmail.com (R.M.); niblackpearl@gmail.com (N.S.)

2 Department of Pediatrics, Faculty of Medical Science, University of Kragujevac, Svetozara Markovica 69, 34000 Kragujevac, Serbia

3 Department of Genetics, Faculty of Medical Sciences, University of Kragujevac, Svetozara Markovica 69, 34000 Kragujevac, Serbia; bljujic74@gmail.com

4 Department of Communication Skills, Ethics and Psychology, Faculty of Medical Science, University of Kragujevac, Svetozara Markovica 69, 34000 Kragujevac, Serbia

* Correspondence: marinagazdic87@gmail.com

Abstract: Background: Monosomy 18p is a chromosomal disorder resulting from the deletion of the short arm of chromosome 18. While a lot of cases result from the partial deletion of 18p, only a few reported cases are caused by the deletion of the whole short arm of chromosome 18 due to unbalanced translocations occurring between chromosomes 13 and 18 (13;18). 18p- monosomy presents with a variety of clinical manifestations, including facial dysmorphism, intellectual disability, and short stature, among others. **Case presentation**: Here, we report a case of a one-year-old girl with 18p- monosomy resulting from an unbalanced translocation between chromosomes 13 and 18 (45, XX, t(13;18) (q12:p11.2)). Our patient had facial dysmorphism and stunted growth. Additionally, she had hypotonia and required thyroxine supplementation from a young age. To our knowledge, this is the first case of astigmatism in a patient with this deletion and an unbalanced translocation between chromosomes 13 and 18. **Conclusions**: The present case demonstrates the phenotypic spectrum of a rare variant of monosomy 18 caused by an unbalanced whole-arm translocation between chromosomes 13 and 18. Our study emphasizes the significance of cytogenetic testing to diagnose this disease, which has been described only five times in the literature.

Keywords: 18p deletion syndrome; 18p monosomy; unbalanced translocation; hypotonia; hypothyroidism; astigmatism

1. Introduction

A chromosomal disorder resulting from the deletion of all or part of the short arm of chromosome 18 is known as 18p deletion syndrome [1]. The majority of cases occur due to de novo deletions, although cases of direct parent-to-child transmission have been reported [2,3]. While most cases result from the terminal deletion of 18p, 16% of the cases that have been reported were as a result of an unbalanced whole-arm translocation resulting in monosomy 18p [2].

The clinical manifestation differs among individuals with different chromosome breakpoints, so patients with monosomy 18p can develop any symptom of 18p deletion syndrome. The most common features of the syndrome are intellectual disability, speech delay, and short stature [4–6]. Patients show facial dysmorphism, including ptosis, round face, microcephaly, a flat and broad nasal bridge, protruding ears, horizontal palpebral fissures, epicanthal folds, and strabismus. Many patients with this condition have refractive errors such as myopia and hyperopia, as well as dental and various skeletal deformities [4,7]. Endocrine abnormalities are also found in these patients, of which growth hormone deficiency is prevalent, isolated, or as a part of hypopituitarism, so growth factor treatment is justified [3,7,8]. Hypotonia is quite common in these patients [5,7]. 18p deletion may result in severe brain malformations such as holoprosencephaly in some cases [9,10]. The most common complications in the neonatal period in patients with complete 18p deletion include jaundice, respiratory difficulties, and feeding problems [6]. Patients may present with dystonia in young adulthood [11–13]. Although cardiac malformations are uncommon, some patents may have septal defects, Tetralogy of Fallot, or situs abnormalities [14,15]. Patients with 18p deletion may also develop autoimmune diseases such as Graves' disease, rheumatoid arthritis, lupus, or psoriasis [7,16–19]. Additionally, a reduced serum level of immunoglobulins, most notably IgA, results in immune dysfunction and may contribute to chronic otitis media [3,7]. A cytogenetic analysis is necessary to make a definite diagnosis of 18p monosomy. Considering the variety of clinical manifestations in these patients, a multidisciplinary approach is needed to provide them with adequate medical care.

Here, we describe the clinical features and diagnostic workup of a patient with monosomy 18p due to unbalanced translocation between 13 and 18 chromosomes. To the best of our knowledge, a total of five patients have been reported so far, and this is the first case of 18p- syndrome in a Serbian patient.

2. Case Description

2.1. Signs and Symptoms

An 11-month-old infant was admitted to the Pediatric Clinic's hematology department because of refractory anemia. The patient was the first child of healthy parents. She was born after a normal full-term pregnancy and delivery, and was small for her gestational age. The birth weight was 2890 g (p3) and length was 47 cm (<p3). During pregnancy, the mother had a urinary infection and used antibiotics. Because of neonatal jaundice, the girl was treated with phototherapy.

At 11 months of age, her weight was 7 kg, height was 67.3 cm, and head circumference was 43 cm, which is 2SDs (standard deviations) under the average. She showed generalized stunted growth and developmental delay. A head examination showed light blonde hair, light complexion, broad forehead, light eyebrows, a depressed and broad nasal bridge with light hyperpigmentation on the nasal tip, upslanting palpebral fissures, epicanthic folds, a deep and long philtrum, an almond-shaped palpebral fissure, a thin upper lip, and a high-arched palate. She had two lower teeth and dentition was delayed.

During a neurological examination, the patient had central hypotonia and assumed frog-leg posture lying down. The girl sat independently, bent forward. She could crawl and stand, but not walk. She had difficulties with swallowing and chewing. An EEG during spontaneous sleeping showed nonspecific bilateral fronto-central abnormalities.

The hematologists were looking for a cause of anemia. The girl came to hospital with a hemoglobin value of 102 g/L and erythrocyte count of 3.64 × 1012/L. The blood tests showed low levels of iron (5.1 µmol/L) with a low total iron-binding capacity (43.4 µmol/L) and low transferrin saturation (11.8%). Hemoglobin electrophoresis revealed no abnormalities for her age. Because of the feeding difficulties and development delay, a gastroenterologist was consulted. We excluded celiac disease by detecting no anti-tissue transglutaminase antibodies in the blood and cystic fibrosis by detecting normal levels of chloride in the sweat. An analysis of her feces showed no blood nor parasites in the stool. Allergy tests for nutritive allergens were negative.

The immunological tests presented a low level of serum IgG antibodies for the patient's age and normal levels of serum IgA and IgM antibodies (IgG = 2.19 g/L, IgA = 0.13 g/L, IgM = 0.86 g/L). The population of mononuclear cells was analyzed by immunophenotyping of the peripheral blood. Mature B lymphocytes comprised 27% of all the mononuclear cells, while T-lymphocytes comprised 52% in a CD4:CD8 ratio = 3:1. NK lymphocytes comprised 10% of the analyzed cells. The absolute number of isotype-switched memory B lymphocytes was marginally reduced compared to the reference range according to age (Table 1).

Table 1. The analysis performed on the population of B lymphocytes determined by the electronic limiter of the flow cytometer based on the lateral scattering of the light beam and the intensity of expression of the CD19 molecule.

Subpopulations of B Lymphocytes (%)		**Reference Values for Age 18 Months–4 Years**
Total memory B lymphocytes (CD19+CD27+)	3.9	7.0–24.3
Naïve B lymphocytes (CD27−IgD+)	95.0	69.2–90.5
Double-negative B lymphocytes (CD27−IgD−)	1.1	1.2–8.3
Memory B lymphocytes without isotype switching (CD27+IgD+)	2.6	4.6–16.3
Isotype-switched memory B lymphocytes (CD27+IgD−)	1.3	2.7–12.5
Subpopulations of B lymphocytes (/μL)		**Reference values for age 18 months–4 years**
Total memory B lymphocytes (CD19+CD27+)	41	45–175
Naïve B lymphocytes (CD27−IgD+)	1007	212–1027
Double-negative B lymphocytes (CD27−IgD−)	12	10–56
Memory B lymphocytes without isotype switching (CD27+IgD+)	28	23–113
Isotype-switched memory B lymphocytes (CD27+IgD−)	14	20–93

Her hormonal status showed low free thyroxine levels (10.99 pmol/L), while the levels of thyroid-stimulating hormone were normal. The level of insulin-like growth factor was 15.0 ng/mL. The cortisol values were normal. An ophthalmological examination revealed astigmatism in both eyes.

A psychologist evaluated the patient when she was 1 year old based on information provided by the patient's mother using the Brunet–Lézine Scale. The results of testing were under the expected norms for her age, with IR = 87, suggesting that the child's psychomotor development was delayed by about 48 days. The developmental delay was most noticeable in the domain of gross and fine motor skills.

The parents gave written consent for the publication of this case report.

2.2. Genotype–Phenotype Correlation

The genotype–phenotype correlation was limited and included feeding difficulties and poor growth, minor facial dysmorphic features, global developmental delay with hypotonia, and speech delay.

2.3. Molecular Cytogenetics

A standard karyotyping analysis performed on peripheral blood lymphocytes using G-banding techniques revealed a female karyotype with an unbalanced translocation between the long arm of one chromosome 13 and the long arm of one chromosome 18, resulting in a karyotype of 45XX, t(13;18) (q12:p11.2).

Molecular karyotyping was carried out using the SurePrint G3 Human CGH array kit 8X60K following the manufacturer's instructions (Agilent Technologies, Santa Calara, CA, USA, UCSC hg19, NCBI Build 37, February 2009) in order to identify the size and location of genetic deletions/gains which often accompany chromosomal abnormalities. The results were analyzed with the CytoGenomic 5.1 (Agilent) program.

The parents' cytogenetic assessment revealed that they had normal karyotypes, indicating that a de novo translocation between the long arms of chromosome 13 and 18 had resulted in 18p- syndrome in this case.

The standard karyotyping analysis detected a female karyotype with an unbalanced translocation between chromosomes 13 and 18: 45XX, t(13;18) (q12:p11.2).

The molecular karyotyping of the patient's genomic DNA taken from peripheral blood revealed a deletion of the short arm from the 18p11.32 to p11.21 region (14.79 Mb) affecting 191 genes, of which 65 were protein-coding genes (Figure 1). Despite the large size of the deletion, its precise size and location had not been detected previously by karyotyping. The results were consistent with chromosome 18p deletion syndrome.

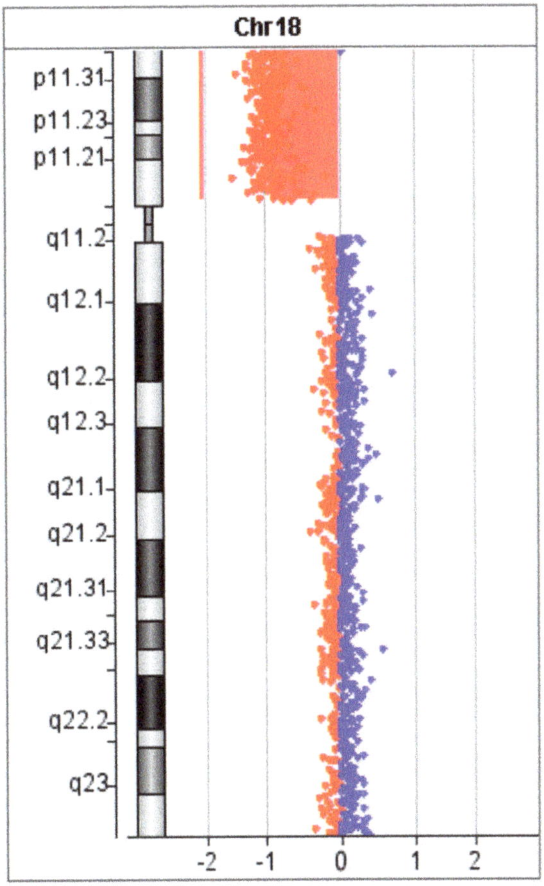

Figure 1. The result of array-CGH of the patient. Zero value indicates equal fluorescence intensity ratio between the sample and reference. Copy number losses shifted the ratio toward left (red) whereas copy number gains towards the right side (blue). Our result showed the deletion of short arm from 18p11.32 to p11.21 region (14.79 Mb).

2.4. Treatment

There is no causative treatment for 18p monosomy. The treatment is directed towards alleviating specific symptoms and depends on clinical manifestations. Early developmental stimulation and treatment from speech therapists and oligophrenologists are very important because of developmental delays. The physiatrist's stimulation treatments must be intensive. This patient should be followed by an ophthalmologist because of the astigmatism. Regular check-ups with an endocrinologist and further monitoring of growth and pituitary function are important because of the patient's hypothyroidism. Lifelong thyroxine therapy is necessary and depends on the blood hormone levels. A neurologist should follow the patient's further development with periodical EEG monitoring because of previous nonspecific changes and potential seizures, which could be a manifestation of this syndrome. Our patient needs regular hematologist and immunologist check-ups because of her anemia, low levels of IgG immunoglobulins, and reduced absolute number of memory B lymphocytes. Her iron deficiency should be corrected with iron supplementation.

3. Discussion

The incidence of monosomy 18p is estimated to be about 1:50,000 live-born infants, with a female to male ratio of 3/2 [5]. To the best of our knowledge, there are only five previously published cases of unbalanced translocations occurring between chromosomes 13 and 18 (13;18) associated with 18p- syndrome [20–24], and there are none in the Serbian population. The first known case in the world was described in a 27-year-old male in 1979 [20]. Herein, we report a rare case of a female infant diagnosed with 18p- syndrome as a consequence of a de novo unbalanced whole-arm translocation between chromosomes 13 and 18 (Supplementary Figure S1). Three previously described patients also had a de novo translocation, and for two of them, there were no data about inheritance. At the time of writing this article, the current patient is the youngest patient diagnosed with this condition, and the second female [20–24].

Our patient had early nonspecific signs of this disorder in the neonatal period. She had neonatal jaundice and generalized hypotonia, which persisted until she was 11 months old and admitted to our hospital [5,7]. While these signs could be the first manifestation of monosomy 18p in the neonatal period, there was no evidence of this feature in five other patients described with this deletion and unbalanced translocation between chromosomes 13 and 18 [5,7,20–24]. On physical examination, we noticed minor facial dysmorphism, stunted growth, and developmental delay [4–6]. Regarding the fact that she was born small for her gestational age, her weight and height were still 2SDs under the average [5,6]. Low levels of insulin-like factor 1 (IGF-1) do not have strong significance at her age. Two previously described patients who had this syndrome had low birth weights [21,22], while all of them had short stature [20–24].

One of the main features of monosomy 18p is facial dysmorphism. In accordance with all the reported patients with this syndrome, together with the unbalanced translocation between chromosome 13 and 18, our patient had some dysmorphic characteristics [4,5,20–24]. There is no pattern which is always presented, but there are some manifestations that are more common. Almost every patient reported with this condition had a different head shape. All of them presented with eye disorders. The most common issue was strabismus, followed by ptosis, epicanthic folds, hypertelorism, and others [20–24]. Ear malformations were described in just two patients, one with posteriorly rotated ears, and another with large low-set ears [20,21]. In patients with an unbalanced translocation between chromosome 13 and 18, a flat nasal bridge was commonly described. A long or broad nose was rarely seen [20–24]. Almost all the patients had dental problems and some of them had a high-arched palate [20–23]. Three of the five previously described patients had a short neck [20,21,24]. Some of them had a large sloping or prominent forehead [21,22]. All of these dysmorphic features are summarized in Table 2.

Table 2. Facial dysmorphism of patients with monosomy 18p and unbalanced translocation between chromosome 13 and 18 based on their karyotype.

Cases	Case 1	Case 2	Case 3	Case 4	Case 5	Our Patient
s	45, XY, −13, 18, +t(13;18) (13qter→cen→18qter)	45, XY, der(13;18) (q10;q10)	45, XX, t(13p;18p)	45, XY, der(13;18) (q10;q10)	45, XY, der(13;18) (q10;q10)	45XX, t(13;18) (q12:p11.2)
Head shape	Normal circumference of head	Triangular broad face	Dolichocephaly	Brachycephaly	Round face	Microcephaly
Eyes	Strabismus	Strabismus, ptosis, epicanthic folds	Strabismus, hypertelorism	Ptosis, hypertelorism, protruding eyes	Strabismus, ptosis, hypertelorism	Almond-shaped upslanting palpebral fissures, epicanthic folds
Ears	Posteriorly rotated	Large low-set	NA	NA	NA	Normal
Nose	NA	Long and broad	Flat nasal bridge	NA	Flat and long	Depressed and broad nasal bridge
Mouth	Dental caries	Disarrayed teeth, dental caries	High arched palate	Hypodontia	NA	Deep and long philtrum, high-arched palate, delayed dentition
Neck	Short and broad	Short	NA	NA	Short	Normal
Other	NA	Large sloping forehead, alopecia	Prominent forehead	NA	NA	Light blonde hair, light complexion, broad forehead, light hyperpigmentation on the nasal tip
References (year)	Moedjono SJ et al. [20] (1979)	de Ravel TJ et al. [21] (2005)	Nema et al. [22] (2016)	Safavi et al. [23] (2019)	Choi et al. [24] (2022)	

Our patient received thyroxine supplements for hypothyroidism, which was reported in only one of five patients in the available published papers [21]. We should also highlight that our patient is the first reported to have hypothyroidism at such a young age. All of these patients had ophthalmological manifestations, but our patient is the only one to have astigmatism and have this as her only ophthalmological manifestation at the time of investigation [7,20–24]. There is no evidence that iron deficiency is related to this condition, although feeding problems and low food intake in these patients can lead to nutritional deficiency. Anemia has not been reported in any other patient described in the literature. However, all the previously described patients had psychomotor development delay [20–24]. Despite the fact that our patient's EEG showed nonspecific changes, she had no seizures, so there was no need for anticonvulsive medicine in contrast to three other patients described before [22–24]. The low levels of serum IgG antibodies for the patient's age, which can be connected to 18p monosomy [7], require further involvement of a hematologist or immunologist. Also, the absolute number of memory B lymphocytes was marginally reduced compared to the reference range according to age, so this should be monitored in the future. One of the previously described patients had IgA deficiency, which is in accordance with the majority of patients with monosomy 18p who presented with immunodeficiency. On the other hand, there are no data about the immunological status of the other patients, just recurrent lower respiratory tract infections in one of the patients [7,20,22]. Like in almost every patient who has 18p monosomy [5,6], and every patient described who, has the unbalanced translocation between chromosomes 13 and 18, but not a deletion, the psychological testing of our patient suggests that the child's psychomotor development was delayed by about 48 days [20–24]. This was mostly in terms of motor skills, but speech delay was present, which is in accordance with all of the other described patients [20–24]. Though a lower IQ was expected in our patient, as it was significantly reduced in four other reported cases, her age was a limiting factor in determining her IQ. Data on a patient's IQ are missing in another paper [20–24]. Also, as skeletal disorders were described in three of the five previously described patients, it is recommended that our patient be closely monitored for that kind of anomaly in the future [20,21,24].

G-banding, a fundamental technique in cytogenetics, provides a clear visualization of the entire karyotype and can detect large-scale chromosomal changes. However, it lacks the resolution to detect small genetic changes (greater than 5–10 Mb). Moreover, high-quality metaphase spreads are necessary, which can be challenging to obtain from some cell types [25]. The most significant disadvantages of microarrays include the large number of probe designs based on sequences of low specificity, as well as the lack of control over the pool of analyzed transcripts [26]. Moreover, due to the targeted nature of microarrays, microarray testing relies on pre-defined probes to detect known genetic variations. Through a deeper exploration of the genes lost in the deletion and their possible roles in the observed phenotype, we can connect the genotype to the phenotype more explicitly. An absence of specific functional genes in the most distal part of 18p causes clinical manifestations of 18p-syndrome such as a round face and short stature. According to the Decipher base, out of a total of 191 genes, 16 genes are disease-associated genes (OMIM morbid genes). AFG3L2 is a candidate gene for hereditary spastic paraplegias or neurodegenerative disorders as well as spastic ataxia–neuropathy syndrome. Mutations in SMCHD1 are causative for the development of facioscapulohumeral muscular dystrophy type 2. Moreover, the PIEZO2 protein has a role in rapidly adapting mechanically activated currents in somatosensory neurons. Its abundant expression was detected in dorsal root ganglia sensory neurons, suggesting a potential role in somatosensory mechanotransduction. Thus, it is possible that the central hypotonia and assumed frog-leg posture lying down seen in our case might have resulted from the deletion of several genes such as AFG3L2, SMCHD1, and PIEZO2. In addition, the MC2R gene plays a role in immune function and glucose metabolism, so we assume that it could be related to our patient's immune profile. For other genes located in the deleted 18p11.32 to p11.21 region (APCDD1, EPB41L3, GNAL, LAMA1, LPIN2, NDUFV2, PSMG2, TGIF1, THOC1, TUBB6, TYMS, and USP14), we could not find a direct correlation with the phenotype. Cytogenetic testing provides us with an opportunity to distinguish 18p- syndrome associated with unbalanced translocation (13;18) from other neurodevelopmental disorders featuring mild intellectual disability and short stature. Since there is no causative treatment for 18p monosomy, a timely diagnosis is crucial for the application of an appropriate treatment in order to alleviate specific symptoms and clinical manifestations. Moreover, parents can be counseled about their expectations of a certain syndrome, and, with them, review the genetic risks. Therefore, a multidisciplinary approach is necessary to identify the expected clinical features and increase our knowledge of 18p- syndrome, all in the aim of improving the patient's quality of life.

A genetic counselor should predict the eventual clinical manifestations of the disease according to the patient's genotype. A multidisciplinary approach is paramount and therapy must be individual. In addition, patients require lifelong monitoring [4,22]. As in our case, psychomotor stimulation is essential and could relieve symptoms and slow down the progression of disease, so a speech therapist, oligophrenologist, and physiatrist should be involved in the patient's therapy from the early stages of their disease. Neurological examination and monitoring is necessary because of the different neurological conditions that these patients may have. Holoprosencephaly is a severe brain malformation, linked with poor prognosis and limited therapy options [4,9,10]. Patients with seizures require EEG monitoring and anticonvulsive therapy [22–24]. The early diagnosis of endocrine disorders like pituitary or thyroid dysfunction can help, especially at an early age, because the hormonal status has a great importance in metabolism and nervous system development and function. Feeding problems and a low food intake sometimes cause nutrient deficiencies or malnutrition; a pediatrician, gastroenterologist, or nutritionist should prescribe adequate supplementation and a diet plan. Refractive errors like myopia and hyperopia, astigmatism, strabismus, and other ophthalmological conditions sometimes need correction and timely interval ophthalmology check-ups. Also, cooperation with an immunologist is important, especially when common infections or autoimmune diseases are reported. Cardiac malformations are uncommon in 18p deletion syndrome, but require special attention and sometimes even surgical treatment [14,15]. Specific orthopedic or other surgical procedures depend on the severity and location of the anatomical abnormalities [22]. Psychological support for the patients and their families can help with dealing with the diagnosis and also coping with effects of treatment.

The prognosis of these patients is unpredictable and depends on their genotype–phenotype correlation [7]. An early diagnosis, an individual approach to every patient, and the timely treatment of specific manifestations can slow down the progression of the disease and improve the patient's quality of life. For those patients with severe brain malformations, the prognosis is poor; otherwise, survival up to the sixth decade has been reported [4,21].

4. Conclusions

The present case report demonstrates the phenotypic spectrum of a rare variant of monosomy 18 caused by an unbalanced whole-arm translocation between chromosomes 13 and 18. Having in mind that this syndrome can be easily overlooked in a clinical setting, our study emphases the significance of cytogenetic testing to diagnose this disease, which has been described only five times in the literature.

Supplementary Materials: The following supporting information can be downloaded at https://www.mdpi.com/article/10.3390/diagnostics15030358/s1: Figure S1: Array-CGH profiles analysis using Agilent CytoGenomic Analytics software.

Author Contributions: Conceptualization, B.M., M.G.J., Z.I. and B.L.; methodology, B.M., R.M. and N.S.; investigation, B.M., R.M. and N.S.; data curation, B.M., M.G.J. and R.M.; writing—original draft preparation, B.M. and M.G.J.; writing—review and editing, Z.I. and B.L.; funding acquisition, B.L. All authors have read and agreed to the published version of the manuscript.

Funding: This study was supported by the Ministry of Education, Science and Technological Development of the Republic of Serbia (Agreement No. 451-03-65/2024-03/200111).

Institutional Review Board Statement: Ethical review and approval were waived for this study. At our institution, the publication of case reports is exempt from requiring approval by our Institutional Review Board.

Informed Consent Statement: Written informed consent was obtained from the patient's parents to publish this paper.

Data Availability Statement: All data are contained within the article.

Conflicts of Interest: The authors declare no conflicts of interest.

References

1. Jin, Q.; Qiang, R.; Cai, B.; Wang, X.; Cai, N.; Zhen, S.; Zhai, W. The genotype and phenotype of chromosome 18p deletion syndrome. *Medicine* **2021**, *100*, e25777. [CrossRef] [PubMed]
2. Qi, H.; Zhu, J.; Zhang, S.; Cai, L.; Wen, X.; Zeng, W.; Tang, G.; Luo, Y. Prenatal diagnosis of de novo monosomy 18p deletion syndrome by chromosome microarray analysis. *Medicine* **2019**, *98*, e15027. [CrossRef]
3. Hasi-Zogaj, M.; Sebold, C.; Heard, P.; Carter, E.; Soileau, B.; Hill, A.; Rupert, D.; Perry, B.; Atkinson, S.; O'Donnell, L.; et al. A review of 18p deletions. *Am. J. Med. Genet. Part C Semin. Med. Genet.* **2015**, *169*, 251–264. [CrossRef] [PubMed]
4. Jain, M.; Goyal, M.; Singhal, S.; Nandimath, K. 18p deletion syndrome: Case report with clinical consideration and management. *Contemp. Clin. Dent.* **2017**, *8*, 632–636. [CrossRef]
5. Turleau, C. Monosomy 18p. *Orphanet J. Rare Dis.* **2008**, *3*, 4. [CrossRef] [PubMed]

6. van Wijngaarden, V.; de Wilde, H.; van der Molen, D.M.; Petter, J.; Stegeman, I.; Gerrits, E.; Smit, A.L.; Boogaard, M.-J.v.D. Genetic outcomes in children with developmental language disorder: A systematic review. *Front. Pediatr.* **2024**, *12*, 1315229. [CrossRef] [PubMed]
7. Sebold, C.; Soileau, B.; Heard, P.; Carter, E.; O'Donnell, L.; Hale, D.E.; Cody, J.D. Whole arm deletions of 18p: Medical and developmental effects. *Am. J. Med. Genet. Part A* **2015**, *167*, 313–323. [CrossRef] [PubMed]
8. Yang, A.; Kim, J.; Cho, S.Y.; Lee, J.-E.; Kim, H.-J.; Jin, D.-K. A case of de novo 18p deletion syndrome with panhypopituitarism. *Ann. Pediatr. Endocrinol. Metab.* **2019**, *24*, 60–63. [CrossRef]
9. Chen, C.-P.; Huang, J.-P.; Chen, Y.-Y.; Chern, S.-R.; Wu, P.-S.; Su, J.-W.; Pan, C.-W.; Wang, W. Chromosome 18p deletion syndrome presenting holoprosencephaly and premaxillary agenesis: Prenatal diagnosis and aCGH characterization using uncultured amniocytes. *Gene* **2013**, *527*, 636–641. [CrossRef]
10. Yin, Z.; Zhang, K.; Ni, B.; Fan, X.; Wu, X. Prenatal diagnosis of monosomy 18p associated with holoprosencephaly: Case report. *J. Obstet. Gynaecol.* **2017**, *37*, 804–806. [CrossRef]
11. Di Rauso, G.; Cavallieri, F.; Monfrini, E.; Fraternali, A.; Fioravanti, V.; Grisanti, S.; Gessani, A.; Campanini, I.; Merlo, A.; Toschi, G.; et al. A Case of 18p Chromosomal Deletion Encompassing GNAL in a Patient with Dystonia-Parkinsonism. *J. Mov. Disord.* **2024**, *17*, 236–238. [CrossRef] [PubMed]
12. Crosiers, D.; Blaumeiser, B.; Van Goethem, G. Spectrum of Movement Disorders in 18p Deletion Syndrome. *Mov. Disord. Clin. Pract.* **2018**, *6*, 70–73. [CrossRef]
13. Nasir, J.; Frima, N.; Pickard, B.; Malloy, M.P.; Zhan, L.; Grünewald, R. Unbalanced whole arm translocation resulting in loss of 18p in dystonia. *Mov. Disord.* **2006**, *21*, 859–863. [CrossRef]
14. Digilio, M.C.; Marino, B.; Giannotti, A.; Di Donato, R.; Dallapiccola, B. Heterotaxy with left atrial isomerism in a patient with deletion 18p. *Am. J. Med. Genet.* **2000**, *94*, 198–200. [CrossRef]
15. Kocaaga, A.; Yimenicioglu, S. Presentation of an Infant with Chromosome 18p Deletion Syndrome and Asymmetric Septal Hypertrophy. *Glob. Med. Genet.* **2022**, *09*, 179–181. [CrossRef] [PubMed]
16. Dolek-Cetinkaya, D.; Demirpence, M.; Gorgel, A.; Salgur, F.; Bahceci, M. A Rare Association of Monosomy 18P Syndrome and Polyglandular Autoimmune Syndrome Type IIIA. *Balk. J. Med. Genet.* **2013**, *16*, 81–83. [CrossRef]
17. Chau, A.; Ramesh, K.H.; Jagannath, A.D.; Arora, S. Rheumatoid arthritis in an adult patient with mosaic distal 18q-, 18p- and ring chromosome 18. *F1000Research* **2017**, *6*, 1940. [CrossRef]
18. Herlin, M.K.; Jensen, J.M.B.; Andreasen, L.; Petersen, M.S.; Lønskov, J.; Thorup, M.B.; Birkebæk, N.; Mogensen, T.H.; Herlin, T.; Deleuran, B.; et al. Monozygotic triplets with juvenile-onset autoimmunity and 18p microdeletion involving PTPRM. *Front. Genet.* **2024**, *15*, 1437566. [CrossRef]
19. Wester, U.; Bondeson, M.; Edeby, C.; Annerén, G. Clinical and molecular characterization of individuals with 18p deletion: A genotype–phenotype correlation. *Am. J. Med. Genet. Part A* **2006**, *140A*, 1164–1171. [CrossRef] [PubMed]
20. Moedjono, S.J.; Funderburk, S.J.; Sparkes, R.S. 18p--syndrome resulting from translocation (13a;18q) in a mildly affected adult male. *J. Med. Genet.* **1979**, *16*, 399–402. [CrossRef]
21. de Ravel, T.J.; Thiry, P.; Fryns, J.-P. Follow-up of adult males with chromosome 18p deletion. *Eur. J. Med. Genet.* **2005**, *48*, 189–193. [CrossRef] [PubMed]
22. Sinha, R.; Nema, D.; Venkatnarayan, K.; Dalal, S.; Sodhi, K. A Rare Association of Monosomy 18 with Translocation 13p 11/18 with Cholelithiasis. *J. Pediatr. Neonatal Care* **2016**, *4*, 1–2. [CrossRef]
23. Safavi, M.; Ashtiani, M.T.H.; Badv, R.S.; Azari-Yam, A.; Vasei, M. A Rare Cytogenetic Variant of Monosomy 18p Syndrome as a Consequence of Whole-Arm Translocation between Chromosomes 13 and 18. *Arch. Iran. Med.* **2019**, *22*, 627–628. [PubMed]
24. Choi, J.Y.; Moon, J.U.; Yoon, D.H.; Yim, J.; Kim, M.; Jung, M.H. 18p Deletion Syndrome Originating from Rare Unbalanced Whole-Arm Translocation between Chromosomes 13 and 18: A Case Report and Literature Review. *Children* **2022**, *9*, 987. [CrossRef]
25. Caleb, E. Molecular Cytogenetics: Bridging the Gap Between G-banding and Next-generation Sequencing. *J. Cytol. Hisol.* **2024**, *15*, 755.
26. Jaksik, R.; Iwanaszko, M.; Rzeszowska-Wolny, J.; Kimmel, M. Microarray experiments and factors which affect their reliability. *Biol. Direct* **2015**, *10*, 46. [CrossRef]

diagnostics

Interesting Images

Plastic Bronchitis: Extensive Cast Expectoration in a 6-Year-Old Boy with Fontan Circulation

Jochen Pfeifer [1,*], Martin Poryo [1], Peter Fries [2] and Hashim Abdul-Khaliq [1]

1 Department of Pediatric Cardiology, Saarland University Medical Center, 66421 Homburg, Germany
2 Clinic for Diagnostic and Interventional Radiology, Saarland University Medical Center, 66421 Homburg, Germany
* Correspondence: jochen.pfeifer@uks.eu; Tel.: +49-6841-1628390

Abstract

We report on a 6-year-old boy with underlying hypoplastic left heart syndrome and a total cavopulmonary connection (Fontan circulation) with a diagnosis of plastic bronchitis. After an initial good response to therapy, his productive cough became significantly stronger again. Four months later, the patient's mother brought a preserving jar containing an extensive bronchial cast to the clinic, the size of which is rarely seen in small children. Plastic bronchitis is a rare but dreaded complication in patients with Fontan circulation as well as in infectious or inflammatory diseases; its treatment is challenging.

Keywords: plastic bronchitis; bronchial cast; expectoration; congenital heart disease; Fontan circulation; cavopulmonary connection; bronchoscopy; complication

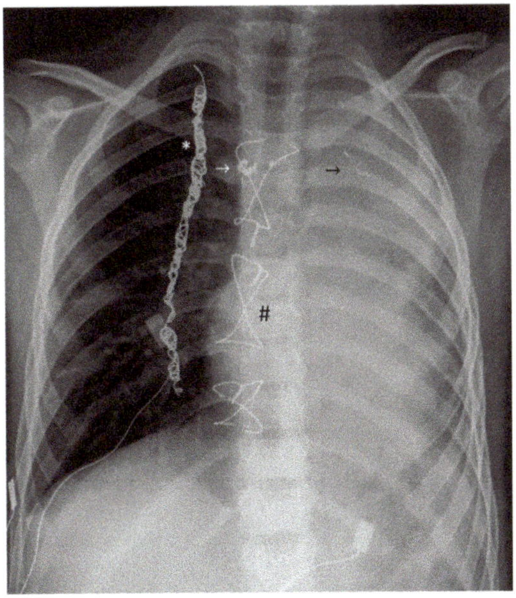

Figure 1. We present a case of a 6-year-old boy with hypoplastic left heart syndrome including mitral and aortic valve atresia, hypoplasia of ascending aorta, left ventricle, and atrium, as well as mild tricuspid regurgitation. At four days of age, a Norwood procedure with modified Blalock–Taussig

https://doi.org/10.3390/diagnostics15222864

shunt was performed. Chylothorax, wound infection, and mediastinitis complicated the postoperative course but were successfully treated. At the age of 5 months, a partial cavopulmonary connection (in the form of a bidirectional Glenn anastomosis) was established, and at the age of 4.5 years, a complete cavopulmonary connection (18 mm extracardiac Fontan conduit, 4 mm fenestration) was established. Due to the occurrence of multiple diffuse systemic-to-pulmonary collaterals originating from the right internal thoracic artery, this vessel was completely embolized with coils. Two more collaterals were selectively embolized using microcoils and a vascular plug. Other diffuse and branched arterial collaterals could not be closed due to their small size and tortuous course. He was treated with sildenafil, propranolol, lisinopril, and diuretics. The invasively measured Fontan circuit pressure was mean 10 mmHg three months earlier. First, the patient showed a good physical performance with a transcutaneous oxygen saturation of approximately 90% throughout. There were no symptoms of hypalbuminemia or protein loss, and serum albumin, immunoglobulin, and protein levels were within the normal range. Finally, the boy was admitted to the clinic with a cough that had been getting worse for several days, severe dyspnea, and reduced oxygen saturation of 55%. Chest X-ray showed extensive dystelectatic and atelectatic areas of the left lung (chest X-ray, anterior–posterior projection, showing extensive dystelectasis and atelectasis of the left lung; previously implanted wire cerclages (#), coils in the right internal thoracic artery (*), as well as microcoils and a vascular plug for embolization of systemic-to-pulmonary collaterals (arrows) are also visible). The echocardiographic examination revealed unchanged, fairly good function of the systemic ventricle with moderate tricuspid valve regurgitation and mild congestion of the inferior vena cava. The laboratory results did not reveal any significant abnormalities. Microbiological tests were negative for both viral and bacterial infections. He underwent bronchoscopy with lavage and removal of several fractions of rubber-like fibrous casts from the left bronchi, which histologically contained mucin, fibrin, lymphocytes, and macrophages, leading to the diagnosis of plastic bronchitis. Subsequent treatment in the pediatric intensive care unit included mechanical ventilation for 10 days, and inhaled mucolytic, fibrinolytic, and bronchodilator therapy, namely dornase alpha, hypertonic saline, recombinant tissue-type plasminogen activator, salbutamol, and ipratropium bromide. In addition, positioning therapy and repeated suctioning of the airways were performed. The boy's condition improved significantly. He was discharged after three weeks and continued with inhaled mucolytic and steroid therapy (saline, aerosolized heparin, budesonide, and dornase intermittently), anticongestive medication, and physiotherapy at home. In addition, treatment for pulmonary arterial hypertension (sildenafil) was continued.

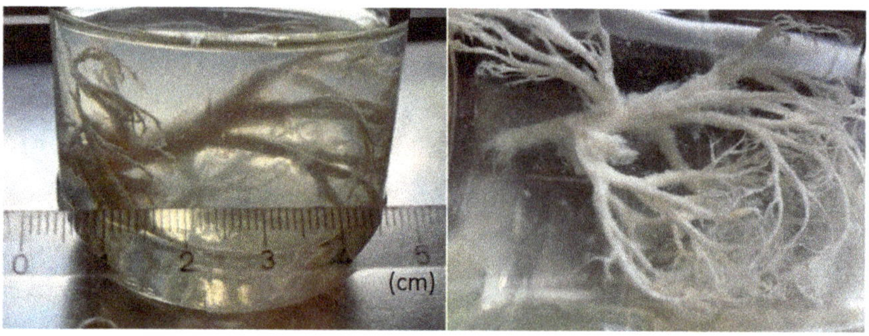

Figure 2. Four months later, the boy's mother presented a preserving jar containing a highly ramified, whitish cast that the boy had expectorated due to persistent plastic bronchitis (photographs (two views) of the jar containing the cast in aqueous solution). The expectoration represented a coherent three-dimensional cast of the bronchial system of almost an entire lung side with a maximum length of approximately 8 cm. Also referred to as cast bronchitis, plastic bronchitis is a rare but severe complication of various diseases with an incidence of about 4% in Fontan patients [1]. Its symptoms are chronic cough, hypoxemia, and expectoration of proteinaceous casts, which mainly consist of fibrin and leucocytes. Cases involving expectoration of extensive bronchial casts have previously been described [2–8], but they are very rare to this extent in young children. In complex congenital heart diseases, failing Fontan circulation and systemic-to-pulmonary collaterals typically promote

the disease. Further risk factors include chylothorax, ascites, and prolonged chest drainage after surgery [9]. Male patients are more frequently affected [10]. The exact etiology of plastic bronchitis is still unknown. The most probable pathophysiological causes are increased systemic venous pressure, lymphostasis, and retrograde intrathoracic lymph flow; increased capillary permeability due to chronic inflammation promotes the leakage of protein-containing fluid into the bronchi and the formation of casts. The loss of intravascular proteins and hypoalbuminemia lead to a vicious circle with a further reduction in oncotic pressure and resulting lymphatic leakage [9,11,12]. Plastic bronchitis in Fontan patients has serious prognostic implications, as the 5-year mortality rate is reportedly up to 50% [13]. Treatment is challenging and not standardized. A combination of anti-obstructive and anti-inflammatory treatment, as well as optimization of the Fontan physiology, appears to be the most promising strategy [14]. In addition to the above-mentioned fibrinolytic and mucolytic medication, which were used in our case, N-acetylcysteine, urokinase, or alpha-chymotrypsin as well as pulmonary vasodilators, octreotide, and low-fat diet are therapeutic options. Surgical and interventional procedures may include the creation of a Fontan fenestration (if missing) or Fontan takedown as well as embolization of systemic-to-pulmonary collateral arteries [14–18]. Selective percutaneous lymphatic embolization, for example, using n-butyl-2-cyanoacrylate, vascular plugs, or microcoils [9,19–21], or surgical ligation of the thoracic duct [22], may be considered in the absence of a therapeutic response. Although precise data are lacking, the risk of refractory or recurrent plastic bronchitis appears to be high. Compared to previously reported pediatric cases, ours is a typical case of plastic bronchitis, as it involves a male Fontan patient who expectorated characteristic casts. Nevertheless, the huge casts described, which the patient's mother presented in a jar, are rarely seen in young children. The altered lymphatic drainage following chylothorax after the first operation, the multiple collaterals, as well as the tricuspid insufficiency may have contributed to the development of plastic bronchitis in our patient. Rigorous embolization of arterial systemic-to-pulmonary collaterals and percutaneous lymph embolization must be considered. However, recurrence despite extensive therapy can occur frequently. Other possible diseases associated with plastic bronchitis are asthma, *Mycoplasma pneumoniae* pneumonia, chronic inflammatory or infectious diseases, previous surgical procedures, and other chronic or severe systemic diseases [15,23,24]. The case presented shows that plastic bronchitis is a very difficult complication to treat in patients with Fontan physiology. Even in young children and during treatment, severe cast expectoration may occur. Combined therapy with inhalation, respiratory therapy, and the optimization of Fontan circulation is the most effective approach.

Author Contributions: Conceptualization, J.P. and H.A.-K.; methodology, J.P. and H.A.-K.; validation, J.P., M.P., P.F. and H.A.-K.; formal analysis, J.P., M.P., P.F. and H.A.-K.; investigation, J.P.; resources, H.A.-K.; data curation, J.P.; writing—original draft preparation, J.P.; writing—review and editing, M.P., P.F. and H.A.-K.; visualization, J.P.; supervision, H.A.-K.; project administration, H.A.-K. All authors have read and agreed to the published version of the manuscript.

Funding: This research received no external funding.

Institutional Review Board Statement: The study was conducted in accordance with the Declaration of Helsinki, and approved by the Institutional Ethics Committee (ethics committee of the medical association of the Saarland, Saarbrücken, Germany; protocol code 151/25. Date: 27 August 2025).

Informed Consent Statement: Written informed consent has been obtained from the patient's parents to publish this paper.

Data Availability Statement: Data are contained within the article.

Conflicts of Interest: The authors declare no conflicts of interest.

References

1. Caruthers, R.L.; Kempa, M.; Loo, A.; Gulbransen, E.; Kelly, E.; Erickson, S.R.; Hirsch, J.C.; Schumacher, K.R.; Stringer, K.A. Demographic characteristics and estimated prevalence of Fontan-associated plastic bronchitis. *Pediatr. Cardiol.* **2013**, *34*, 256–261. [CrossRef] [PubMed] [PubMed Central]

2. Maqsood, A.; Imel, L.R. Plastic Bronchitis. *N. Engl. J. Med.* **2022**, *386*, 780. [CrossRef] [PubMed]
3. Mehta, I.; Patel, K. Lymphatic Plastic Bronchitis. *N. Engl. J. Med.* **2022**, *386*, e19. [CrossRef] [PubMed]
4. Wei, P.; Song, H.; Li, J.; Ren, Y. Plastic Bronchitis in a Child. *Indian J. Pediatr.* **2023**, *90*, 829–830. [CrossRef] [PubMed]
5. Chaudhari, M.; Stumper, O. Plastic bronchitis after Fontan operation: Treatment with stent fenestration of the Fontan circuit. *Heart* **2004**, *90*, 801. [CrossRef] [PubMed] [PubMed Central]
6. Singhi, A.K.; Vinoth, B.; Kuruvilla, S.; Sivakumar, K. Plastic bronchitis. *Ann. Pediatr. Cardiol.* **2015**, *8*, 246–248. [CrossRef] [PubMed]
7. Verghese, S.; Jackson, M.; Vaughns, J.; Preciado, D. Plastic bronchitis in a child with Fontan's physiology presenting for urgent rigid bronchoscopy. *Anesth. Analg.* **2008**, *107*, 1446–1447. [CrossRef] [PubMed]
8. Tzifa, A.; Robards, M.; Simpson, J.M. Plastic bronchitis; a serious complication of the Fontan operation. *Int. J. Cardiol.* **2005**, *101*, 513–514. [CrossRef] [PubMed]
9. Mackie, A.S.; Veldtman, G.R.; Thorup, L.; Hjortdal, V.E.; Dori, Y. Plastic Bronchitis and Protein-Losing Enteropathy in the Fontan Patient: Evolving Understanding and Emerging Therapies. *Can. J. Cardiol.* **2022**, *38*, 988–1001. [CrossRef] [PubMed]
10. Nayır Büyükşahin, H.; Emiralioglu, N.; Sekerel, B.E.; Soyer, T.; Oguz, B.; Güzelkaş, I.; Sunman, B.; Alboğa, D.; Akgül Erdal, M.; Yalcın, E.; et al. Plastic bronchitis during childhood: Diversity of presentation, etiology, treatment, and outcomes. *Pediatr. Pulmonol.* **2023**, *58*, 2559–2567. [CrossRef] [PubMed]
11. Mazza, G.A.; Gribaudo, E.; Agnoletti, G. The pathophysiology and complications of Fontan circulation. *Acta Biomed.* **2021**, *92*, e2021260. [CrossRef] [PubMed] [PubMed Central]
12. RochéRodríguez, M.; DiNardo, J.A. The Lymphatic System in the Fontan Patient-Pathophysiology, Imaging, and Interventions: What the Anesthesiologist Should Know. *J. Cardiothorac. Vasc. Anesth.* **2022**, *36 Pt A*, 2669–2678. [CrossRef] [PubMed]
13. Schumacher, K.R.; Singh, T.P.; Kuebler, J.; Aprile, K.; O'Brien, M.; Blume, E.D. Risk factors and outcome of Fontan-associated plastic bronchitis: A case-control study. *J. Am. Heart Assoc.* **2014**, *3*, e000865. [CrossRef] [PubMed] [PubMed Central]
14. Harteveld, L.M.; Blom, N.A.; Hazekamp, M.G.; Ten Harkel, A.D.J. Treatment and outcome of plastic bronchitis in single ventricle patients: A systematic review. *Interact. Cardiovasc. Thorac. Surg.* **2020**, *30*, 846–853. [CrossRef] [PubMed]
15. Patel, N.; Patel, M.; Inja, R.; Krvavac, A.; Lechner, A.J. Plastic Bronchitis in Adult and Pediatric Patients: A Review of its Presentation, Diagnosis, and Treatment. *Mo. Med.* **2021**, *118*, 363–373. [PubMed] [PubMed Central]
16. Xiong, L.; Rao, X.; Peng, X.; Zhang, G.; Liu, H. Management of Plastic Bronchitis Using α-Chymotrypsin: A Novel Treatment Modality. *Cureus* **2021**, *13*, e13551. [CrossRef] [PubMed] [PubMed Central]
17. Pfeifer, J.; Poryo, M.; Gheibeh, A.; Rentzsch, A.; Abdul-Khaliq, H. Transcatheter Embolization of Systemic-to-Pulmonary Collaterals: A New Approach Using Concerto™ Helix Nylon-Fibered Microcoils. *J. Clin. Med.* **2024**, *14*, 113. [CrossRef] [PubMed] [PubMed Central]
18. Pfeifer, J.; Gheibeh, A.; Fries, P.; Poryo, M.; Rentzsch, A.; Abdul-Khaliq, H. Transcatheter Embolization in Congenital Cardiovascular Malformations-Variable Use of Vascular Plugs. *Cardiovasc. Ther.* **2024**, *2024*, 4778469. [CrossRef] [PubMed] [PubMed Central]
19. Maleux, G.; Storme, E.; Cools, B.; Heying, R.; Boshoff, D.; Louw, J.J.; Frerich, S.; Malekzadeh-Milanii, S.; Hubrechts, J.; Brown, S.C.; et al. Percutaneous embolization of lymphatic fistulae as treatment for protein-losing enteropathy and plastic bronchitis in patients with failing Fontan circulation. *Catheter. Cardiovasc. Interv.* **2019**, *94*, 996–1002. [CrossRef] [PubMed]
20. Dori, Y.; Keller, M.S.; Rome, J.J.; Gillespie, M.J.; Glatz, A.C.; Dodds, K.; Goldberg, D.J.; Goldfarb, S.; Rychik, J.; Itkin, M. Percutaneous Lymphatic Embolization of Abnormal Pulmonary Lymphatic Flow as Treatment of Plastic Bronchitis in Patients with Congenital Heart Disease. *Circulation* **2016**, *133*, 1160–1170. [CrossRef] [PubMed]
21. Haddad, R.N.; Dautry, R.; Bonnet, D.; Malekzadeh-Milani, S. Transvenous retrograde thoracic duct embolization for effective treatment of recurrent plastic bronchitis after fontan palliation. *Catheter. Cardiovasc. Interv.* **2023**, *101*, 863–869. [CrossRef] [PubMed]
22. Shah, S.S.; Drinkwater, D.C.; Christian, K.G. Plastic bronchitis: Is thoracic duct ligation a real surgical option? *Ann. Thorac. Surg.* **2006**, *81*, 2281–2283. [CrossRef] [PubMed]
23. Sharifi, A.; Rahbar, R.; Fynn-Thompson, F.; Farasat, E.; Pugi, J.; Samadizadeh, S.; Mohammadi-Brenjegani, A.; Ghaedsharaf, S.; Zojaji, M. Plastic bronchitis in pediatrics: A systematic review of etiologies, clinical presentations, treatments, and prognosis. *Int. J. Pediatr. Otorhinolaryngol.* **2025**, *195*, 112422. [CrossRef] [PubMed]
24. Yang, L.; Zhang, Y.; Shen, C.; Lu, Z.; Hou, T.; Niu, F.; Wang, Y.; Ning, J.; Liu, R. Clinical features and risk factors of plastic bronchitis caused by *Mycoplasma pneumoniae* pneumonia in children. *BMC Pulm. Med.* **2023**, *23*, 468, Erratum in *BMC Pulm. Med.* **2023**, *23*, 499. [CrossRef] [PubMed] [PubMed Central]

MDPI AG
Grosspeteranlage 5
4052 Basel
Switzerland
Tel.: +41 61 683 77 34

Diagnostics Editorial Office
E-mail: diagnostics@mdpi.com
www.mdpi.com/journal/diagnostics